WAKING
the GLOBAL
HEART

Published by

B O O K S

Santa Rosa, CA 95403
www.EliteBooks.biz

Library of Congress Cataloging-in-Publication Data:

Judith, Anodea, 1952-
Waking the global heart / Anodea Judith.-- 1st ed.
p. cm.
Includes bibliographical references (p. 354) and index.
ISBN 0-9720028-6-3 (hard cover)

1. Civilization, Modern--21st century. 2. Love--Social aspects.
3. Civilization--Philosophy. 4. Social evolution--Psychological
aspects. I. Title.
CB430.J83 2006
909.82-dc22

2006006706

Cover and Interior design by Ursa Minor & Alian Design
Typeset in Perpetua
Printed in USA by Bang Printing
First Edition

10   9   8   7   6   5   4   3   2   1

Waking the GLOBAL HEART

HUMANITY'S RITE OF PASSAGE FROM THE LOVE OF POWER TO THE POWER OF LOVE

ANODEA JUDITH, PH.D.

www.WakingtheGlobalHeart.com

Elite
BOOKS

Santa Rosa

Praise for
WAKING *the* GLOBAL HEART

Waking the Global Heart has been written for our day in history. In Anodea Judith's brilliant weaving of the inner world of spiritual reality and mythic power with the world we now see daily teetering on the edge of chaos, she reminds us that transformation lies ahead. When you put this book down you will see that a heart centered civilization is an evolutionary stage that awaits us. She reminds us that we cannot resist the beauty that lies in the heart of humanity and that the heart will ever draw us to our truest purpose.

—**James O'Dea President,**
Institute of Noetic Sciences

Waking the Global Heart is a powerful guide through the violence and brilliance of the past up to the present and beyond. She sets our potential for transformation in this evolutionary, historical context and really opens the doors of possibility wide. It's a beautiful piece of work."

—**Barbara Marx Hubbard,**
author of *Conscious Evolution, Emergence*

"With compassion and insight, Anodea Judith explores one of humanity's most critical questions: Where are we on the human journey? She looks at the monumental challenges now facing the human family and sees a hopeful rite of passage ahead—one that will enable us to move from our adolescence as a species and into our early adulthood. She offers a large, mythic story to guide humanity into our initial maturity—a compelling archetype of humanity's compassionate heart that can enable us to pull together on behalf of a promising future."

—**Duane Elgin, author of** *Awakening Earth,*
Promise Ahead **and** *Voluntary Simplicity,*

Evolution is the gods' way
of making more gods.

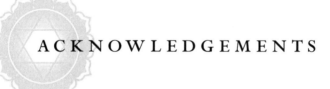

ACKNOWLEDGEMENTS

Everything that comes into being begins in relationship. Over the many years that I have worked on this manuscript, there have been countless relationships that contributed to my thinking, and many who helped to bring this project to completion. Firstly, my long time partner, Richard Ely, who created the historical charts in the chapters ahead, and whose knowledge in these matters was a continual resource and sounding board. Secondly, my current co-heart, Lion Goodman, who keeps my heart open to new possibilities and keeps me laughing. I thank them both for their love.

In praying for the right publisher, Dawson Church at Elite Books appeared like an angel. He has been a delight to work with, along with his assistant, Jeanne House. Thanks to Cynthia Smith, who worked as my office and research assistant during the latter stages of the manuscript. Hunter Roberts stimulated and challenged many ideas in our treasured walks and talks. I would like to thank Debora Hammond for her consultation on the history of science and on systems theory, and Dana Wimmer and Jan C. Vaessen for their consultation on Christianity. Thanks to Hari Meyers and Oberon Zell-Ravenheart for their expertise in mythology. Thanks to Brooks Cole for his understanding of human-technology interfaces. I am especially grateful for the lively discussions that flew across the dinner table at our many salons, and for all the various guests that attended over the years.

I would like to thank Gareth Hill for his inspiration on the static and dynamic aspects of masculine and feminine around which I organize much of this material—and thank him as well for giving me permission to put my own spin on it as I apply it to humanity's collective childhood.

For the inside pictures and cover, I would like to thank Ian Szymkowiak at Alian Design and to the folks at Ursa Minor: Zack Darling, for implementation, and Ben Flax for the diagrams. Thanks also to Susan Edwards for the indexing. Thanks to my son, Alex Wayne, who created the website for this book, and to my publicist Adrienne Biggs. Thanks to all of you for your support and creative contributions.

And lastly, I would like to express my gratitude for this incredible world we live in and all its countless blessings. May we awaken our hearts and cherish and protect all that we have been given.

–Anodea Judith, Ph.D.

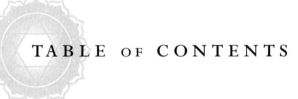

TABLE of CONTENTS

PREFACE.. 10

PART ONE: Who Are We?

1 THE CURTAIN RISES: *The Drama of Our Time*............................ 17
2 THE CALL: *Unsuspected Longings*..................................... 39
3 PREPARATION: *The Underworld Journey* 45

PART TWO: Where Did We Come From?

4 IN THE BEGINNING: *The Realm of the Mother* 57
5 WATERING THE SOUL: *The Neolithic*............................. 71
6 FROM WILL TO POWER: *The Dynamic Masculine*......................... 87
7 BIRTH OF THE HERO: *Bronze and Iron Ages* 109
8 FROM ARCHETYPES TO IDEAS: *The Dawn of the Static Masculine*.. 127
9 LIKE FATHER, LIKE SON: *Early Christianity and the Biblical Myth* ... 141
10 SHEDDING LIGHT ON THE DARKNESS:
   The Dark Ages to the Reformation 161
11 FROM FAITH TO REASON: *The Enlightenment* 179
12 SPIRALING INTO ECSTASY: *The Dynamic Feminine*................... 199
13 NO TIME LIKE THE PRESENT: *The Power of Now*....................... 219

PART THREE: Where Are We Going?

14 DON'T AGONIZE, SELF ORGANIZE:
   Better Living through Living Systems................................ 237
15 I, THOU AND WE: *Joining X, Y, and Z* 256
16 REALMS OF THE HEART: *Opening the Global Chambers*............... 287
17 WEAVING A NEW STORY: *The Coming Age of the Heart* 313

TIMELINE 330
END NOTES 342
BIBLIOGRAPHY 354
INDEX 360

PREFACE

When I was a young child, my parents had an impossibly messy drawer in the kitchen that held string, cord, wire, and various kinds of fasteners. Whenever someone reached into the drawer to use one of these things, the contents came out in a great tangled blob, only to get thrown back again with frustration. One of my favorite things to do—and one that kept me happily occupied for hours—was to empty the drawer and untangle the strings. I would patiently follow all the threads through their maze, untying the knots, until the tangle was neatly separated into usable little piles. It gave me a great deal of satisfaction and, of course, pleased my mother to no end. I have been following threads in one way or another ever since. In this book, I attempt to untangle the collective threads of our human story and reweave them into a vision that can guide us to the future.

If it weren't for the certain knowing that everyone who is aware of today's global challenges feels small in the face of them, I would never have had the *chutzpah* to write this book. In fact, over the many years I've worked on this manuscript, I tried to give it up many times, but somehow never got away with it. I told myself that it was out of my reach, over my head, beyond my subject of expertise—that other people wrote books like these, but not I, a mere woman who is wildly in love with this world. It is this love that wouldn't release me from my task; that kept me awake at night; that compelled me to pour through texts and sit at my keyboard to bring you these words.

So much for using this preface to convince you of my qualifications.

What is more important, however, and the method to my madness in this humble beginning, is that most people stay out of the kitchen, not because they can't take the heat, but because they think they don't know how to cook. Most people are stopped by beliefs in their own inadequacy—thinking they don't have the tools, the experience, or the education to make a suitable offering.

I challenge that belief. I instead insist that the new world that we are creating needs *everyone.* Passion and dedication are as important as skills. Help can be found and skills can be obtained if the passion and dedication exist. But there are innumerable skills going to waste for lack of dedication. Amateurs built the Ark, while professionals built the *Titanic.*

I didn't have all the skills I needed when I began this book. I am a psychotherapist by training, a writer and workshop presenter by profession, and a visionary philosopher by heart. My talent is recognizing patterns in the psyche—both individual and collective—and my claim to fame is my articulation of the Eastern system of the chakras as an archetype for wholeness and a template for transformation. Having spent thirty years looking at life through the lens of the chakra system, which has long been regarded as a path to personal evolution, I became aware of how this system offers us a potent map for our collective evolution. This path makes sense of our past, guides us through the present, and illuminates a positive future. It is this vision I wish to share.

In my role as a psychotherapist, I spent over twenty years watching individuals struggle with the shrapnel lodged in each of their souls from the collective gestalt of our human follies. Wrongs that never should have been committed, beliefs that serve no positive purpose, and suffering that could have been avoided—these were the constant realities tugging at my heart. As I handed over the tissues hour after hour, year after year, I came to the conclusion that it is not enough to bandage the wounds—*we have to stand up and address the slaughter.* For it is clear to me that unless we unravel the threads of the archetypal patterns that govern our collective lives, we will never evolve beyond bandaging the wounds. Those threads will be used for bandages rather than weaving a new tapestry.

I confess that I am not a historian by training, but only by interest. Historians typically focus their expertise on a particular area of history, and are expected to stick to the facts and refrain from speculation. As a result, one does not get the overview that puts these facts into a broad—and admittedly conjectural—evolutionary perspective. I instead regard myself as a storyteller. Like a therapist, I am interested in the formative experiences of our collective childhood that lead to the beliefs and complexes that feed our present social imbalances and environmental crises. This storytelling begins with the prehistory of our common beginnings and leads through the present and into a visionary framework for the future.

As the past only comprises half of this book, in order to leave room for the future, I had to be very selective in what I chose to write about. For that reason, it is primarily the story of *Western* history that I tell in this book, and in sweeping broad strokes that illustrate the archetypal dynamics and inner psychology of our common ancestral childhood. This is partly to keep the storytelling down to a manageable size, but also because it is the *values* of Western culture, despite its enlightened sophistication, that pose the greatest threat—and promise—to our collective world. And while this is changing rapidly as Third World countries enter the global playing field, it is primarily the Western world that has the technological capacity to change the trajectory that is now aiming squarely toward a mass extinction of everything we hold dear.

We can only take the reins of the future into our own hands by understanding how those reins got hitched onto the animal that is now leading us astray. For this reason, we need to understand the past from our earliest social beginnings in the wilds of the Earth—far predating the beginning of masculine rationality—in order to fully comprehend where we are now. I ask you, beloved reader, to review with me the unfolding human mystery play for the sole reason that I believe that each of you has a part to play in the next act.

Looking at the programs we were given for this drama, we see that our current time is usually referred to as the post-modern era. If that is so, then what's next? The post-post-modern era? And then the post-post-post era? What if we instead regard our time as the *pre-dawn era,* that liminal realm between the wee hours of the night and the new day? It is always darkest before the dawn, yet that does not mean that I believe we are yet at the darkest point. Instead I wish to light some lamps in preparation for that darkest point—so that we don't get lost in the dark when and if it does arrive, and that we don't *lose heart* in the depths of the trials that I believe lie ahead of us.

To say that things will likely get darker before the new dawn may sound alarmist to some and I have no objection to that term. If the cancer is spreading, the ship is sinking, or the building is burning, then sounding an alarm is one of the sanest things we can do. But even more important when sounding an alarm is to propose an alternative. To yell fire in a crowded theatre with no exit sign, or to watch the *Titanic* go down without enough lifeboats only leads to despair.

There are many people today who are sounding alarms about our environment, our economy, our governments, and our social injustices. And there are many people getting lost in despair. What I believe is needed at this time is not only a realistic evaluation of our collective situation, but a story of hope. Not the kind of hope that says to a child, "Don't worry, it will all be OK, just go back to sleep," but the kind of hope that employs all of our efforts in creating a mature vision of what's possible. For in my many years of attending to the wounds of the human heart, only the presence of hope could lighten and heal the heart. When hope arises, there is a deeper opening to new possibilities— and to love.

A viable vision of the future can only be created by all of us. I offer here both the dark and light sides of our collective story, which I hope will ignite your own love for this glorious world, for the incredible beings that live in it, and for your part in the astounding future that awaits us all.

—Anodea Judith, 2006

PART ONE

Who Are We?

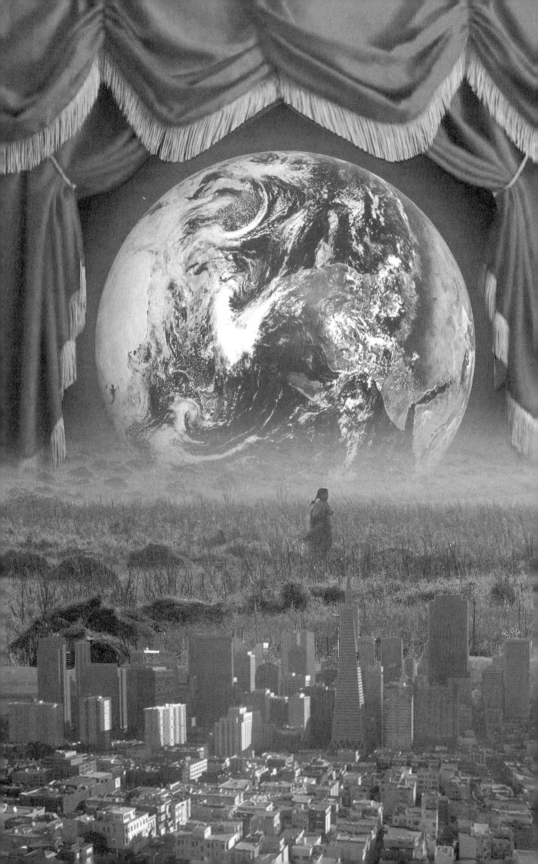

CHAPTER 1

THE CURTAIN RISES
The Drama of Our Time

> *The only myth that is going to be worth talking about in the immediate*
> *future is one that is talking about the planet, not this city, not these people,*
> *but the planet and everybody on it. And what it will have to deal with will be*
> *exactly what all myths have dealt with—the maturation of the individual,*
> *from dependency through adulthood, through maturity, and then to the exit;*
> *and then how to relate this society to the world of nature and the cosmos...*
> *And until that gets going, you don't have anything.*[1]

—Joseph Campbell

The human drama is nearing its denouement. The great unveiling is approaching, a time when the power structures of the world begin to crumble and people of the heart sing out a new truth. Many voices are joining the chorus, many feet are walking the path, many minds are dreaming possibilities for a magnificent future. For beneath the crises that are looming at every level of civilization, the global heart is awakening, beating out the rhythm of a new and glorious dance, calling us to a better way of living.

You who are dreamers and poets, executives and laborers, healers and teachers, artists and visionaries, parents and lovers—each of you plays a part in bringing forth the new dawn. You are the ones who will be leading humanity's rite of passage into the next age. For the awakening of the global heart occurs as each of its many cells opens to the power of love in its own heart and joins together to pump life and breath into every corner of the globe. Physically, the heart is an organ that keeps us alive through a coordinated network of cells beating together. Spiritually, the heart is the center of love, the primordial force that calls things into relationship, the force that makes our lives worthwhile. Globally, the heart is a symbol of a new organizing principle for how to live together on this finite jewel of a planet.

The cultural transformation from the *love of power* to the *power of love* is the drama of our time. Ours is an era that future historians will look back upon, marveling at the magnitude of the challenges and changes we are now experiencing. They will call it a time of Great Awakening, a time when the best and the worst of humanity played their parts in the fate of human evolution. But if future generations are alive to tell this story, it will only be because the best of humanity prevailed and pulled together with a love so profound that the seemingly impossible was achieved.

Human consciousness is being drawn inexorably toward the same issues, the gaze of collective attention focused like never before. Center stage is now everywhere, broadcast from living rooms, automobiles, airports, and cell phones, from radios, newspapers, magazines, and the Internet. Increasing numbers of people watch the unfolding events with bated breath. Some have been watching for quite some time, with growing concern. Others are just waking up, rubbing their eyes in confusion. Still others prefer to remain asleep, doing their best to ignore the signs that point to an impending and massive shift at every level of civilization.

As we meet for coffee, for dinner, for business meetings, or for romantic dates, the conversation buzzes like an audience murmuring between acts. Where's it all going? What will happen next? What's wrong? Who's right? What should we do? What *can* we do? And most frightening of all—especially among the youth today—are those who wonder if we will even survive into the next age. For the emerging generation is watching in despair as the adults in charge recklessly spend their inheritance with little regard for the future.

In the theatre of our world, we are simultaneously audience and cast, playing to an instantaneous feedback system that continually shows us our reflection. But rather than the image of a single character, we are witness to a global tapestry, weaving itself into a new picture. Its threads were spun from archaic forces long ago, woven together by the myths, legends, and heroic deeds of our ancestors. To weave a new picture, we must engage with these forces and take them into our own hands—with maturity, with consciousness, and most of all, *with heart*. For we who are alive at this time—whether we like it or not—are entering *a rite of passage into the future*. This rite is both personal and collective. We are no longer separate strands in the web of life, but the very weavers of the web that holds us all.

We stand at the dawn of a new era. Immersed in technology, yet hungry for the sacred, there is deep longing for a story that balances masculine and feminine, progress and sustainability, order and freedom, power and love. The stories we tell ourselves shape our world. They guide our relationships to each other, to the environment, and to the future. Life in the twenty-first century is spinning a new myth. It is time to listen to the growing chorus of voices that make up this story. Together, we are discovering and inventing a way to the future.

To weave a new story, we must inquire into the essential questions asked by myths and legends of all ages: *Who are we? Where do we come from? Where are we going?* It is these questions that give meaning to the drama, and define the parts that each of us has to play. It is to these questions, wrapped around the unfolding human mystery play, that this book is addressed. Here we find guidance for the mythic journey, not only as individuals, but also for the emerging story of what we are becoming together.

WHO ARE WE?

In the drama thus far, humans have become an astounding species unlike any other. Birthed from the primal womb of nature, billions of years in gestation, we have risen out of Stone Age infancy, crawled across the land in teeming toddlerhood, and labored through thousands of years of sibling rivalry, to arrive at the present time—in the tumultuous throes of adolescence. Some are just entering this adolescent period, others are right in the middle of it, while an increasing number are transitioning to adulthood, undergoing the rite of passage from power to love.

With technological power that far surpasses our maturity, our species stands poised between epic creation and potential annihilation, equally capable of either. Whether through genius or lunacy, our actions today affect the future of us all. Issues of power and love, war and peace, poverty and prosperity, tyranny and freedom, individual rights and community needs hang unresolved in our story thus far. In the past, these issues were local affairs—but now they have global proportions. Though our time is one of unprecedented change, major players in this drama still read from outdated scripts that fail to address the needs of the present, let alone those of the future. The next act has not yet been written. It is about to begin.

ADOLESCENT INITIATION

As the curtain rises, we see an adolescent culture entering into a monumental rite of passage into adulthood. The elders who have been in charge are no longer showing us the way—for the way is so different, they truly don't know what it is. They can only go along the roads they know best, even when these roads appear to be leading us in the wrong direction. Those roads took us to where we are now and they have formed a deep groove in the collective psyche. Yet their linear routes have taken us so far from the center that they are now leading us astray. The old maps can't tell us how to get to the future.

In this rite of passage, then, there are are no figureheads to lead the way, no authority figures who will solve the big problems for us. For the task of initiation is to awaken our own authority. Where most previous religions have posited a Mother Goddess or Father God, the current trend in spirituality is to awaken the divinity found within, through practices that open a direct connection to higher and deeper states of consciousness. Not only are we "on our own" in terms of parental guidance, we are simultaneously the first few generations saddled with the responsibility of saving the entire world. Our ancestors worked to save their tribe, expand their empire, or defend their country. Now the protection of the planet itself is at stake.

Power no longer resides outside of ourselves, but awakens when we speak the truth within our own hearts. The root of the word *authority* is *author*, which means that we are all writing this story together through the collective speaking of our truth. Gandhi used the term *satyagraha*, from the Sanskrit word meaning "force of truth." This force has the power to change the world.

Duane Elgin reports that in his questioning of people across cultures—from India to Japan, England to Brazil—over two-thirds agree that humanity is in its adolescence.[2] It's easy to see why. We need only turn on the television to see adolescent behavior raging through all ages, races, creeds, and genders. Creative but disrespectful, powerful but reckless, narcissisticly obsessed with our looks, and bursting with teenage libido, we are sorely lacking in social and environmental conscience. We are fascinated by flashy gadgets and fast changes. We are driven by the whimsy of our desires. Like teenagers thoughtlessly cleaning out the refrigerator while entertaining their friends, human populations are insatiably consuming the once vast cupboards of oceans and forests in the attempt to satisfy their voracious appetites.

And why not? Hasn't Mother Nature always kept the cupboards well stocked in the past, free to her children, just for the asking? Hasn't our sole responsibility been to take in resources, to grow and to learn? Did we ever think it was possible that Mom's cupboards could run out?

Adolescence is a time when physical growth comes to a halt. It's the time when we take that prodigious life force and learn to grow in a new dimension. At best, this dimension is spiritual, growing towards deeper understanding of ourselves and our world. But if this passage is blocked, adolescents act out recklessly, often harming themselves and their environment—even before they know what they are losing.

To become adults, adolescents who have previously been nurtured, cared for, and educated by elders must learn to provide for themselves, and others in turn. They must learn about the meaning of life, the structure and order of the world, and their purpose within it. Yet they are also compelled—by the unique life force within them—to question and change that structure as they grow into it. It is a tumultuous time, as any parent knows, and there are days when we may look at our teenagers with exasperation and wonder if they will ever grow up. Yet we have no choice but to move forward as best we can, and hold a container for their process.

Just as adolescence marks the end of physical growth, *our human population has grown to its adult size and can no longer continue to expand in a physical dimension.* We have reached (if not surpassed) the carrying capacity of our biosphere. World population has doubled in the last half-century, climbing from 2.5 billion in 1950 to 6.3 billion in 2005.[3] Just for perspective, this means there has been more population growth in the last half-century than in the four million years since the earliest humans walked on their hind legs! If not checked, this number could double again in the next fifty years. From the depletion of top soil and underground aquifers used to grow our food, to the diminishing oil reserves that bring our groceries to the table; from the disappearing forests and the creatures who live there, to the greenhouse gases that are raising global temperatures; from urban smog, to waste disposal; from the billions who live in poverty to the epidemic diseases that threaten life—every facet of human and non-human society is impacted by our unchecked population growth. What Malthus predicted back in 1798 is now a reality:

> "...I say, that the power of population is indefinitely greater than the power in the earth to produce subsistence for man. Population, when unchecked, increases in a geometrical ratio. Subsistence increases only in an arithmetical ratio. A slight acquaintance with numbers will show the immensity of the first power in comparison of the second."[4]

CHILDREN	ADOLESCENTS	ADULTS
Dependent	Independent	Interdependent
Continuous growth	Growth spurt	Growth stabilized
Lives in present	Rebels against past	Plans for future
Parents are Gods	Parents fall from grace	Become parents
Obedient	Rebellious	Cooperative
No power	Reckless power	Shared power
Needs help	Resists help	Gives help

It is not only population growth that must be curbed, but the way that we view progress and success. Ever since the Industrial Revolution, progress has been measured by growth. The success of a company is usually defined by its expansion, not its social contribution. Growth is measured in terms of more products, bigger markets, larger infrastructure, and ultimately greater profits. Whether that means building more housing developments, expanding roads and highways, infiltrating indigenous cultures with Western products and lifestyles, or simply crafting a way to make more with less—our "industrial growth society" must place its value on something other than growth before we exhaust our life support systems. That the word "downsizing" has entered our vernacular shows that much of this expansion is already reaching its limit. We are quickly discovering that growth-based futures have no sustainable future.

Yet, just like an adolescent, growth has been the driving force of our biology since its earliest beginnings. Prehistoric nomads focused on images pertaining to birth. The Bible tells us to go forth and multiply. In our earlier eras, this was entirely appropriate. Yet it created a force that has its own momentum. Like the infamous ship, *Titanic,* it's not easy to turn such a colossal system around—even when we see the iceberg up ahead. In order to survive, we must harness that creative urge to multiply and point the evolutionary arrow in a new direction.

Let's face it: Mother Nature is stressed out. Our days are numbered as innocent children living in the ever-abundant Garden of Eden, where divine parents supply every need and whim without replenishment. No longer can we be the semi-conscious parents of unlimited offspring, overpopulating the planet while remaining ourselves as indulged children in an illusory garden of delights. It's time we outgrew our adolescent war games of sibling rivalry, where we leave Mother Nature to clean up the ravages of our destruction. No longer can we define ourselves as isolated individuals, seeing ourselves as uniquely entitled to take whatever we want from wherever we find it, while social malaise and growing poverty crawl in the shadows of the wealthy few— whom we regard as heroes.

The culmination of four billion years of evolution now rests in our hands. With the ability to permanently change climate through global warming, the potential of mass destruction through nuclear warfare, with gene-splicing and cloning occurring in our laboratories, we are the first race of creatures with the capacity to influence the direction of evolution and the future of life on this planet. Such potential has never occurred before in our evolutionary history. It signals an extraordinary need for responsibility and a driving imperative to wake up. At the very least, it requires the maturity of adult wisdom and behavior. But even more, it calls for an awakening of the heart. For love is the key to that which endures.

We are now facing a collective adolescent identity crisis. Our challenge is to foster a new identity, as elements of a larger matrix, and as parents of a new millennium. But we are not yet adults. We are, as Jean Houston has said, "people of the parentheses,"[5] living in the nebulous ground between the old age and the new, neither child nor grown-up, undergoing the tremendous changes of adolescent transformation. In one way or another this transformation will eventually come to us all. We may resist the call and remain stubbornly attached to the old ways, or we can surrender to the transformation, and advance to the other side. We cannot remain the same and still survive.

GLOBAL RITE OF PASSAGE

A rite of passage is an initiation into an unknown world. The instigators of our current initiation are not individuals, but the combined results of human civiliziation. These initiating elements bring us into blinding paradox at every turn. They parade across television screens that bombard us with images of father figures granting the illusion of safety—while feeding the rise of terrorism through aggressive military actions. They come from the capacity to witness the birth of galaxies in the macrocosm, to the manipulation of tiny genes in the microcosm. Initiating factors appear as data that tell us our world is in danger, and a news media that keeps us preoccupied with stories of mass distraction. They come from instantaneous access to the world's knowledge base—and gross ignorance about our collective reality. Both positive and negative, these factors are the by-products of the values that shape our society. They are the wake up call emanating from the possibility of environmental and economic collapse, epidemic diseases, nuclear disaster, and a technology that is loading real time Technicolor into the global brain and taking it to the stars.

The time has come. The rite of passage has begun. We must enter the mystery to emerge on the other side.

What does it mean to "come of age" as a species? How do we outgrow dependent childhood and adolescent rebellion to grow into sustainable maturity? How do we weather the coming storms and create the necessary transformation? And how do we make sense of what we've done in the past, so as to better understand what we must do now?

WHERE DO WE COME FROM?

This question might be more appropriately framed as, "How did we get into this mess?" How did we get to a place where we can fly to the stars, but not feed the children? How did we get to a place where we fight wars over oil, so we can pollute our air sitting in traffic jams? How did we create a world in which we don't know our neighbors, have little time for our friends, and abuse our children? How is it that we have discovered and learned so much about the world around us, yet still seem to be dangerously lost on our path to the future?

In tribal cultures, an essential part of a rite of passage was to teach *the history of the tribe from the beginning of time.* Only initiated men and women who understood this history and the sacred forces that shaped it were allowed to become elders in the tribe. This is not to inhibit innovation by binding the initiate to an inflexible tradition, but to *ground* their actions in an understanding and experience of the sacred realm. We must understand our history to harvest its energy for the future.

In working with a client in crisis, a good therapist not only tries to mitigate the crisis itself, but also examines the client's past, to identify the events, beliefs, and assumptions that created the client's situation. With a world in crisis, we must do the same self-examination on a collective level. We must examine our history and expose the assumptions and beliefs that have led to the current situation. We must understand the preceding acts of the human story from an archetypal perspective, in order to keep from repeating our mistakes and perpetuating our traumas. From this examination, we can rise into wisdom.

For this reason, our story will begin by examining the childhood of our collective history as the roots for our collective future. To argue that we are, indeed, adolescents that are "coming of age in the heart," the stages of childhood development will be mapped onto the eras of history. This history is largely Western, because it is Western culture that has the greatest influence on the shaping of the global tapestry right now—for better or worse. But this history also goes back to pre-historic roots that are common to us all. Because any viable vision of the future must integrate both masculine and feminine values, these historical stages will also be viewed in light of the archetypal masculine and feminine valences that shaped each era. This is not to blame either gender for events along the way, but to better illuminate the dynamic interplay that defines our future roles together.

An equally important thread that runs through my telling of this tale comes from the Eastern mystical tradition of yoga, through the map described by the ancient system of energy centers known as the *chakras*. As a comprehensive system, the *chakras* form a profound formula for wholeness, not only for individual awakening, but for the evolution of society as a whole. As a result of my life's work in this area, my deep understanding of the chakra system has illuminated a pattern that leads me to believe that we are moving from a culture based largely on the third chakra, which is associated with power and the emergence of ego-based consciousness, to the fourth chakra, whose focus is love, relatedness, and a more transcendent consciousness. In my previous book, *Eastern Body, Western Mind: Psychology and the Chakra System as a Path to the Self,* (Celestial Arts, 1997) I chart the correlation between the chakras and stages of individual development. In the book you now hold, I map this pattern onto our collective development. A simple chart showing how these stages map onto the chakras, appears on pages 30 and 31. A more complex chart, featuring elements discussed in the pages ahead, appears on pages 214 and 215).

The progression through the chakras begins at the survival-oriented root chakra of our ancestral beginnings, and moves steadily upward, through the socialization of early cultures (second chakra), into the struggle for power and empire (third chakra), and partly into the fourth chakra, associated with love, compassion, and relationship. It is argued here that we have not fully arrived in the heart, having gotten trapped in the ego's love of power and the masculine rigidity of imperial power structures. The result is a fragmented society divided against itself: men against women, civilization against Nature, and war within ourselves and between each other. A divided world cannot fully enter the heart. Nor can it find peace.

In chakra theory, *it is only by embracing the full spectrum of human consciousness that we can bring about a true awakening of the heart.* This involves developing the upper chakra realms of communication, vision, and spirituality, and *integrating* them with the lower chakra attributes of the body, the emotions, and personal power—attributes that have been largely repressed by the predominant spiritual tradtions. Modern technology has only recently opened the upper chakras on a planetary scale, through the ability to communicate words and images through mass media and the Internet. Simultaneously, we are entering a spiritual revolution, one that focuses more on the process of individual awakening – through such practices as meditation, yoga, fasting, and a smorgasbord of self-help techniques. Because we have the capacity to organize humanity through a world-wide technological network, we are—for the first time in history—ready to awaken the global heart as an organizing principle for a planetary society.

WHERE ARE WE GOING?

In the body, heart cells beat together, coordinating their actions. When heart cells are separated, they beat independently at different rhythms. When they make contact with each other, they beat in unison, pumping oxygen and nutrients throughout the entire system, nourishing every cell. It is through contact and connectedness that we coordinate our rhythms and beat together. It is time for the many parts of our world to come together and awaken the global heart, beating in unison with love for our world. These parts include genders, races, religions, and nations, as well as the many aspects of civilization such as economics, education, technology, media, government, science, and philosophy.

To *come of age in the heart* is to enter a rite of passage that transforms ego-centered self-interest into an embodied expression of love. Guilt, fear, or manipulation will never produce lasting evolutionary change, but what is inspired by love is fueled by natural willingness, even excitement, to serve a higher purpose. Think of the efforts we put forth for the people and things we love. What else but love could get us up in the middle of the night to change a soiled diaper? What else but love could keep an activist woman in a redwood tree through two hard winters, in defiance of loggers and timber corporations? What else but love makes us care for things that we value, and do the work of that caring willingly, even joyfully?

Yet it seems too many of us have fallen out of love with the world. Like a bad marriage, we have forgotten the once-shining beauty of our partner, forgotten even that we are engaged in a partnership. Disenchanted, we use and abuse our environment, spinning without anchor through a life of destruction and disconnection, broadcasting this destruction through our newscasts, and simultaneously distracting ourselves with addictive consumption of cheap substitutes to fill the emptiness. In an estranged relationship, we have forgotten the sanctity and rights of the other person. As we dishonor them, we are no longer engaged with a "thou" but are instead acting out against an "it." We lose touch with the numinosity, power, and beauty of the Sacred Other.

CHAKRA CORRESPONDENCES AND AGES

CHAKRA	ONE	TWO	THREE
Sanskrit Name meaning	Muladhara root support	Swadhisthana One's own place	Manipura lustrous gem, jeweled citadel
Location	base of spine	sacral area	solar plexus
Element	earth	water	fire
Psychological association	grounding security	pleasure sexuality	power and will
Individual developmental phase	womb to 1 year	6 months to 2 years	18 months to 3-4 years
Historical Time period	Paleolithic	Neolithic	Bronze and Iron Ages

In both individual and cultural development, the opening of a particular chakra does not mean that its development is completed in that phase. Often higher levels of realization are necessary in order to consolidate a previous chakra phase.

In the maturation of the individual, the heart phase is early childhood, while adolescence is equated with the opening of the sixth chakra. The reason we are now at our adolescence culturally, yet still not consolidated in the

FOUR	FIVE	SIX	SEVEN
Anahata unstruck unhurt	Vissudha purification	Ajna to perceive and to command	Sahasrara thousandfold lotus
heart	throat	brow	top of head
air	sound	light	thought
love relationship	communication creativity	intuition imagination	consciousness intelligence
4 – 7 years	7-12 years	adolescence*	adulthood
Began c. 600 B.C.E.	Began in Renaissance	Began 20th century	Now dawning

heart, is that we are suffering from arrested development, a topic dealt with fully in these pages.

In the collective tasks, it can be seen that we have achieved, at least partly, the tasks of the upper chakras, yet have not yet arrived at peace and freedom for all. It is argued that global communications in the fifth, sixth, and seventh chakra realms are necessary to achieve a global awakening in the heart.

To come of age in the heart is to *fall back in love with the world,* to find that our world is subject, not object; to realize that, yes, the self *is* sacred, but so is the entire web of life. In the realm of the heart, we reconstitute the archetype of sacred partnership: balanced, respectful, and mutually enhancing. Here we are inspired to act from passionate dedication, not spineless obedience; to be repossessed by the sacred, rather than dispossessed by its lack; to be pulled forward by an evolving vision from the future, rather than held back by the decaying patterns of the past.

This coming of age transformation is simultaneously individual and collective. In our private lives, many of us are being forced by the acceleration of events around us to face our own depths, examine unconscious motives, and upgrade our values and belief systems to meet the pace of a rapidly changing world. But these individual changes are small compared to what is being asked of us collectively: to not only change ourselves, but to transform the world in which we live. We are products of this world. We think with its forms, depend on its products, breathe its very air.

The path toward wholeness, which Jung called the archetype of *individuation,* is now being thrust upon the collective psyche. Individuation is the soul's process of maturing and awakening to its true nature. It often begins in a crisis that forces deeper self-examination. Here we find forgotten selves, reclaim disconnected parts, such as our shadow or wounded child, and bring our inner masculine and feminine into balance and relationship. This process calls us to break the confines of cultural conformity and begin to live authentic and embodied lives.

Just as it occurs for individuals, our task is to *collectively* face our hidden shadow of violence, greed, and domination and stop projecting it onto others. We must balance the powers of masculine and feminine not only in socio-economic status, but also in terms of our innate values, making emotional intelligence as necessary as cognitive genius, nurturance as important as accomplishment, receptive wisdom as valuable as creative expression. Only through this integration of values will we transform our larger cultural systems.

Such transformation begins with a shift in the archetypal framework that tells the story of who we are and why we're here. Our current age of power has delivered vast knowledge, sophisticated technology, and personal freedom, greater than at any time in our history. Yet the shadow side of our power has created pollution and tyranny. Power and domination, where one part rules over another—such as mind over body, male over female, white over black, civilization over nature, or personal gratification over the needs of others—has typified our world for the last several millennia. The Age of Power brought us the initial steps of individuation from an undifferentiated tribal unity, much as our personal autonomy emerges from an initial fusion with our mother. Separating from the archetypal Mother and giving birth to the ego brought us the Heroic Age. The heroic journey has been a rightful quest for power, but this quest has now overshot its mark.

The Hero's journey mirrors the initiation process: heeding a call to serve something greater, separating from what is known and dissolving the structures of one's individual consciousness, entering the belly of the underworld, facing trials and ordeals, meeting and merging with archetypal forces, opening to new vision, then rebirth and return. We are all at different stages of this journey. Some of us are experiencing dissolution; some of us are in the underworld. Others are battling their ordeals, and many are discovering and opening to archetypal forces, returning with new vision. We are all a part of this initiation, each in our own way.

Sometimes the most demanding task of the Hero's quest is the *return home,* where the fruits of the quest—the elixir of healing or the enlightened vision—are brought back to a broken and ailing world. The Hero's quest begins with the striving of an individual—but ends in the healing of community. The quest illuminates our power, but the return is an act of love.

The return is seldom easy. Who wants to leave their new-found paradise to return to an ailing world? Who wants to have doors slammed in their face, or confront the apathy of a world that wants to remain in denial? Who wants to return a hero but be treated like the child that left? Sometimes the Hero chooses not to return.

Others, like Galileo, who dared to suggest that the Earth just might be traveling around the sun, are locked up, censored and punished. Mahatma Gandhi and Martin Luther King were murdered, while Nelson Mandela spent most of his life in jail. Yet, if we understand this archetypal drive—*and longing*—to come home again, we can open the passage for our heroes to return, and embrace the gifts they bring with an open mind.

EVOLUTION IS THE GODS' WAY OF MAKING MORE GODS

This is a basic premise of this book. You can replace the concept of God with whatever term, gender, or pantheon you like, but the point is that evolution proceeds, not only toward greater complexity and freedom, but also towards ever more potent god-like powers of creation and destruction. When we can influence the course of life on our planet through global warming, species extinction, or gene splicing—to say nothing of nuclear warfare—we are approaching the power of gods. But have we evolved the wisdom and grace equal to that power? If not, what does it take for us to get there?

Some say it will take a global disaster for humanity to wake up. They may well be right, for we know that rites of passage include *some* kind of death. There are values and behaviors that are so deeply embedded in Western culture, and are so pointedly unsustainable, that clearly *something* needs to die. Do we need to go through a global "detox" in order to remain healthy? And while natural and man-made disasters have always occurred, the difference today is one of scale. Because of Earth's population density, disasters now affect millions. On some level, they affect us all.

Disasters do open our hearts. This was evident in the outpouring of public support following the destruction of the World Trade Center on September 11, 2001, the Tsunami of 2004, and the flooding of New Orleans in 2005. Earthquakes and hurricanes, floods and droughts, all break down the isolation of individuals, and awaken a sense of community. Disasters are one form of initiation. However, a proper initiation can also *mitigate* disaster by awakening a guiding vision. Without that vision, we are stuck in old belief systems, with only guilt to guide our current behavior. We know we shouldn't drive so much, use so much, waste so much. But most people feel they have little alternative. Others are not even aware of their impact. Nor is it easy to give up privileges we have come to rely upon.

By contrast, a guiding vision can give us something to move *toward* instead of something to move *away from*. No disaster was necessary to switch from an electric typewriter to a word processing computer; it was simply a better idea. It didn't require a failure of the telephone system to make room for cell phones. When a better way becomes apparent, we choose it naturally. *A destructive lifestyle is simply ignorant of a better way.* What's needed is a vision of the future as an organizing principle, much as the blueprints for a house organize the laborers who build it. Without something positive to move toward, we are much like an adolescent who is acting out, suffering from lack of guidance.

Yet the public media broadcasts information that is often more destructive than creative, attacking or destroying innovation before it has time to mature. Progressive ideas in politics, new discoveries in science and medicine, the leading edges of social movements, and alternative spiritualities—these frontiers are often dismissed as unrealistic elements of a fringe society. When new ideas are so blatantly necessary, one has to wonder why this is so. Our collective vision of what is possible is the organizing principle for our transformation. But none of us can create this alone, for that is part of the old way, and is, by nature, counter to the vision of collective awakening.

The evolutionary biologist, Elizabet Sahtouris, has popularized a metaphor for transformation based on the metamorphosis of the caterpillar into the butterfly. This process has so many parallels to our collective rite of passage that we will refer to it again and again throughout these pages, as a guiding image for our collective changes.

When a caterpillar nears its transformation time, it begins to eat ravenously, consuming everything in sight. (It is interesting to note that individuals are often called "consumers" and one of the largest manufacturers of heavy construction machinery is called "Caterpillar, Inc.") The caterpillar body then becomes heavy, outgrowing its own skin many times, until it is too bloated to move. Attaching to a branch (upside down, we might add, where everything is turned on its head) it forms a chrysalis—an enclosing shell that limits the caterpillar's freedom for the duration of the transformation.

Within the chrysalis a miracle occurs. Tiny cells, called "imaginal cells," begin to appear. These cells are wholly different from caterpillar cells, carrying different information, vibrating to a different frequency–the frequency of the emerging butterfly. At first, the caterpillar's immune system perceives these new cells as enemies, and attacks them, much as new ideas are called radical, and viciously denounced by the powers now holding center stage. But the imaginal cells are not deterred. They continue to appear, increasing in numbers until the new cells are numerous enough to organize into clumps. When enough cells have formed to make structures along the *new* organizational lines, the caterpillar's immune system is overwhelmed. The cells of the original body then become a nutritious soup for the growth of the butterfly.

When the butterfly is ready to hatch, the chrysalis becomes transparent (much as the Internet is making many hidden actions transparent). The need for restriction has been outgrown, yet the struggle toward freedom is part of the process. Were the chrysalis opened too soon, the butterfly would die. As the butterfly emerges, it fills its wings with liquid, (a "right wing" and a "left wing," we might note), and then flies away to dance among the flowers.

The awakening of the global heart results from transforming the body politic from the unconscious, over-consuming bloat of the caterpillar into a creature of exquisite beauty, grace, and freedom. This coming of age process takes us to a new mythic reality, a larger story, ripe with meaning and direction. It takes us from the naïve egocentricity of childhood into a larger reality of interdependent reciprocity. It is not a passage that ends in the gray grimness of adult responsibility, denying the colorful spirituality of childhood innocence. Rather, it is a reclaiming of wholeness that denies little, and embraces all.

It is from this abundance that we can love and cherish our world.

This book is the story of that passage. It examines the beginning stages of the Hero's journey of dissolution and darkness. It takes us back to the beginnings of humanity, to our ancient birth from the Great Mother, where we reclaim our roots. It takes us through the twists and turns of our collective infancy into early childhood, and then through the struggle for power and freedom, the attempts and failures at unity, the development of technology and communication, and the hunger for a new vision at this time. We will examine the archetypal Mother and Father, with their Son's and Daughter's emancipation from oppression and dependence, finally leading into the budding maturity of both men and women capable—perhaps for the first time—of truly egalitarian relationships. This takes us historically from a basic *thesis,* into its complete *antithesis,* for the purpose of finally creating a new and dynamic *synthesis.*

From the love of power to the power of love, this rite of passage is the emerging myth of our time.

ESSENTIAL POINTS

• We live at a time of unprecedented challenge and opportunity.

• Our power to affect the future of life on Earth is dangerously more developed than our emotional and spiritual maturity.

• We are culturally like adolescents, undergoing an initiatory rite of passage into adulthood and the next era of civilization.

• This passage marks the transition from the love of power to the power of love as an organizing principle for society.

• Our cultural values are formed by an ongoing play of archetypal energies that have definable patterns. These patterns have been woven through history and make us what we are today. Part of the initiation process is to learn the archetypal patterns of the past.

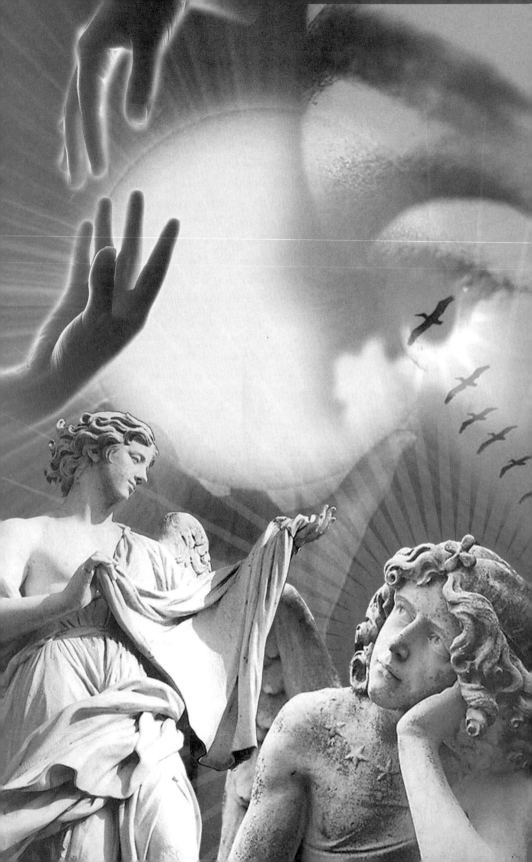

CHAPTER 2

THE CALL
Unsuspected Longings

What we do not love, we will not save.

—Wendell Berry

When fate arrives at your door, there is no lock strong enough to hold it back. It may find you asleep, unprepared, too busy, or defiant, but these states are no deterrent. Destiny does not wait for your mood to change. When the time is ripe, the rite of passage begins. Such rites eventually come to us all.

Initiation begins when we listen to the call tugging at our hearts. Rainer Maria Rilke says, "What goes on in your innermost being is worthy of your whole love; you must somehow keep working at it."[1] That inner being is unconsciously connected to something larger. It longs to move the petty distractions out of the way, to dissolve the separations that keep us isolated, and to belong to something that inspires pride – whether it be a project, a community, or a country. It is this pull, emanating from the deep unconscious, that acts as a "strange attractor," invisibly guiding our lives toward greater meaning and purpose.

This is known as *the call* and it comes in many forms. It may begin as a restless dissatisfaction with your daily life, or a deep depression. It may result from the churning in your gut over the daily news, or an inspiring story told to you by a friend. It may come from a tragic loss, or an unexpected boon. But however the call finds its way into your private chambers, it changes the course of your life.

Most commonly, such calls begin with a blunder: a simple lapse of attention that lets unconscious urges rise to the surface just long enough to take over the reins and steer the journey in a new direction. Joseph Campbell described these blunders as the result of suppressed longings, "ripples on the surface of life, produced by unsuspected springs,"[2] This might be an affair that snares the psyche in relentless passion, revealing the unacknowledged limitations of your marriage. It might be a sudden injury that makes a dead-end job impossible to perform, or a pregnancy that binds you to a relationship you were wanting to end. It may seem like a random quirk of fate, but looking back upon it later, you find that the hand of destiny was clearly marked by your own fingerprints.

If you are one of the lucky ones, it appears as an unexpected boon—landing that big part, receiving a financial windfall, or sudden recognition in your field. A new love may call you to a deeper level of awakening. Maybe you are just leaving home for the first time, going off to school, leaving a dead marriage, or graduating from decades of raising children. The life unfolding before you will be different from the one you were leading.

Fate is not always a welcome visitor, however. Sometimes she is clothed in darker colors. A piercing phone call in the middle of the night announces the death of a loved one; a life-threatening illness forces you to re-examine all your assumptions. Perhaps an innocent blunder brings disgrace in your career, or someone you trusted turns out to be a thief who bankrupts your business. You might wake up to discover a note pinned to your pillow that says your marriage is over, or that your child has run away. These, too, will change the course of your life and hopefully awaken a deeper awareness. As we move closer toward humanity's collective rite of passage, more and more individuals will be facing these difficult challenges.

Yet there are some who experience neither the highs nor the lows of fate's intervention, and simply bide their time *waiting* for fate to intervene, restless and dissatisfied with their life. They secretly hope that some unexpected event will create changes they can't seem to make on their own. And sooner or later it will—but not always in the way they might have wished. Others take this dissatisfaction as an impetus to reach for something greater than themselves.

Everything in life prepares you for answering the call—yet it seems that nothing you know fits the new challenge—for its very purpose is to bring you to a new realm. Like the caterpillar wrapped in a chrysalis, you cannot know who you are becoming when the process begins. It is only in hindsight, looking back from the other side of the transformation, that you finally understand. You can resist the process and remain as a common larva, or you can relinquish control and emerge as a butterfly. But once you begin, you cannot remain the same.

When the old world is stripped away, it reveals another world hidden beneath. A reluctant mother, bent on pursuing an adult career, discovers the magical world of children. The homeowner ravaged by fire or flood discovers the freedom of living without possessions. The lover who engages in a secret affair discovers vital parts of herself coming back to life. Each loss, though difficult, brings a new awakening. Each cloud has a silver lining.

As modern culture continues its ecologically destructive path into the future, we can see that in many parts of the world, whole villages and cities, even countries, are facing these tragic wake up calls. Earthquakes and tsunamis, hurricanes and floods, droughts, disease, economic collapse, wars, political oppression, and acts of terrorism, are disturbing or destroying lives by the millions. As we continue our destructive behavior toward Nature and each other, these events will only increase in frequency and severity. Dense populations incur high casualties when natural disasters occur.

Such tragedies are initiatory wounds. They cause us to lose our childhood innocence and wake up to the necessity of protecting our future. They open the heart to compassion. They break through isolation, and force us into community and cooperation.

The destruction of the World Trade Center in September 2001 is a prime example of a collective initiatory wound, at least for Americans. Like ritual circumcision or loss of a digit, the loss of the two towers of power that proudly scraped the skyline of New York City awakened the whole world to an unexpected and horrendous tragedy. America's proud invincibility was made vulnerable, and the U.S. was stripped of its inno-cence. In the months that followed, the forgotten land of Afghanistan, starving from the effects of drought, and suffering under a violent, tyran-nical regime, suddenly received global attention. Issues of prosperity and poverty, freedom and tyranny, war and peace, were brought before us all, begging for a new story.

Beneath the cries for vengeance and the aerial bombers that flew to Afghanistan, the September 11th tragedy stimulated an unparalleled wave of love and solidarity around the world. Vigils were set, prayers were uttered, peace marches were held, and nations that had been ene-mies formed coalitions. Even children sent their allowances to relief funds. Beneath the war drums and cluster bombs, a global humanity was revealed. Over sixty-five nations and every major faith were rep-resented in those towers. As we looked outward to see where to aim our hurt and anger, we found that our own faces stared back at us from every corner. The lines between us and them, here and there, right and wrong, were blurred. The three thousand deaths of those in the towers was an atrocity, but America, too, had blood on its hands. We killed unknown numbers of Afghanis in the bloodbath that followed, and even more in the war in Iraq that still rages as I write. That blood cuts across cultures, and goes back through the millennia as a *very old story,* one that is in desperate need of revision.

Initiation is a series of stress tests in which our character is challenged. Which will we choose: vengeance or negotiation, war or peace, opposi-tion or synthesis? When we consistently choose peace, we will move out of the testing phase of this initiation and truly begin the next round of civilization. Initiation is a way of bridging the past and the future, elders and youth. To initiate is to begin. Yet this beginning is anchored in the wisdom of elders, who carry and protect sacred traditions from the past, even as they remain hidden while we face our trials unaided. Without initiation, there is no continuity between the generations, no meaning-ful communication, nothing that demands respect for sustaining a cul-ture. In some tribal societies, it is believed that failure to initiate their youth will create a generation that will destroy their culture, and this important continuity will be lost. Whether this results in active rebellion and destructive activities, or merely a generation that is so lost that they meekly follow the politician with the largest campaign fund, the failure to initiate creates a tragedy for the future of us all.

Since we do not live in a culture that has consciously created "wisdom" initiations, we have far too many people, both in and out of power, who are incomplete adults with arrested development—in short, an adolescent society. These half-grown adults have no way to face their wounds, so instead these wounds are passed on to others, who in turn pass it on further. Consequently, the initiatory process finds a back door into our lives—with nervous breakdowns, chronic health issues, midlife crises, drug addiction, military indoctrination, and neighborhood gang wars. While exceptional individuals may find their way through this morass to some kind of spiritual awakening, none of these situations are an optimal way to achieve that goal. When we miss taking our lessons at the proper time, they become more difficult later.

If a sudden seminal event calls you to the path of initiation, know that you are not alone. But know that the event itself is not the transforming factor in your life. No, this is just the beginning. This is merely the *call* to change. The change itself is the more difficult and lengthy process. You can resist the call until it beckons again louder, or you can heed its message and hope that it treats you gently.

The times that are now upon us are initiating the race of humans into a new era. Many are hearing the call. Many are awakening from slumber. We have our longings, our urges, our visions, and our hopes, but we do not yet know just where they will take us. The call of the heart will take us into the mystery.

ESSENTIAL POINTS

• Rites of passage often begin with a call.

• This call may come from within or be forced by circumstances, but it often comes from unsuspected longings stirring in the unconscious.

• The call takes us into the mystery of initiation.

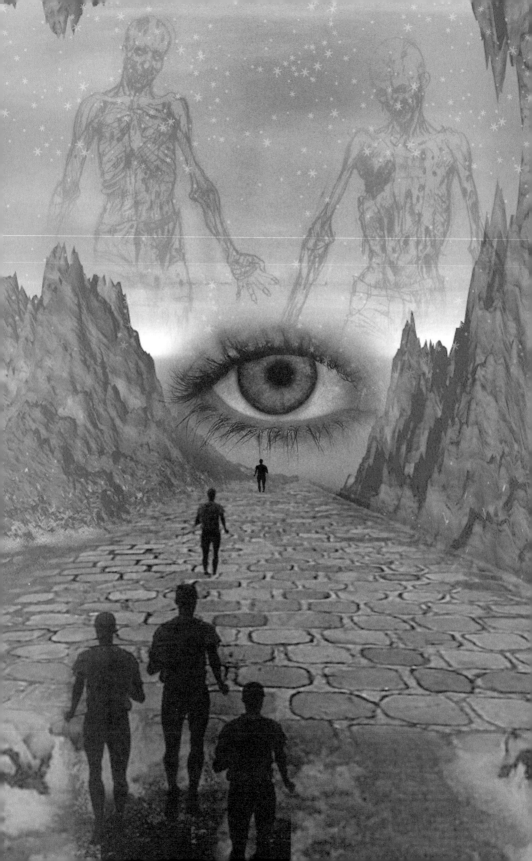

CHAPTER 3

PREPARATION
The Underworld Journey

All true things must change and only that which changes remains true.

—C. G. Jung

Rites of passage: ancient, mysterious, alluring. Whether the call comes as a whisper or a command, a yearning or a sentence, how shall we answer? How do we face this numinous passage? How do we prepare for entry into sacred realms? And what kind of process can we expect?

Initiation is characterized, not only by learning the history of the tribe, but also by challenging ordeals. In many cultures, past and present, adolescent rites of passage involve challenges that are arduous, frightening, and frequently painful. Separation from one's parents and community, sensory deprivation, breaking or filing a tooth, scourging, scarification, burnings, circumcision with a sharp rock, or dangerous acts such as hunting a totem animal or killing an enemy—these were common elements of such rituals. There are countless variations from many cultures, but they all had at least one thing in common: they were designed to break down the smaller ego-self in order to embrace a larger web of life. From this wider perspective, one's own life can then take on deeper meaning and purpose, one that is in alignment—and therefore in service—to the greater whole. In these societies—as it should be in all—only initiates who have embraced the web of life are empowered to take its threads into their own hands and direct the future of their communities.

Carl Jung said: "Only that which can destroy itself is truly alive."[1] In some cultures, the possibility of death was a very real element in their rites of passage. Initiates often understood that failure to pass the test could end their life. Is it so different for us as a species? To naïvely continue in the same direction of mindless consumption, and fail to initiate necessary changes, could bring life as we know it to a tragic end. The ultimatum is written on our many walls: *transform or die.*

Transformation (from *trans* meaning across or over, and *formation,* meaning the making of form) is the journey one takes to find a new form. To emerge into this new form, the old form must be irrevocably altered—even destroyed. This is no easy process. Our lives are embedded in the old form. We are made from it, dependent upon it. We think with its images, judge ourselves with its values, unconsciously respond to its programming. This is why there is always some kind of death in the process of transformation. It is this very death that we fight with such intensity, that we run from in our dreams, that we try to escape through chemical obliteration. But it is this very death that brings us to rebirth.

Breaking the old form is necessary. It creates the fertile ground for a new emergence, much as plowing prepares the soil, or decaying compost fertilizes a garden. But the passage itself—that liminal state between the loss of the old and the beginning of the new—is a frightening and mysterious process. It cannot be predicted, controlled, or outsmarted. It can only be experienced. We must go through it to get to the other side.

Finding entrance into the realm of the sacred is the first mystery that must be probed. This entrance is not a physical place, but an attitude of openness within the psyche. Without that openness, the unfamiliar is rejected and its mysteries remain undiscovered. Without that openness, you will certainly fail the initiation. Breakdown is usually required before breakthrough can occur. The more one resists that which is new, the greater the breakdown must be. We must undo who we think we are and get down to our basic essence in order to build a new structure.

Both ascendent and descendent spiritual paths agree on this point, though their approach is vastly different. Ascendant spirituality includes those paths that seek salvation through transcendence, by moving upward into etheric, intellectual, and meditative realms, leaving the heavier, earthly concerns behind in order to find ultimate truth. Such paths try to dissolve attachment to the earthly, egoic self and its limitations, in order to pierce through the illusion of *maya* and open to a more inclusive reality. Here, ego death is voluntary, or hopes to be, but it may take many years (or lifetimes) of dedication before the last sticky vestiges of our attachments are extinguished. Buddhism, Zen, yoga, most forms of Christianity, Islam, many New Age philosophies, (as well as most interpretations of the chakras), all tend to focus primarily on ascending paths of consciousness. This transcendence is the central tenet of what is considered to be the world's perennial wisdom.

The descending path, though brutal, is faster and less equivocal. The death phase of initiation is one of separation, loss, and dissolution, mythically represented as a journey to the Underworld. This unpleasant downward journey strips a person of all false props and hopes, including those sought in the ascendant practices. In the Underworld, you don't relinquish your attachments—they are pried from your dead, cold hands, destroyed before your very eyes, amputated without anaesthesia. Descending paths strip you down—not only to your foundation, but to the core upon which such a foundation is built. Only then can you truly find roots that are solid; nourished by the deep, hidden layers of the collective unconscious. These instinctual roots are indestructible, and give strength for the journey ahead. Only by getting all the way down to our foundation are we really free to create a new reality, straight from the underground up. Such a path may not grace the top of our fun list, but it is, nonetheless, tremendously effective.

To survive this journey, we must learn the rules of the Underworld.

The story of the goddess Inanna's descent to the Underworld is believed to be one the oldest written myths, preserved on fragments of clay tablets from ancient Sumer that have been dated around 1750 B.C.E. [2] The story tells how Inanna, tender of the great World Tree, traveled to the Underworld to attend a funeral, something that even a goddess cannot do without fundamental sacrifice. When she arrives at the Underworld gate and knocks at the portal, the gatekeeper, Neti, sends a message to Ereshkigal, the ruler of that dark realm, that the Queen of Heaven has arrived.

"A maid, as tall as heaven, as wide as the earth, as strong as the foundations of the city wall, waits outside the gates," cries Neti. [3]

Ereshkigal replies: "Bolt the seven gates of the Underworld. Then, one by one, open each gate a crack. Let Inanna enter. As she enters, remove her royal garments. Let the holy priestess of heaven enter bowed low."

As each gate opens, something vital is demanded from her: her royal crown, the beads at her neck, the beads at her breast, her breast plate (called "come man come,") her gold ring, her lapis measuring rod and line, and her royal robe. [4]

At each gate, Inanna protests adamantly, "What is this?" Each time the gatekeeper, Neti, scolds her: "Quiet Inanna! The ways of the Underworld are perfect. They may not be questioned!"

Oh, how we protest when we tumble into darkness! How we shake our fists at whatever we believe in, how we whine to anyone who will listen, and failing to find sympathy, how much we pay our therapists! Little good does it do. Better to surrender to the darkness and get on with it than to curse the sputtering candle. In that surrender, sweet and dark as it is, lies the humility that opens us to receive something new.

Herein lies the purpose of the Underworld journey. R. J. Stewart, in his book, *The Underworld Initiation,* describes this explicitly:

> "The breaking down of the personality, therefore, is regarded as inevitable and essential in magical growth. The growth cannot occur without the clarifying breakdown; hence the old term 'twice born' for initiates. During dissolution, the constituent elements of the personality, both superficial and long-term, are reduced. What remains are the individual archetypes, resonating in harmonic pattern attuned to the Life Source." [5]

It is from these harmonic threads that we weave our future. The urge to survive is the indelible bottom line, the connecting link to all life, the fundamental trajectory of evolution. It is only when we face death and surmount it that the tremendous power of the survival instinct shows its true strength. All fears tumble in the face of this mighty one. It is this aspect of Underworld initiations that brings the initiate unmitigated strength.

This principle is the very core of the most enduring initiatory experiences known. The Eleusinian Mysteries, held annually in ancient Greece for about two thousand years, were famous in the ancient world for granting initiates an unwavering optimism in the power of life. While the secret core of the ritual was never revealed, the story it enacted is one of the best-known myths today. Demeter, the grain goddess, loses her daughter, Kore, the spring maiden, to the foreboding figure of Hades, King of the Underworld and Lord of Death. As any mother can understand, Demeter's loss is profound, yet none will console her. So extreme is her grief and rage at the abduction of her daughter, she refuses to let the crops grow. Without food, humans die, and without humans, who will worship the gods? This is a serious matter for all!

Alas, even a mother's love—and a goddess at that—is too weak to change the hands of fate. Kore must experience the mystery in order to grow from mere daughter and Maiden to Queen and Goddess. Soil that is bleached dry by the burning sun has no fertility. Without a refuge of cool and quiet darkness in our soul, we "burn out." Kore must learn to embrace the darkness in the Land of the Dead in order to contain within herself the dark fecundity of Earth. Only through union with darkness can she later be penetrated by sunlight and contain the polarities that bring forth life. Thus we find Kore's maturation from Maiden to Mother follows a period of darkness and loss.

R. J. Stewart again comments:

> "The UnderWorld Initiation fulfills the mediating role of humankind. Only when the individual has been through the Underworld can he or she mediate the solar energies into the land, or bring the Light and the Dark together." [6]

The Underworld initiation prepares one to integrate Earth and Heaven, dark and light, soul and spirit. If getting to the heart involves healing the many divorced polarities that have split our world and snared it by the teeth of antagonistic struggle, then the Underworld foray into quiet and darkness is an essential step for integrating the light of transcendence.

That doesn't mean it's easy. Remember: the caterpillar in the chrysalis experiences a complete dissolution of its original body on the way to becoming a butterfly. In the beginning of this process, the imaginal cells of the butterfly are so threatening, they are attacked by the immune system of the dying caterpillar.

In the same way, our psychological defenses may rally fiercely against the initial phases of any initiatory forces that enter our lives. We may attack a new idea that threatens our old way of thinking, or protest adamantly when failure of a career, marriage, or physical health brings us that impending sense of doom. Often we blame ourselves, looking for what we did wrong to "deserve" such misfortune, ("What did I do to make him leave me?") or looking to blame others ("If only Dad had paid attention to me!"), when in fact, it may simply be a sign that we are ready for the dubious distinction of life's *advanced* lessons. The fruits of such dark lessons are the hardy morsels that prepare us to receive the light of realization.

The Underworld journey is about dissolution, the necessary breakdown that precedes breakthrough. The purpose of this dissolution is surrender. Our current paradigm of power is based, among other things, on willed effort. Western culture operates under the myth that anything can be achieved if the will is strong enough and we just try hard enough. But the paradigm of the heart is based on a deeper principle, one that informs the will but is not ruled by it. This requires surrendering our will to a larger matrix.

But when all is dissolving, how do we keep from losing hope? How do we find an anchor to get us through? If we are to truly dissolve our being down to the immortal essence at the core, there must be some larger structure holding us while we fall apart. The caterpillar is held by the chrysalis, just as the broken bone is protected by the cast. In the Hero's journey, the belly of the beast, trapping its prisoner in his or her darkest hour, becomes the very womb of rebirth.

The belly of the beast represents a limit. The fetus in the womb grows prodigiously until the limit of the uterus is reached, and this stimulates birth. A fetus cannot continue to grow, or even survive beyond this point, unless it descends through the birth canal, and enters the larger world.

Collectively, the parameters of our planet pose just such a limit on our cultural transformation, forcing society into a new birth. Butting up against the limits of our resources, we are forced to change our ways. Since it is not our first birth, it has all the earmarks of being a rebirth, and hopefully one that will bring us great joy. But first we have to go through the Underworld.

Underworld journeys can be personal, impersonal, or transpersonal. Our individual journeys are quite personal, and our cries of "Woe is me!" echo this fact. The hand of fate that deals our losses can seem, by contrast, incredibly *impersonal*. Earthquakes and floods do not choose individuals. Those who lost their lives in the World Trade Center, the 2004 tsunami, or the New Orleans flood were innocent victims of impersonal fate.

There is also a transpersonal level—one that destroys the ego to awaken a more transcendent state. The ancient Hindu god Shiva destroys illusion with a lightning bolt from his third eye so that we may better see what is real. Lion Goodman, in his story, "A Shot in the Light"[7] discovered transcendence as a result of getting shot in the head by a hitchhiker he had befriended. Loss can open us wider, letting go of the finite in order to perceive the infinite.

MAGNIFYING THE DARKNESS

Collectively, we are entering a kind of Underworld state, even as many signs of transformation are taking place. Public media broadcasts violence through the cultural nervous system on a daily basis, enlarging these issues to excess. Why this unbalanced broadcast of Underworld conditions at a time when breakthroughs are also occurring? And why are innovations and positive trends buried in the back pages of the newspaper?

In my years of pondering the human condition, I have long puzzled over the public proclivity for violence over love—in stories, movies, television, news, and even children's video games. Why is it that sex, which at its best is an act of love and pleasure, is forbidden–while pain and violence are not only featured but glorified? We build monuments to military heroes. We create video games whose central goal is to kill as many as you can in the shortest time possible. Statistics tell us that crime rates have declined by over fifty per cent since 1993,[8] yet the reporting of crime dominates the media. The motto of front page journalism is, "If it bleeds, it leads." Why do we do this?

I offer two possible answers, and they both dance around the same pivotal point in the death-rebirth process. The first is that we *are* going through a massive dissolution process in our culture–the breakdown that precedes breakthrough. This is our shared Underworld experience. As environmental imbalances increase, more and more people will be facing painful losses. Unlike Inanna, who protests adamantly to no avail, the voices of objection about these matters are still too few. Our culture's prevailing tendency is to avoid and deny. We distract ourselves with sensationalist stories, with sales at shopping malls, with insipid television shows, and with the acquisition of more and more *stuff.* Things are dissolving all around us, but we simply change the channel and turn our attention elsewhere. *As long as we are distracting ourselves, the darker issues must be magnified to get our attention.*

Furthermore, the new structures arising, like the imaginal cells in the chrysalis, are outwardly attacked by old system—the very pillars of tradition that are in the process of dissolving. New discoveries in science are attacked by traditionalists, alternative medicine is attacked as quackery by most doctors, and spiritual diversity is attacked by religious fundamentalists of all stripes. Each of these has been vehemently assaulted during their first emergence by the powers that want to remain on center stage. Is it any wonder that our cultural immune system, armed as it is with the planetary antibiotics of nuclear weapons, is poised to fire at any possible moment? Are we approaching an auto-immune disease, where our defenses will turn and attack the very structures of our collective body? It is at least encouraging to remember that the butterfly undergoes the same process and lives through it. Perhaps we will, too.

So what happens when we truly face our dissolution, when we turn our face to the collective Underworld of violence and destruction?

We begin to turn things around.

When television broadcasted real-time scenes of carnage from the Vietnam war, a passionate peace movement was born. (The Bush administration knows this, which is why pictures of war and destruction in Iraq are repressed.) Rather than some intellectual concept of horror that was happening *over there,* it came home to U.S. living rooms and spawned the largest antiwar movement of the 20th century. For many reasons, including the pressure from the peace movement, the Vietnam war ended before its logical and horrific conclusion.

Now, the Internet brings images of killings and torture in Afghanistan, Iraq, the Middle East, and other war-torn areas. These pictures awaken us to our collective Underworld. However, on the Internet, they are only seen by those who have already become aware of the issue, whereas during the Vietnam war, the broadcast came to homes without viewers seeking it out, waking up many who were not yet aware of the horrors of warfare.[9]

The second reason I believe violence holds such a spell over the priests of the media and their countless parishioners is that we are unconsciously hungry for that primal push of survival that makes us feel so incredibly *alive.* Removed from the natural environment by the many wonders of modern living, our innate survival instincts, wired as they are for extreme situations, go dormant. Our nervous systems, however, having not changed much in 150,000 years, are wired for more primal experiences.

Awakening our core survival instinct is the vital turn-around from death into life. This floods the system with power and aliveness, a necessary ingredient for survival—both as individuals and as a species. In realizing we can blow ourselves to bits with nuclear weapons, we give birth to a peace movement. The failures of allopathic medicine are generating an alternative healing movement. The threat of environmental destruction fuels the ecology movement. Facing our shadow is the beginning of transforming our demons.

The mere instinct for survival isn't enough, however. The germinating seed that yearns for the future must be in the process of becoming something. For this we need intention, understanding, and information. The zygote needs the information encoded in the DNA. The builder needs blueprints. *To rise from the dead we need a reason to live.*

That reason *in*forms us, gives us "form inside." It builds our structure and makes us strong and solid. Form gives us direction, sparks the will, and gets us determinedly through that ridiculously tight birth passage—a passage any sensible logic would hold impossible.

In the dark of the Underworld, removed from our normal way of seeing, we begin to create a vision. But for that vision to be sustaining, it must have deep roots. Those roots dig down into the Earth, into our past, into that which came before. Here we enter the womb of Nature, the belly of the Great Mother. It is from this sustenance that the stalk grows tall and strong, with roots deep enough to support our reach for the stars.

ESSENTIAL POINTS

• The cycle of symbolic death and Underworld journey, followed by rebirth, is common to many ancient myths and most initiation rites.

• Initiates face death in the form of dissolution of their normal way of thinking and being. This usually involves some kind of separation and loss.

• To keep from losing hope in the darkness of the dissolution period, it is helpful to have a vision for life. This vision helps the initiate reform on the other side of the ordeal.

PART TWO

Where Did We Come From?

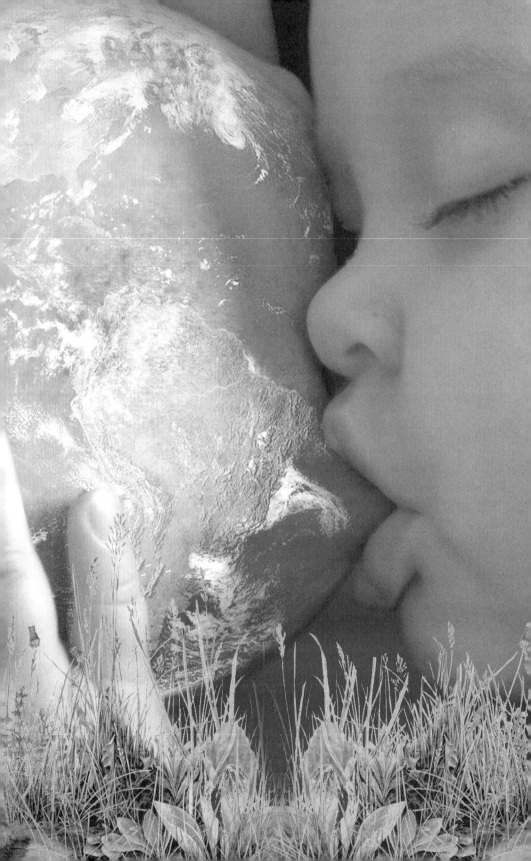

IN THE REALM OF THE MOTHER

The Static Feminine

> *Every threshold passage...is comparable to a birth*
> *and has been ritually represented, practically everywhere,*
> *through an imagery of re-entry into the womb.*[1]

—Joseph Campbell

Out of the womb of the Underworld comes birth. Birth is our ultimate beginning, the primary initiation. After that, the first order of business is simply to stay in the game, in short: *to survive.* This is evolution's primary rule. It must be met for evolution to occur. In preparing for a cultural rebirth, it is essential to understand the archetypal dynamics of our original birth.

Survival instincts comprise the most fundamental level of sentient awareness. They are the basis of the collective unconscious, that shared realm of awareness of which we are mostly unaware. They are hard-wired into everything with a nervous system—or even without one—if we consider the way bacteria mutate to resist medicines. Survival instincts are the ground of consciousness, the foundation, and the roots of our being. They are the expression of Nature's powerful urge to *continue,* for unless something can establish itself and exist through time, it has no hope of evolving.

This is true for an organism, for a relationship, for a species, for an ecosystem and for a culture. If humanity is to evolve on this planet—

if we are to survive the current initiation and grow into a thriving global community—we must master the challenge of survival, not just individually, but together.

This was the prime directive of the earliest humans, so it is here we look to the ancestral beginnings of our culture. Having taken the daring step of walking upright on two feet, humans entered a dangerous world. We could only survive together in cooperative groups or clans. To be cast out from the group meant certain death. To join cooperatively with others in the task of survival necessitated a particular development of consciousnes. It required skills, tools, language, and rules—*strict rules.*

These rules of survival were dictated by the Earth. They were absolute. To live in the severity of Ice Age conditions, and hunt dangerous animals, was to understand the unequivocal power of Mother Nature. She was the Mother that provided everything–but Her rules were not to be trifled with. Breaking the rules could threaten the tribe's magical relationship with its surroundings, and hence its survival. Mother was all-giving, and all-powerful, but She could kill as well as bring forth life. In fact, to early human consciousness, She was All.

Much like the mother of an infant.

Survival instincts, handed down from mother to child, father to son, and our ancestors through the ages, are deeply embedded within our nervous system, honed from millions, if not billions, of years of evolution. Called *innate releasing mechanisms* by Joseph Campbell, these survival instincts appear as inherent tendencies in the psyche that form the fundamental building blocks of consciousness. Such instincts cannot be erased. They can, however be dominated. The cost is putting ourselves at odds with both Mother Nature and our own inner nature.

In the ancient Yogic system of chakras, survival instincts comprise the level of consciousness related to the first chakra, forming the foundation of the entire chakra system. The first chakra is associated with the element *earth,* our holy and sacred ground of being— with Mother Nature. She is the mother of us all, the origin of life, the enveloping field that nourishes us as we grow, the foundation of life.

And a most beautiful Mother she is. Her verdant hills and valleys, mountains of snow that melt into rivers of life, abundant tapestries of color and grace, to say nothing of her unfathomable complexity, are proof enough that She is divine. She is the primal beginning, the sustaining middle, and the holy ground that reabsorbs us all when it is time for the end.

As the first chakra's element is earth, its Sanskrit name, *muladhara,* means "root support." Roots of living things move downward, into the earth, where they provide support for the plant to grow upward. They are the place we come *from,* and therefore symbolize our origin and our past, as in exploring the roots of a belief, a problem, or a cultural tradition. Roots are the primal source from which all things grow. We do not help a plant to grow faster by pulling up on its roots.

In the individual, the *muladhara,* or root chakra, awakens at birth, when the task of consciousness is to learn how to operate a physical body and deal effectively with the physical world. To achieve this, an infant must learn to cope with earth's inherent force—gravity—a challenge that develops such skills as grasping and holding, sitting up, and achieving verticality on its own tiny feet. During this stage of sensory motor development, a child wakes and sleeps frequently, lapsing in and out of alert consciousness. While asleep, he or she surrenders to gravity and returns to an oceanic state, a sea of unity without differentiation. When awake, awareness is busy coping with the challenges of the physical world and learning how to maintain the continuity of its physical form.

The primary caregiver during this time is usually the mother. The mother is the most immediate root, the last place we inhabited before birth, and therefore the original ground of our being. The mother is our first interface to the physical world, the supplier of our needs, the prime protector. She is is the first archetype we experience, our primary matrix, our first teacher.

THE BIRTH OF CULTURE

Few people actively remember the circumstances of their birth. Yet it still has a profound effect on the psyche. Fortunately, a little research into our birth records or talking with family members can bring to light the factors that formed the ground of our earliest beginnings. Likewise, our culture seems to have forgotten that we originated from the feminine womb. The Mother Goddess has been all but erased from collective awareness. Only through recent archaeological research is her reality slowly regaining a foothold in the mythological framework that makes up our society.

The infant phase of human civilizaton corresponds to the Upper Paleolithic, a time known as the Wurm Glaciation, when glaciers up to a mile thick covered the northern part of Europe, Asia, and North America. This era lasted from about 80,000 to 10,000 years ago. Our present human iteration, *Homo sapiens sapiens*, began far south of the ice, originating in Africa more than 100,000 years ago, as descendants of the first proto-humans, nearly four to six million years earlier. It was only about 40,000 years ago that our Cro-Magnon ancestors migrated into Europe, though the frigid climate may make us wonder why. Surviving the long winters at the edge of the ice would have forced our ancestors to direct their developing intelligence toward cooperative survival skills—skills which became fundamental to the foundation of civilization.

It was during the latter part of this last Ice Age that we see the first proliferation of prehistoric art, seen in the elaborate cave paintings such as Lascaux and Altamira, and numerous small sculptures of mother figures found all across Europe and Asia. This is described as a mysteriously revolutionary period of history, an explosion of symbolic thinking and creative behavior, revealing widespread mythological beliefs. In parallel to the beginnings of individual human life, the primary focus of this earliest art focused on images of animals and the Mother archetype. Elaborately painted animals danced on the walls of caves, deep in the womb of the Earth. These images signified the sacredness of the hunt and were probably part of an intiation rite for men.

Reaching out across 30,000 years of dust and ashes, images of the Great Mother, with her round, pregnant belly, remind us that deep within our collective consciousness was another time, another reality, characterized by a sacred regard for women's role in the creation of life. From over 3,000 archaeological sites, scattered across more than a thousand miles, from Western France to central Siberia, some 30,000 sculptures of clay, marble, bone, copper, or gold have been found, all attesting to an apparent reverence of the divine feminine as a fundamental aspect of the miracle of life. While these figurines are not identical, they all share common characteristics: they are small and portable, three to six inches high, have featureless faces, accentuated breasts, bellies, and buttocks, and pointed legs that could be stuck in the ground. It is obvious these are not individual likenesses, but are symbolic in nature. Nor are they limited to a single tribe or area, but represent a widespread sacred symbol of worship.

These figurines symbolize the icons of humanity's first religion—the era of the Great Mother. Her fertility and abundance were linked with that of the Earth itself—the plants that return each year, the young animals that are born in the spring, and the renewal through pregnancy from the all-too-common presence of death during a time when life expectancy was less than thirty years. There is a reason we speak of the Earth as Mother Nature. Marija Gimbutas, the late archaeologist and pioneer in this realm, states:

> "It was the sovereign mystery and creative power of the female as the source of life that developed into the earliest religious experiences. The Great Mother Goddess who gives birth to all creation out of the holy darkness of her womb became a metaphor for Nature herself, the cosmic giver and taker of life, ever able to renew herself within the eternal cycle of life, death, and rebirth."[2]

THE PRIMAL THESIS

Anthropologist, Richard Leakey writes that "The basis of all primate social groups is the bond between mother and infant. That bond constitutes the social unit out of which all higher orders of society are constructed." [3] Like the individual child whose primary world is the mother, our original embeddedness in Nature represents a state of collective consciousness completely centered around the archetype of the Great Mother: mother as environment, mother as food supplier, mother as birth-giver and life-taker. This ground of Nature forms our collective primal thesis, the original backdrop of human existence. It forms the fundamental ground of human evolution: the *participation mystique* or fused identity that links culture and environment with the same inseparable bond as mother and infant child. Just as early humans could not escape the narrow confines of Nature's rule, an infant child cannot survive on its own outside the realm of a mother or nurturing caretaker. It is no wonder that the most abundant art images of the time were those of ample, pregnant women.

In the fused dynamic between infant and mother, and between early humans and Nature, it is conjectured that there is very little awareness of self as separate from the environment. As it is the primal matrix from which we began, our surroundings are an indivisible part of experience, just like the air that we breathe, something we take for granted. Maturation is a gradual separation from the mother, as we grow strong enough to claim our independence.

Our ancestors would have had no idea how big the planet was, or even that it was a planet. They didn't know where they had come from or what would happen in the future. Life emerged from Nature in a unified stream. All was an eternal unfolding of the here and now.

This original thesis of infant and mother—whether as an individual child or a primitive culture—can be called the era of the *Static Feminine,* the first of four combinations of archetypal forces that we will visit in our journey through time. Gareth Hill writes about these archetypal dynamics most beautifully in his book, *Masculine and Feminine: The Flow of Opposites in the Psyche,* where they are applied to the evolution of the personal psyche. [4] My presentation here is my own extrapolation from his work.

Hill symbolizes the Static Feminine as an enclosing circle, a limit that is simultaneously cyclic and eternal. We can see this symbol as the original wheel of life onto which we climb with each birth, the primordial first chakra of physical existence. It is the cell with a nucleus and membrane, the sun surrounded by a planetary orbit, the cycles of Nature beyond which survival is not possible. An infant cannot go too far from the mother and still live. The circle represents that boundary.

The circle is the most basic and universal symbol we have. It is the unified field, the undifferentiated whole, sometimes correlated to Uroboros, the primordial serpent that bites its own tail. As such it represents what philosophers and psychologists have called a pre-personal, undifferentiated consciousness, that sleepy realm of awareness that has not yet awakened to the possibilities of an individuated self, not even to the concept of difference at all. Symbolically, the circle is the symbol of ultimate wholeness, the original perfection, the place we begin. It is the original unity of opposites, the self-contained completion, without begining or end, the original cell. More literally, the circle is the roundness of the pregnant belly, the nourishing breast, and the gentle curve that is so characteristically woman. The circle is the cycle of seasons, the self-renewing generative force that brings us birth, life, death, and birth again, in its eternal cycle.

The boundaries of the circle represent the natural limitations of the field of life. Early humans could not transcend light and dark with the flick of a switch. They could not transcend distance with an airplane, nor shield against cold with thermopane windows and push-button heat. Rarely do we escape the gravity of earth itself. We are still bound to this mortal sphere, to the Earth itself for our survival.

Though Gareth Hill mentions only the form of the circle itself, I see each circle as defined by a center. For the breast, it is the nipple; for the child, it is the mother; for the solar system, the sun. For our ancestors, it would have been the clan mother.

Each one of us is the middle of our own circle, expanding outward to the edges of our bodies, relationships, and communities. If we are bound by fear, our circle remains small and closed. If we are too expansive, the energy within the circle becomes diffuse. Some of us keep those boundaries closer than others, inviting or withstanding limitation, depending upon your point of view.

It is this circular boundary that defines both the positive and negative aspects of the Static Feminine.

The positive aspect of the Static Feminine is that it is nurturing, containing, generative, and maternal. It fosters life, and keeps life protected. Respect its boundaries and you will be safe, cared for, nurtured, and protected. It is stable, solid, and familiar.

The negative aspect is that it is indeed *static*—stable, but limiting, solid but unchanging, familiar but stagnant. Things in stasis continue just as they always have, without innovation. Limiting oneself to the cycles of the Static Feminine can be boring, repetitive, and menial. In a woman's life, it is that stage when she is bound to her infant—cooking, eating, cleaning, feeding, changing diapers, cooking, eating and cleaning again.

The Static Feminine occurs for men as well. It is found in the work of a farmer, always cyclic, bound to the fixed seasonal timing of sowing and reaping, and the many repetitive chores involved. It is found in most menial jobs, where one follows a parental boss without question, sticking to the rules without much room for creativity or expansion. In social groups, the Static Feminine psyche can be seen in fundamentalism—the need to conform exactly to the beliefs and behaviors defined by the group. It could be argued that denial of our fundamental ground in Nature creates the shadow form of religious fundamentalism today, an attempt to find the comfort of the Static Feminine values of family and simplicity.

There is little freedom in the realm of the Static Feminine. What exists remains just as it is. Biology is destiny. Its rule is, as Sam Keen has stated: "Never do anything for the first time."[5] If each age is characterized by an act of heroism, then the ability to uphold tradition and remain totally faithful to the laws of Nature, is the heroic act of the Static Feminine. This forms the basis of our traditions and our unquestioned assumptions. It rears its head in that all-too-common statement, "But we've always done it this way," or "That's just the way it is."

In every person's life, there are times of beginnings: a new job, a new relationship, family or business. It is essential during these times to find elements of the Static Feminine structure to nourish and support these tender beginnings. This can be found by going to conferences, universities, ashrams, health retreats, a therapist's office, or any other means of enfolding oneself in a kind of maternal support. The limitation of this support, however, is that all too often, we are required to mimic the party line, and we forfeit the ability to think critically. Cult mentality, religious or political fundamentalism, or the enforced conformity dictated by group identity all comprise the shadow side of what is initially a drive toward nourishment and support. We suffer from arrested development if we cling too tightly to this support, much as a child fails to grow up when it can't differentiate and gain independence from its mother. Yet we weaken our roots, hence our vitality, if we move too far from this essential foundation.

As our pre-dawn society reaps the accumulated consequences of ignoring Mother Nature's limits, we find that the Static Feminine has been largely obscured, for reasons we will explore in great detail further on in our story. Meanwhile, through the rise of feminism and the archeological discovery of ancient goddess figurines, there has been a new glorification of the Static Feminine. Women are reclaiming their right to ample bodies, their divinity as mothers and nurturers, and their connection with the divine in a feminine form. Many indulge in the fantasy that this period was an idyllic golden age, forgetting that life was hard, with little concept of freedom.

The deep ecology movement rightly stresses the need to return to the obedience of Nature's laws—or reap the consequences. Yet today's culture has moved so far beyond this state of simplicity that returning to it *en masse* is literally impossible, and would certainly kill much of the population. We cannot go back to the breast and suckle an unlimited supply of mother's milk. We have long outgrown our infancy, with our needs having grown beyond the Mother's ability to provide. It is not likely that humans will voluntarily give up cars, airplanes, or technology in general. But we can embrace the sacred ground of Nature as the fundamental value of a healthy society—not as a commodity to be packaged and sold, regarded only for its monetary value.

The Static Feminine is an essential part of our heritage and our wholeness. It is where we began, the primal thesis from which we emerged. We must embrace it to be whole, but we need not be bound by its limitations. Though the child at this stage may have the ideal of everything provided for him without effort, he is still a helpless and dependent child. Though Nature is bountiful and beautiful, survival depends, in part, on being able to transcend the impersonal nature of the cold and dark, and live beyond the life span of our Paleolithic ancestors. It is this challenge which develops intelligence, creativity and cooperation.

In the world of the Paleolithic, it was men who hunted the large game and women who gave birth. Both are essential acts, critical to the survival of the tribe. Both aspects were regarded as sacred roles. Yet their duties were separate: one centered around birth, the other around death. This basic difference is important—not that one was good and the other bad, as we could easily suppose—but that both are necessary elements of survival, mirrors of the essential unity of the circle of the Static Feminine. As Michael Meade has said, "Death is not the opposite of life, it is the opposite of birth. Both are aspects of life."[6]

Understanding the challenges we face today requires our comprehension of this balance between life and death, for we stand at a time when creation and destruction rest equally within our hands. Indeed these are the forces of the gods, and to become gods we must learn to wield both wisely. Both are essential elements in the continuation of any successful species. Both are constantly occurring in Nature. To create life without limits is to court death. To wage war without limits is to threaten life. As we move forward in time, we will witness the continuing cosmic dance of life and death in the unfolding drama of the human mystery play.

ESSENTIAL POINTS

• Humans were born from the primal world of Nature. This was the infancy of our collective beginnings.

• We were merged with Nature the way an infant child is merged with its mother.

• This period is known as the era of the Great Mother and corresponds to humanity's first chakra development, ruled by the values of the Static Feminine—cyclic, stable, and unchanging.

• This formed the primal thesis of our archetypal development and the ground of our collective psyche.

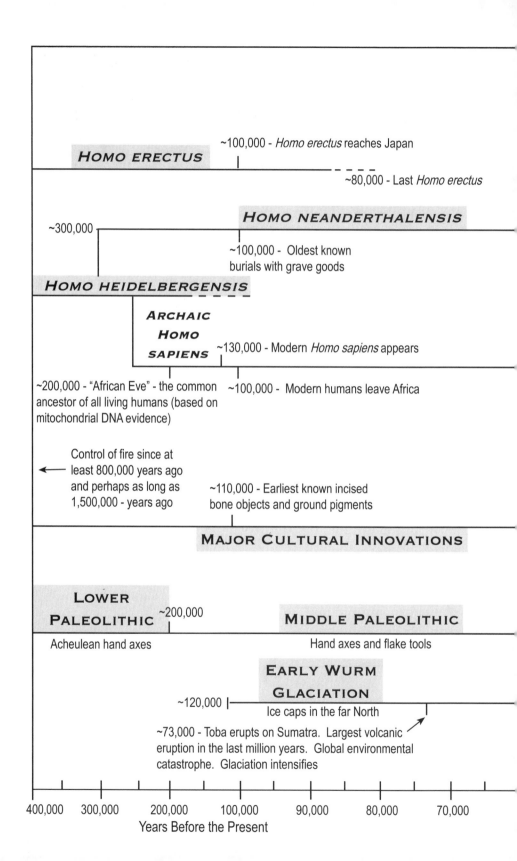

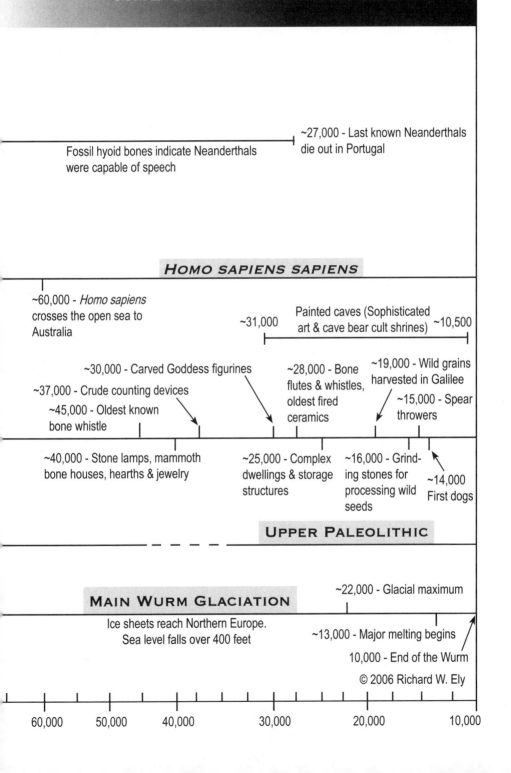

Time Chart 1 - The Paleolithic

~27,000 - Last known Neanderthals die out in Portugal

Fossil hyoid bones indicate Neanderthals were capable of speech

Homo sapiens sapiens

~60,000 - *Homo sapiens* crosses the open sea to Australia

~31,000

Painted caves (Sophisticated art & cave bear cult shrines) ~10,500

~30,000 - Carved Goddess figurines

~37,000 - Crude counting devices

~45,000 - Oldest known bone whistle

~28,000 - Bone flutes & whistles, oldest fired ceramics

~19,000 - Wild grains harvested in Galilee

~15,000 - Spear throwers

~40,000 - Stone lamps, mammoth bone houses, hearths & jewelry

~25,000 - Complex dwellings & storage structures

~16,000 - Grinding stones for processing wild seeds

~14,000 First dogs

Upper Paleolithic

Main Wurm Glaciation

~22,000 - Glacial maximum

Ice sheets reach Northern Europe. Sea level falls over 400 feet

~13,000 - Major melting begins

10,000 - End of the Wurm

© 2006 Richard W. Ely

60,000   50,000   40,000   30,000   20,000   10,000

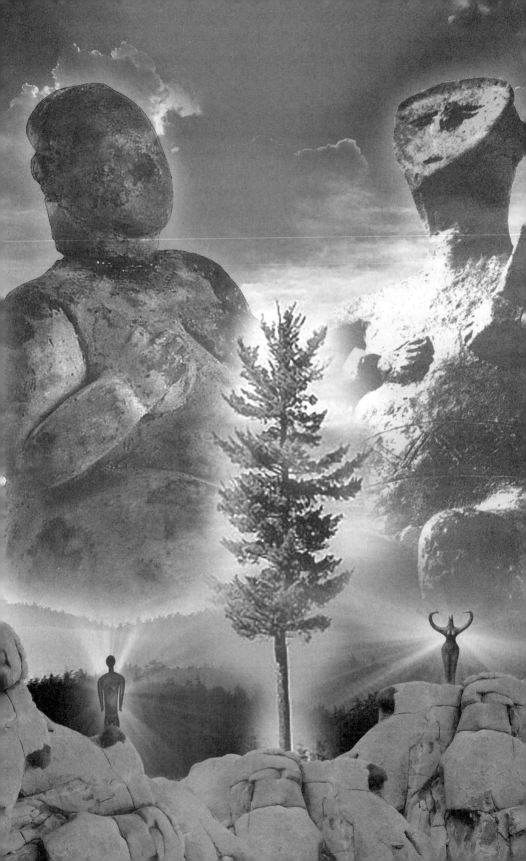

WATERING THE SOUL
The Neolithic

> *Change can erupt like a river, undammed
> from the shifting of psychic ground.*[1]

—Michael Meade

In the initiatory process, there are both masculine, fiery initiations, and watery, feminine ones.[2] The masculine initiations teach a boy to become a man through trials, challenges, ordeals, and intimidations. The soul that overcomes these difficulties learns to conquer fear, discovers the power of its own strength, and develops the confidence and bravery necessary for adulthood. This is essential for both men and women, but traditionally, in the ancestral world of the hunt, such stoic courage was a necessity for the men. A man would be a liability for all concerned if he couldn't be counted on to hold onto his wits and perform well in the face of danger.

The watery initiations, however, are of another order indeed, for they are the initiations into beauty, pleasure, feeling, and, most of all, into mystery. It is the watery initiations that bring us to the heights and the depths of experience, and inspire heroic deeds—not by fear, but by devotion. Fiery initiations teach us strength and courage, watery initiations open the soul to feeling and love. They occur through encounters with a Sacred Other.

To move from first chakra to second, is to move from the element of *earth* to the element of *water*. Where earth is still, predictable, measurable and quantifiable, water is moving, ever-changing, and elusive, as it melts from snowy peaks, and makes its journey to the sea. Water carves the earth with infinite patience, teaching us the first language of time as it reveals millions of years of geologic history, exposing the layers beneath the surface. Following the path of least resistance, water flows in the grooves created by a prior journey. In this way, water is passive and surrendering. Yet it has great power: the power to sculpt mountains and carve valleys, to tumble sharp stones into smooth cobbles, and to produce an entire ecosystem from the soil it has carried down from the fiery peaks of volcanoes.

As a symbolic element of the soul, water is the liquid medium that cools, nurtures, and cleanses. It carries the molecules of emotion from inner experience to outer expression. It cools and tempers the fires of anger; it releases the grief of underlying wounds. Before we can open the heart, our wounds must cleansed by the waters of the soul.

Water is connected to the feeling function–that mysterious bridge between the mind and the body that connects conscious and unconscious. Feelings arise of their own accord, unbidden, from the unconscious. We find that we are angry, depressed, or afraid, regardless of whether or not we desire these states. Yet the mind has ways of covering over feelings and shutting off watery emotions when they are unpleasant, or deemed inappropriate. Such feelings do not die; they are merely suppressed and buried.

When the mind chooses to block emotions, they are carried by the body. We may think we're not afraid, but our belly is knotted into a hard ball. We may try to deny our anger, but our jaw clenches. We grind our teeth at night, during those times when the unconscious holds the upper hand.

To nourish the waters of the soul, one must reclaim the function of *feeling*. Without feeling, there is no ground for empathy, a quality that is essential to the heart's awakening to compassion. The senses stimulate feelings–whether of pleasure or pain, enjoyment or disgust. The five senses are a gateway through which the outer world enters into consciousness. By honoring our senses, we become sensible, instead of senseless.

And what stirs the senses more deeply than beauty and pleasure?

Beauty is an essential but unsung spiritual value. One of the hallmarks of the divine—so evident in the natural world—is its remarkable beauty. The silhouette of mountains against a luminous sunset, the scent of a forest after a rain, the abundant display of wildflowers on a hillside, the sound of a bubbling stream, all reflect a divine beauty that abounds in the natural world. If we are to build a world of the future, it must not only be functional. It must appeal to the senses with beauty as well.

Beauty invites the heart to open and love; it attracts us, enthralls us, casts a sensuous spell that can inspire us to great heights. We set aside the great treasures of our national parks because of their exquisite beauty. For the artistry of Nature acts as a balm to the soul. For beauty's sake we will treasure and care for our world. True beauty reminds us that we are close to the sacred.

EROS AND THE SACRED OTHER

Eros is an ancient god. As the universal principle of attraction—that which brings things into relationship–he is the instigator of the heart's longing for another. To the Greeks, he was the force of desire born from the split between Heaven and Earth, as Chaos and Gaea.[3] In Hindu mythology, he is called Kama. In the Artharva Veda, among India's oldest set of texts, he is referred to as a supreme deity: "Kama was there first. Neither gods nor ancestors nor men can equal him."[4] He is the god of beauty and youth, the impeller of creation, springing from the heart of the Immense-Being (Brahma) and from the primeval Waters.

It is not enough to merely satisfy survival in chakra one. We must satisfy an equally archaic longing–the insistent urge to merge with another. This longing brings us into our first ecstatic encounter with difference–with the consciousness of another soul. Indeed, such an encounter is its own initiation. One does not fully grow from boy to man, girl to woman, or child to adult, without discovering the incredible power of the archetypal *Other.*

The pleasures of sexuality are the perfect seduction into this second level of initiation, and the second chakra is typically associated with the realms of desire, passion, and sexuality. Just as survival consciousness forms the primary challenge of existence, it is the sexual drive of the second chakra that multiplies that existence and extends it beyond ourselves. Through evolution's innate wisdom, it is pleasure that urges the inner current of the soul to connect and bond with another. The insistent pull of the erotic to experience ecstasy—to release, to join, to bond, to spawn, and to love—is all part of the watery realms of the second chakra. Without the waters of pleasure, life is dry, boring, and stagnant. Water helps things move along; it makes life juicy. Without watering the roots so painfully planted in the first chakra, there is no growth, and there will be no sweet fruit to eat. Pleasure, beauty, and erotic allurement invite the heart to open.

But the realm of Eros also brings us into duality: self and other, satisfaction and frustration, pleasure and pain. To reach for another is to risk rejection, to unite with another is to risk loss. Desire is both sweet and dangerous. We discover this when we first explore the world through our senses.

As an infant child grows, her consciousness gradually expands beyond total immersion with the mother as she grows into her toddler stage. As she finds security in her own ground, she begins to explore and expand outward. In this way, she learns about the world. She learns about the dualities of black and white, hot and cold, pleasure and pain. She is starting to move from the nipple at the center of the breast, to explore the outer confines of the circle of the Static Feminine. Yet, she is still unable to survive on her own. She cannot yet move beyond the limits of that circle.

It is the mother who enforces those limits. The natural urge of a toddler in this stage is to expand, yet the naive child does not know where the limits should be.

Until that is internalized, it is the mother who must say "no." With this powerful word of negation, the first experience of conflict arises. As desires awaken, they meet the frustration of limits imposed by others.

Here we come into the dilemma that psychologists refer to as the archetypal split between Good Mother and Bad Mother. The Good Mother is the one who feeds us, picks us up when we cry, and satisfies our every need with kind, patient nurturing. Through her we develop trust, safety, security, and the feeling of being loved.

The Bad Mother is the one who says "no," who slaps our backside for running into the street, who takes away the candy or the toy. She is the one who feels too tired to pay attention to our needs, who is unavailable or angry. She is the mother bird that pushes her baby out of the nest to force it to fly. She is the disciplinarian that makes you do your homework. She is the edge and the limit that may appear cruel, uncaring, or selfish, but whose ultimate nature is also to protect. In fairy tales, she appears as the crone or hag, who threatens to cut off your head. As older women face the loss of their youth and beauty, they often receive projections of Bad Mother and are shunned.

To a child, who is still developmentally in the realm of the Static Feminine and totally dependent on its own mother, this presents an agonizing choice. Who will appear if I do this or that? The Good Mother or the Bad Mother? It is this experience of *choice* that provides the foundation for developing the *will*. Once we choose, it is the will that acts upon that choice.

In this learning, the first distinctions a child makes are binary: hot-cold, light-dark, pleasure-pain, good mommy-bad mommy. This even extends to one's growing sense of self, through the feedback of love and rejection. We start to experience ourselves as a good girl or bad girl, good boy or bad. These distinctions are essential, but incomplete. Most things in life are not quite so black and white, but contain many shades of gray. Greater maturity learns to make subtler distinctions, but the ability to detect differences begins in primitive, binary ways.

Later, as adults, sexuality (also associated with chakra two) is equally charged by the binary conflict between biological imperative and cultural taboos. Not only do we face the possibility of rejection when we reach out to another, but for many the pull of the body involves "going against the rules" set down for us, verbally and nonverbally, since we were first old enough to reach our own genitals. Conditioning goes deep, but biology even deeper. To go against the rules of conditioning is to risk exile, but to go against the self is to enter a deeper abandonment.

This conflict promotes yet another level of awakening. To form relationship, which is the warp and woof of the heart chakra's tapestry, we must first be able to encounter difference and endure conflict. Sexuality is a certain realm for this to happen, for the Sacred Other is most assuredly different. Merging with another inevitably produces some kind of conflict.

The introduction of difference, and its tendency to create conflict, is the next essential element of evolution, after survival. Without difference, nothing will ever change. We will remain in the Static Feminine forever, endlessly following the same circle, without evolving or moving forward. Yet the inertia of the Static Feminine runs deep. In the eternal stability of the Static Feminine era, what caused us to break that bond with the Mother and create something new?

ENTERING THE NEOLITHIC

To answer that question, we now move forward in time from our nomadic ancestors of the Paleolithic Era to the settled agricultural villages of the Neolithic. This change occurred as the last vestiges of the former Ice Age melted away, approximately 10,000 years ago, resulting in a revolution that transformed the culture of humanity and its relationship to Nature.

For several million years—since the begining of our species, really—we were helpless to do anything but follow Mother Nature in her many moods. We followed game wherever it roamed; we ate well or starved according to the times. We lived in caves when we could find them; we collected grasses and plants where they naturally grew. If game was sparse, if winters were hard, if plants were insufficient, there was little we could do about it, except to gather our small tribes and move onward, searching for better conditions and hoping to find a suitable cave to go with them.

Then we discovered the miracle of the seed.

Here began the first steps of taking destiny into human hands. Where Nature's whim could provide or withhold, our ancestors found a means to provide for themselves. Where families had been nomadic, now they could stay in one place, building homes, temples, and villages. Where once we hunted free-running game, animals could now be kept in captivity. Close to home, animals provided eggs, milk, and meat. They were bred and slaughtered as needed, without the dangerous hunt, and without taking the men far away for days or weeks at a time. Where once winters were severe, warming temperatures brought abundant forests, teeming grasslands, and the many creatures that inhabit them. Though still immersed in Nature's cycles, we had gained more than a small shred of independence. We took one small step away from our dependence and enmeshment with Nature as Mother.

To take this step of impregnating the ground and begin farming was a major evolutionary step, one which forever changed the fabric of life on Earth. We can only imagine how it might have happened: A tribe returning to a place inhabited in a previous year finds a new abundance of plants growing near their former hearth. An innovative mind might make the connection, remembering the night her child spilled the seeds outside the cooking area. Or maybe she decided to bury seeds on her own and see what would happen. Or while foraging for roots with a digging stick, another might notice seeds partially sprouted and realize that some conditions were more favorable than others for an abundant return, such as loose ground, prior rainfall, or certain seasons.

Since it is likely that it was women who gathered the plants and tended to the hearth and cooking, while the men hunted, it is conjectured that the mystery of the seed would have first been discovered by women. Preparing the food and making the gourds to carry water, it would have been the women who nurtured the fertility of the fields as a natural part of their duties with home and children, and their association with fertility in general. The mystery of agriculture would have been a natural extension of women's earliler mysteries of birth, life, and death. This does not mean that men were left out of the picture–far from it–especially once the principles of farming became an established community effort. Still, the cycles of sowing, cultivating and reaping were intimately connected with the round of the seasons, and the many moods of the Great Mother. She had, after all, been the central supreme deity of human consciousness since our ancestral emergence from the apes. Such archetypal icons of the psyche are not easily vanquished.

With the melting of the ice, the Neolithic flowered as a true springtime for humanity. While it may not have lightened the workload, it nonetheless eased the struggles of survival from the uncertain conditions of a nomadic life, allowing a more stationary existence. With permanent dwellings, our ancestors could acquire possessions, and build houses and temples.

As the ice melted, there was a dramatic rise in sea level, another aspect of moving from the element of earth (chakra one) to the element water (chakra two). We built ships and traveled by water, which enabled tribes to expand their horizons by contact with people different than themselves, as well as by trading possessions that increased their wealth and skills. With this geological movement of water across the land, and the conscious act of irrigating fields, the roots of civilization were well watered. They not only sprouted, but spread, intertwining and interbreeding, especially along the banks of great rivers and the shores of the seas. It may be that early myths of flooding waters were a metaphor for both the rise in sea level and the flood of irrigation that occurred at this time.

With a means to provide food and shelter, the harsh conditions of survival softened considerably. Fewer babies died while lifespan incrased. Population expanded, while people stayed in one place. From 10,000 B.C.E. to 3,000 B.C.E., global population grew from 5 million to 100 million[5] with the larger Neolithic settlements, such as Çatal Hüyük or Jericho, housing 7,000 - 8,000 people–a very different situation from nomadic tribes that kept their numbers in the low hundreds, hiving off when they grew too large.

The Great Mother had children, and her children grew up to have more children–both daughters and sons, female and male, who mated with each other and added their numbers to the community. The once sole deity of the Great Mother, now accompanied by her divine children, was no longer monotheistic. Her children would eventually grow up to become gods and goddesses in their own right, reflecting both masculine and feminine archetypes arising within the psyche.

The original thesis of the Static Feminine, with its Great Mother archetype, evolved to reflect that of Mother and Child. The Great Mother was no longer simply an elemental breast, but became the sustaining mother that sang her hymns and rocked the cradle of civilization from its helpless infancy into its walking and talking toddlerhood. But even for toddlers, the mother is still central.

Temples were numerous in the old world of the Neolithic. The excavation of Çatal Hüyük in central Anatolia, for example, has given us a glimpse into the largest settlement of its time, housing up to 8,000 people around the 7th millennium B.C. It was a town wealthy from trading and farming, with polished obsidian mirrors, detailed carvings, metallurgy, weaving, and woodworking, all of sophisticated craftsmanship.

Houses in Çatal Hüyük were densely grouped, built on top of each other, with entrances in the roofs. They were made of timber and mud, most of them with temple areas, showing how important religion was to the inhabitant's daily life. Nearly a third of the rooms excavated have large (12 - 18 meters long) multi-colored murals on their walls, many of which were painted, plastered over, and painted again as the need arose. Their images reflected the Life/Death/Regeneration theme of the Great Mother, with pictures of a frog-shaped woman giving birth, surrounded by the symbols of the vulture (who picks the bones clean after death) and the bull's head. Interpretations of the bull's head vary. Some say it resembles the uterus and ovaries; others see it as a masculine procreative force. In the temples of Çatal Hüyük, human skulls, believed to be the abode of the soul, were brought back to the temple for rebirth after the vultures had picked the bones clean. In fact, these temples were so important that small clay models of temples were often found in the homes–miniature buildings with a goddess head on the top, as if the temple were her body.[6] This reflected the idea that the female body was the very temple of the goddess—the abode of fertility and the doorway to life.

FROM GODDESS TO DIVINE COUPLE

Goddess figurines in multiple forms existed throughout the Neolithic period and were common across a wide geographic area: Eastern Europe, Southern Turkey, Egypt, Palestine, Mesopotamia and the Indus Valley of India, such that they were a universally worshipped symbol, recognizable to travelers and strangers. The Static Feminine, which had been but a vague concept in the Paleolithic, became firmly established as the accepted spiritual foundation of the Neolithic culture. It even remains alive today, where Neopagan rituals honor the cycle of the seasons and the inherent dance of life and death within them.

By all indications, this was a peaceful, egalitarian culture. Weapons were not found in Neolithic art, nor were these ancient villages fortified with the defensive walls that would soon appear in cities across the land. By examining the burial remains, it appears that women and men were equally respected. Both shared in the business of life, working together cooperatively. But did they share equal status in their view of the divine?

As time passed and culture developed, the male aspect of the divine—as both lover and son—began to appear. In the heart of the Neolithic—around 5,000 B.C.E., we begin to see not only goddess statues, but gods as well. However, as with any new trend, the god figures were fewer, smaller, and younger, often in postures of submission. While it was clear that the son was gaining entry into the collective consciousness, he still had a long way to go to equal the stature of the Great Mother, who after all, had singlehandedly occupied the center of the psyche since the dawn of human awakening.

Where did this leave men, we might ask? If women were keepers of the mystery of birth, and the Great Goddess was still the primary object of worship, what, then, was the sacred role for the male?

Providing meat through the hunt had given men sacred status during the Paleolithic times. Hunting and gathering were the two essential parts of survival, each with their own mysteries, challenges, and rewards. But as culture progressed into farming and domestication of animals, the importance of the hunt diminished. Yet the realm of birth and the eternal cycles of nature, so connected to the feminine, still held sacred prominence. This produced what Mircea Eliade called a crisis in values, where the sacred relations with the animal world are supplanted by the mystical solidarity between humans and vegetation.[7] He goes on to state that this raises women and feminine sacrality to the first rank:

> "Since women played a decisive part in the domestication of plants, they become the owners of the cultivated fields, which raises their social position and creates characteristic institutions, such as for example, matrilocation, the husband being obliged to live in his wife's house. [8]

This erosion of equality occurred so gradually as to be hardly noticed, taking some 5,000 years while the mystery of the hunt slowly retreated to forgotten realms of the past, or was delegated to small, select groups.

Social inequalities tend to be unstable, and sooner or later breed resentments and counter-movements. If men had lost their original sacred role, it would not be long before that dialectical imbalance would emerge from the collective unconscious to be addressed and corrected. We were not yet playing with a full deck of mature archetypes, in fact far from it.

Differentiation from an essential unity is the beginning stage of an evolution in consciousness, for it takes a step in a new direction. For the child, this stage occurs when she begins to move away from the mother and discover the world on her own, even if only briefly at first. This loss of wholeness, though necessary, is, as Erich Neumann has stated: "experienced as the primary loss—it is the original deprivation which occurs at the very outset of the ego's evolution."[9]

In the archeological remains of Old Europe, between the 6th and 7th millennia B.C.E., the goddess figurines, with phallic neck and egg-shaped body, begin to separate into masculine and feminine symbols. The male becomes the fertilizing force, with the female as the gestating womb. He may appear in the image of a horned animal or phallic serpent, or, as was first seen in the cave murals, a figure of half-man, half beast. Later myths from Sumer, Egypt, and Greece dramatize the bull as the son of the mother goddess, and an actual bull was often sacrificed as the epiphany of the son returning to the mother for rebirth.[10] One striking sculpture from 5800 B.C.E. (from Çatal Hüyük) is of the Goddess and God embracing each other on one side, and the Goddess holding her child on the other. This may represent an understanding of the male role in conception, and it may show the evolution from son to lover.[11] In other sculptures around this time, the god was shown as a full-grown man in various postures: seated with erect phallus, holding his head like Rodin's "Thinker," or with his head bowed in mourning. What was he mourning, we might ask? Was it the loss of innocence? Was he crying for the Mother Goddess, or from his own loss of importance?

As time continued its inevitable march, the phallic forms of the male would loom ever larger in the megalithic uprising of stones, which began to appear sometime after the 5th millenium B.C.E. These standing stones reflected important solar or lunar events. With astounding precision, they required considerable skill in engineering, mathematics, cosmology, and long-range planning—often taking place over the course of many generations, revealing a capacity for abstract thinking and an expanded sense of time. Stonehenge is the most widely known of these megalithic monuments, and is presumed to have been built over a period of 1300 years[12]—a true testament to intergenerational planning. France has as many as 5,000 megalithic sites, while 900 have survived in Britain and over 500 in Ireland.

So we see that in the cradle of civilization the young god was slowly growing up. Still a child to the ancient and primordial Goddess, he became her lover long before becoming her master. But soon the tables would turn, as we will see in the next act of the human drama: the dawning of the *Age of Power.*

ESSENTIAL POINTS

• Water is the element of the second chakra, oriented to emotions, sexuality, and procreation.

• The watery initiations are centered around beauty and the erotic, with a strong emphasis on fertility and procreation.

• Historically this period coincides with the melting of the last glaciation and the discovery and spread of agriculture.

• This is known as the Neolithic period of history, where humans learned to farm, domesticate animals, and develop village life.

• Though still part of the era of the Great Mother, ruled by the Static Feminine, images of male gods started to appear.

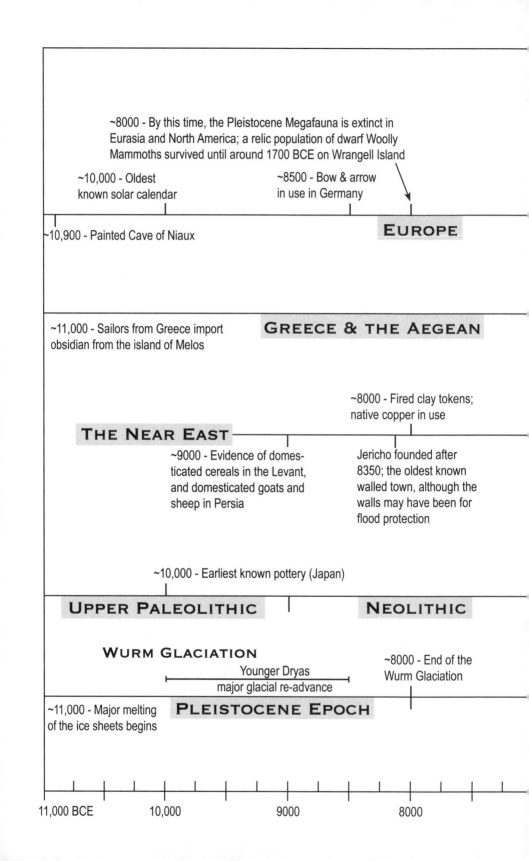

~8000 - By this time, the Pleistocene Megafauna is extinct in Eurasia and North America; a relic population of dwarf Woolly Mammoths survived until around 1700 BCE on Wrangell Island

~10,000 - Oldest known solar calendar

~8500 - Bow & arrow in use in Germany

EUROPE

~10,900 - Painted Cave of Niaux

~11,000 - Sailors from Greece import obsidian from the island of Melos

GREECE & THE AEGEAN

~8000 - Fired clay tokens; native copper in use

THE NEAR EAST

~9000 - Evidence of domesticated cereals in the Levant, and domesticated goats and sheep in Persia

Jericho founded after 8350; the oldest known walled town, although the walls may have been for flood protection

~10,000 - Earliest known pottery (Japan)

UPPER PALEOLITHIC

NEOLITHIC

WURM GLACIATION

Younger Dryas
major glacial re-advance

~8000 - End of the Wurm Glaciation

~11,000 - Major melting of the ice sheets begins

PLEISTOCENE EPOCH

11,000 BCE   10,000   9000   8000

TIME CHART 2 - THE NEOLITHIC

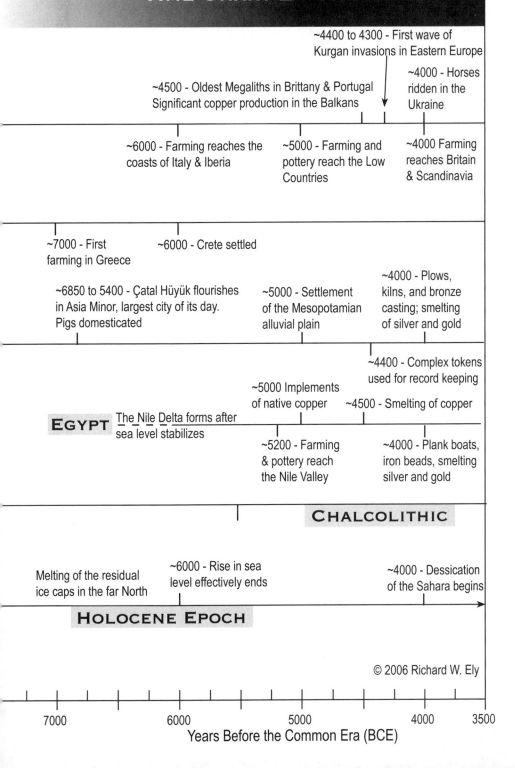

~4400 to 4300 - First wave of Kurgan invasions in Eastern Europe

~4000 - Horses ridden in the Ukraine

~4500 - Oldest Megaliths in Brittany & Portugal Significant copper production in the Balkans

~6000 - Farming reaches the coasts of Italy & Iberia

~5000 - Farming and pottery reach the Low Countries

~4000 Farming reaches Britain & Scandinavia

~7000 - First farming in Greece

~6000 - Crete settled

~6850 to 5400 - Çatal Hüyük flourishes in Asia Minor, largest city of its day. Pigs domesticated

~5000 - Settlement of the Mesopotamian alluvial plain

~4000 - Plows, kilns, and bronze casting; smelting of silver and gold

~4400 - Complex tokens used for record keeping

~5000 Implements of native copper

~4500 - Smelting of copper

EGYPT The Nile Delta forms after sea level stabilizes

~5200 - Farming & pottery reach the Nile Valley

~4000 - Plank boats, iron beads, smelting silver and gold

CHALCOLITHIC

Melting of the residual ice caps in the far North

~6000 - Rise in sea level effectively ends

~4000 - Dessication of the Sahara begins

HOLOCENE EPOCH

© 2006 Richard W. Ely

7000   6000   5000   4000   3500
Years Before the Common Era (BCE)

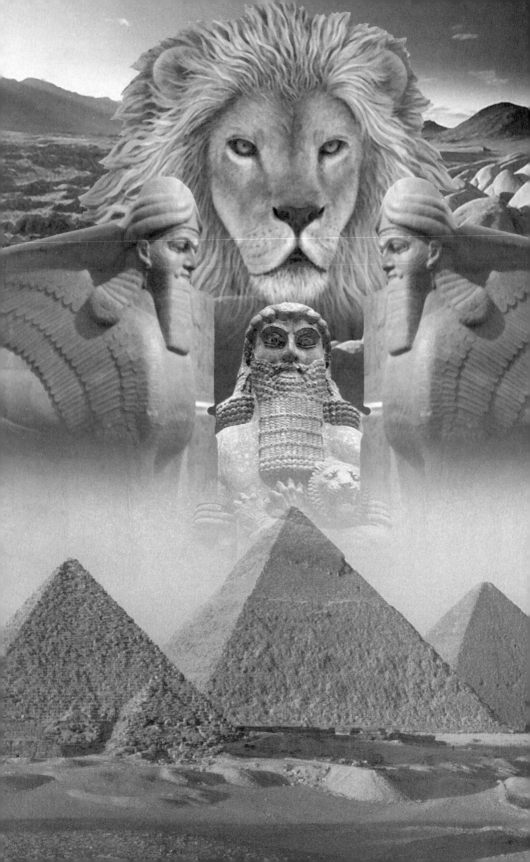

FROM WILL TO POWER

The Dynamic Masculine

> *Our object is not to restore the primordial goddess,*
> *but to emancipate ourselves from the effects of a culture*
> *based on emancipation from her.*[1]
>
> —Catherine Keller

Whatever is worshipped proliferates. If a culture worships birth, there will be babies. If it glorifies killing, there will be wars. If God is the almighty dollar, we will build an economic empire. If art is holy, as it was in the Renaissance, there will be great masterpieces.

The abundance of pregnant-bellied Goddess figurines from the Paleolithic and Neolithic implies that their cultures worshipped the miracle of birth. Supported by the development of farming and the ability to stay in one place and build permanent dwellings, the worship of fertility coincided with an exponential growth in population. Expanding population created new challenges, requiring more food, water, land, and most of all, greater social organization.

Such was the challenge that stimulated the awakening of the next cultural era: the third chakra phase of power and will, out of whose bloody clutches emerged the heroic, ego-identified, individual self. To move from an obedient infant and toddler culture, where power exists outside oneself in the unequivocal rules of Mother Nature, to the birth of individual power, is a necessary step in the process of maturation. Without the awakening of personal power, we would be destined to flow in the eternal circularity of the Static Feminine forever, much like our animal ancestors. No doubt the environment would fare better, but the human race would remain in a helpless, infantile state, unfulfilled in the potential made possible by our opposable thumbs and swollen forebrains.

As an infant child matures into a toddler, his increased motor development allows him to move outward, from symbiosis with the mother into the world at large. Through this process of "hatching" a child develops a sense of individuality, and awakens his personal will. For an individual, it may begin by a chance action such as breaking a lamp while playing. Mother rushes in, saying: "What have you done?" The child stares at the result and knows—perhaps for the first time—that his own action caused the lamp to fall. In this moment he gains an inkling that his impulses and actions affect the world. This is a gradual awakening of self as a causative agent. We spend the rest of our lives learning to control or enhance that influence.

Soon after this realization, at a stage we commonly call the "terrible twos," the typical child actively rebels against the mother and the established order she represents. If she says, "Yes!" the child says, "No!" If she says, "No!" the child will test his limits and do it anyway. This is a stage that psychologists call *differentiation*— the act of differentiating from what is, in order to create and define something new. This struggle is essential for the development of personal autonomy and will.

In correlating Gareth Hill's schema of masculine and feminine valences, the rebellion against the mother would correspond to the awakening of the *Dynamic Masculine*. This occurs for both men and women. The masculine urge to expand beyond the static limits of the mother is represented by an arrow that shoots out from the original circle. Power, once limited to the circle, is now projected outward. The arrow is different from the circle in every way, showing the move from static to dynamic, from cyclic to linear, from inclusive to directive. The linear arrow well symbolizes the willful, penetrating force of the Dynamic Masculine, and its goal-directed initiative.

THE OVERTHROW OF THE MOTHER

Human children have an exceptionally long period of dependence compared to other animals. This creates a strong archetypal bond between mother and child. It takes a great deal of confidence and inner strength to overthrow this bond and claim one's autonomy, a strength gained, in fact, by a solid bonding with the mother as an infant and toddler. This early support forms a firm foundation for the child that makes it feel safe enough to develop will and autonomy.

What happens when an entire culture enters this stage of rebellious differentiation?

Fertility produces babies of both genders. Girls are more likely to imitate their mothers as they grow up—especially in a culture where goddesses are worshipped and the feminine held as sacred. There would be little reason for girls to differentiate. Boy children, however, must differentiate from the mother in order to develop their own masculine nature. *It thus falls to the masculine side of things to carry the initial differentiation from the mother culture into the emerging age of power.*

Imagine the strength required for a culture to overthrow the Great Mother! Her numinous presence would have been the central archetype of worship since the dawn of human consciousness. Her power would have deep roots in the psyche. She was the very land people lived upon, the field that gave them life. It would take a very potent force indeed to overthrow such a power, one that would have to be equal in strength, yet profoundly different. What was this ominous power?

We have stated that the first act of differentiating is one of negation. The mother provides a primal ground, the basic thesis of embeddedness in nature. The differentiating masculine forms an antithesis to that basic thesis, and its values and dynamics turn into their opposite. As it occurs in the child, it also occurs in cultural shifts. Alfred North Whitehead put it bluntly when he said, "Each new epoch enters upon its career by waging unrelenting war upon the aesthetic gods of its immediate predecessor."[2] Joseph Campbell simply called it history's "Great Reversal."[3]

But it was a long, slow turning. It took thousands of years before this initial rebellion crystallized into its own thesis, for the power of the Mother holds strong, due to the excessively long period of bonding. The primacy of the Great Mother extended from the very first glimmerings of spiritual worship, anywhere from 200,000 to 30,000 years ago, to the period in which this reversal began to dominate civilization, beginning with the first Kurgan invasions around 4400 B.C.E., but clearly established in most regions by 3000 B.C.E. This is certainly a long time, and we need only look at the influence of a religion like Christianity, 2,000 years young, to imagine how powerfully the archetype of the Great Mother might have loomed in the collective consciousness of our ancestors.

The overthrow of the mother, singly or collectively, represents a powerful act of rebellion against everything that represents survival and security. It was only the ability to provide for our own survival that made this risk possible. By taking nature into our own hands, through successful planting, harvesting, and building of shelters, humanity gained enough freedom from nature's absolute rules to create a new set of values. Like most achievements, this success, combined as it was with exponential population growth, created exciting freedoms and possibilities, as well as new challenges and problems.

To pull the roots of survival out of their earthen bed and wrap them instead around the clouds of heaven took a force equal in powerf to birth. What cosmic power could possibly break the archaic spell of the Mother and the seamless unity with nature? Only the fear generated by *death* was potent enough to rally consciousness in a new direction. Not that this choice was made consciously—for who in their right mind would choose death over life, violence over peace, and fear over security? Yet, for reasons we would do well to understand, history has made it abundantly clear that humans have made such choices repeatedly. We still do today.

At its beginning, an instinctive rebellion is immature and therefore destructive. New movements take little care to preserve what precedes them, but focus instead on establishing their own values, even at the cost of destroying the base upon which they stand.

Like the action of a frustrated toddler with a new toy just beyond its abilities, social behavior was still based in primitive instincts, shaped by ancestral memories of Ice Age survival. This movement knew not what it was doing or where it was going; an inner imperative simply reached out for power against the helplessness of its infant dependence.

As the locus of power fell to the male side of the population, the *reverence for birth* was replaced by its opposite: the *fear of death*. Earth mysteries were replaced by the worship of sky gods, whose power thundered in the heavens with threats of angry retribution. Cultures that had been peaceful began training armies for defense, protecting themselves with walls and fortifications. As civilization became militarized, death was glorified.

But surely we run ahead of ourselves. For the rulers and kings, governments and armies that stockpile weapons today are the products of an ancient battle over darkness that reigns in the ancestral memory of us all. If we are to rise beyond this dangerously outdated system to enter the age of the heart, we must ask ourselves why humans, alone among Earth's creatures, were given control over the element of fire.

THE DAWNING OF PERSONAL WILL

> *Never doubt that a single person alone can change the world. For indeed it is the only thing that ever has.*   —Margaret Mead

To say, "I will" is to create the future. It is an intention that has a direct effect on coming events. Without the capacity to exert will, we have no control over our future, but remain as children, passive to the effects of larger forces. The process of differentiating awakens the spark of individual will, and in fact, can't be completed without will. This aspect of consciousness has only recently appeared in the evolutionary mix, relatively speaking, meaning that lower animal forms don't seem to have it. This point is essential to understand.

Plants have a life force, but little capability to move on their own. Animals can initiate their own movements, but these actions are largely instinctual, capable of only the most elementary forms of planning. In sharp distinction to our animal ancestors, humans have the capacity to rise above their instincts and exhibit conscious choice, be it wise or foolish. We alone have the ability to control fire, to create and use complex tools, and to do things that have never been done before, even things that threaten our own survival. If we are to move from childhood to adulthood, knowledge of how to use our will, both individually and collectively, is essential. If evolution is the gods' way of making more gods, then mastery of the will in relation to the powers of creation and destruction is an essential lesson within this development.

Will corresponds to the third chakra, located in the solar plexus. This chakra is classically associated with the element fire, in both its benevolent and destructive aspects. The use of fire marks an unequivocal difference between humans and our animal ancestors. Such use started long before the third chakra era began, some say as far back as 800,000 years ago.[4] Yet in the larger scheme of things, this is still relatively recent.

Fire gave us our first power over Nature, enabling us to create an *opposite* condition to what Nature presented. With fire, humans could create light when it was dark, make warmth when it was cold, cook food to make it edible. We could gather around a common source of energy and share stories, fashioning tools as we talked, sang, laughed or loved. But with fire, we also had a greater potential for destruction. Fire could consume the forest and lay it waste, were it not carefully tended and contained.

Tool-making goes back even farther than fire, with the first simple choppers dating back nearly three million years, fashioned by *Homo habilis*. The ability to pick up a stick to defend oneself, to tie a rock to that stick, to sharpen that rock to a point, to make a needle to sew, a hollow a gourd to carry water, to weave a basket to hold plants—each of these discoveries gave us a little more power over the helplessness of infancy. We could move ever so slightly away from the totalitarian control by Mother Nature, and gain some small degree of freedom from the relentless demands of survival. It was the fashioning of *metal* tools by fire, however, with the advent of the Bronze Age, that really mark the beginning of the third chakra era (circa 3150 B.C.E).

The awakening of individual will is harder to pinpoint. At its most basic level, the ability of humans, like other animals, to move about freely has always been present. But the ability to actively rebel against the awesome power of "what is," and take a step in a new direction, requires at least a moderate amount of maturity, only supplied by a solid foundation of knowledge about how to survive. It is this foundation, forged in the eras of chakras one and two, that permits enough security to even conceive of such a thing as *free will*.

It is my conjecture that the awakening of *individual* will—defined as the ability of an individual to act outside of the cultural grooves of his time—was a gradual process which occurred over thousands of years. It would have arisen in some people before others (a disparity that is still evident today). As individual will awakens, it is initially revealed by *choosing to go in a new direction*. As this creates difference, it tends to create conflict. Which, of course, it did. *Solving these conflicts became a central impetus to the organization of civilization as we know it.*

It is logical to see how a growing population would require either increased production or territorial expansion to meet its needs. To increase production and distribute food and goods to the masses would require both administrative skill and labor specialization—setting the stage for class distinctions. Control of production would produce economic disparities, and with it classes of peasants and rulers. Territorial expansion and defense against invasions would create militarism, and with it a warrior class. Hierarchies developed, with gross discrepancies in power and wealth.

The need to keep track of the production and distribution of goods was the impetus for one of the greatest fruits of civilization: the invention of writing. Around 3100 B.C.E. , as symbols pressed into clay, the first cuneiform writing appeared in Mesopotamia. Humans learned to let patterned marks on clay represent something real—thus maturing into symbolic thinking. This marks the beginning of recorded history, for now great deeds and battles could be written down—frozen in time for future generations to ponder.[5] Consciousness extended from the immediacy of the moment toward a wider sense of time.

Evidence from Mesopotamia in 3000 B.C.E. indicates that coordinated projects, such as building a vast irrigation system, were conducted by a temple bureaucracy. It controlled the payment of rations, the development of crafts, and the production of exports.[6] In fact the word *hierarchy* actually means "rule of the sacred," an order of nested powers extending downward from the temple priests. The conquests from militarism produced captive slaves, who provided cheap labor force for these projects, increasing the wealth of their masters. Leonard Shlain, in his book, *Alphabet vs. the Goddess,* points out that the establishment of writing coincides—wherever it occurs throughout the globe—with the appearance of hierarchical societies, loss of status for women, and increased aggression. But which is cause and which is result?

Institutionalized slavery and the unequal distribution of wealth led to a class society, where temple bureaucrats formed an alliance—if not a dependence—with the military. The more wealth a community had, the more it needed to be defended and protected. The more the military plundered other villages and brought home the spoils of war, the wealthier it became. *From the earliest dawn of historical times, we can see how wealth and war became hearty bedfellows.* Their alliance gave power to the few who managed to control the many. And we must remember that it is from this sector of society that our collective history was written.

SUBDUING NATURE AND SEXUALITY

Another important spoil of war is the rape and capture of women, which results in children sired by the dominant tribe. Women, who are biologically and socially programmed to nurture their children, would then be subsumed into the dominant culture, forced to abide by its rules in order to survive and protect their young. Once again, the successful tribes produced more bodies for their armies and workforce. The trading and enslavement of women as multiple wives fed directly into the economic welfare of a community.

It is here that we can trace the beginnings of social control of women's sexuality. While a child's mother is always apparent, the identity of the father is questionable. It can only be made certain by the strict control of a woman's sexual encounters. It was her disgrace, not the man's, that would result from sexual promiscuity. In these cases a woman's very life and welfare of her children depended on her obedience to patriarchal laws.

This era marked a profound change in every facet of Old Europe, one that has continued to the present day. An edict of Urukagina, c. 2350 B.C.E., stated: "Women of former times each married two men, but women of today have been made to give up this crime."[7] Where women had once held property, married more than one man, and were revered as priestesses, ruling over the complete cycle of life, death, and rebirth, societies changed to a masculine ruling elite, typified by the creation of temple bureaucracies, the worship of sky gods, the control of women, and an endless cycle of military conquests.

During this transition, our ancestors shifted from a culture in which people were dominated by Nature to one in which people dominated each other. Moving from rural villages to larger cities, their lives were filled with the stimulus of a human social milieu rather than the flow of Nature. Defending against Nature—whether by building walls for protection, or defending against the sexual urges of human nature—became the dominant theme of the time.

Whether we view this change as inevitable progress or an unfortunate turn of events, there is no doubt that it produced two notable currents in the cultural stream. The first was a tremendous leap in human consciousness through the development of writing, mathematics, irrigation technology, architecture, and crafts. The second was a long period of social and environmental chaos, due to constant wars and numerous natural disasters, such as droughts and floods.

With the advent of writing at the beginning of the Bronze Age, we have for the first time a record of the myths and laws that allow us to witness the archetypal meanderings of history. Whatever conjecture we might make from the burials and artifacts of the Neolithic, written language has the ability to portray a detailed story. The Bronze Age was a transitional time, whose myths tell of the revolving paradigms of Mother to Son, myths that were no doubt passed down orally for many generations before they could be written. Here we find stories of initial separation and the eventual triumph of one part over another. These involve the separation of the World Parents, the slaying of the Mother, the rescue of the Maiden, and the rise of the Hero, all of which set the stage for a unified Father God, who rescues his children from the suffering and chaos that result from this tumultuous and violent period of human history.

Myths of separation also represent the ability to make distinctions, a primary aspect of a budding intellect. The first elements to be separated were the Earth and the Sky, archetypally, the earth *Mother* and the sky *Father*. The separation of the world parents represents the first separation of masculine and feminine, the archetypal divorce from which we all became children of a broken home. This can be seen in many mythologies of the time: The Egyptian Star Goddess Nut and the Earth God Geb who can never quite reach her; the Greek Goddess Gaia and the heavenly chaos of Ouranos, whose separation brings forth Eros or desire; the Japanese Sun Goddess Amaterasu who is sent to a cave by her mate Susanowo; the Maori Mother Poppa and Father Rongi.

The Sumerians provide us with the oldest written myths, which undoubtedly represent an even older oral tradition. They tell of the great goddess Nammu, representing the primal waters of the void, who created the sky god An, and the earth goddess Ki. An and Ki gave birth to a son, Enlil (God of Air or Breath) who separated his parents and then married Ki, repeating the motif of the great mother and her son-lover, long predating Oedipus. In this separation of the world parents, consciousness makes a clear distinction between basic polarities: Heaven and Earth, above and below, spirit and matter, father and mother:

"Enlil, who brings up the seed of the land from the earth,
Took care to move away Heaven from Earth.
Took care to move away Earth from Heaven."[8]

In Egypt, the primal waters of chaos were said to contain a conscious principle of wholeness called Atum, who alone created Shu and Tefnut, air and moisture. Shu, in turn, gave birth to Nut, the star goddess, and Geb, the earth god, and then stood between them as the atmosphere. In Babylonian myth, Marduk cuts Tiamat in half and separates her body into sky and earth, a myth we will revisit in detail further on.

Here we see a repeated theme of the original unity breaking into duality, with the prodigal child, usually a son, standing triumphantly between them. In this way, a single male entity, be it a god or a man, *achieves the heroic task of creating differentiation and then order.* But this order is believed to come from his own decree, rather than the order that exists in Nature. Thus "revealed religions," whose order orients from a human prophet deciphering the word of God, are often diametrically opposed to the natural order, whose scripture is written in the living tissue of the biosphere.

Erich Neumann, in *The Origins and History of Consciousness,* suggests that this original separation created guilt and loss, a feeling of isolation that happens whenever we separate from a source of love and protection. We can see how this suffering and loss was then projected outward to the next set of "separation" myths, which feature a grieving goddess, separated from her child or consort, who wanders the Earth in a kind of exile, searching for her lost loved one. These wanderings eventually take her down into the abyss of the Underworld, where she enters the forgotten realms of the collective unconscious while her son takes center stage as the carrier of light. From this dynamic, the male is often equated with light as the realm of awakened consciousness, while the feminine is associated with the darker, unconscious realm of the soul.

In the Sumerian myth of Inanna, which we visited in chapter three, we see both the separation and the shift in power. Innana was forced to marry the shepherd, not the farmer—perhaps a man from the invading tribe rather than her own pastoral tribe. After she enters the last of seven gates to the Underworld, she finds her sister, Ereshkigal, giving birth in a sweaty and dirty bed. Meanwhile Inanna's consort, Dumuzi, celebrates in her temple above, having taken over her abandoned throne.

In Greece, the story differs very little. The grain mother, Demeter, loses her daughter Kore to Hades, god of the dead. In Demeter's grief and anger against the power of Zeus to make such a deal without mother or daughter's consent, Demeter halts all growth. Here we see the ancient goddess of agriculture raging against the sky god's triumphant power to alter the normal chain of events. Whereas a rightful passage may have been for the daughter to assume her mother's divine station as grain giver, she instead becomes queen of the dead.

In Egypt, it is Isis who loses her brother and consort, Osiris, who is cut to pieces by his dark brother Set. As a result, Isis must search the countryside, looking for the pieces to resurrect her mate. Even mother Mary of Biblical myth loses her son Jesus to the crucifixion, and weeps powerlessly. A mother archetype, without a child to love, is a bereaved goddess indeed. But it gets even worse.

In other myths of the time, the child who has separated his parents now faces the task of slaying the monster of his past, who often appears as a dragon or serpent. The monster, larger than life and replete with animal characteristics, is said to represent the terrible aspect of the Great Mother, whose anger has been incurred by the rebelliousness of her child. She now represents the darkness of the prepersonal unconscious, which will douse the light of the emerging ego at the slightest lapse of attention, requiring constant vigilance. But perhaps this monster is also the chaos one faces with the first experience of standing alone in a world whose established order has been turned upside down in the battle for power. For to keep that power, the chaos must be vanquished. The establishment of order became a major theme in the Iron Age, whose meteoric "metal from the sky" locked the slain goddess into her iron-clad tomb and solidified its new paradigm with iron resolve.

Meanwhile, peoples of the Bronze Age struggled with the constant strife of invading tribes, competing pantheons, and the struggle of growing empires to advance their own civilization and dominate others. To the Assyrians, one of the bloodiest of ancient peoples, conquest was a divine mission of their kings—the initiatory challenge of the rich and powerful. From the Hebrews and the Aryans, one can follow a path of destruction that moves outward from the fertile crescent, into the Indus Valley of India, North Africa, Greece, and Northern Europe, violently fragmenting the fabric of civilization, even as it was being built.

As a defensive strategy, cities built ever-larger fortified walls, circles around their nucleic temple center, much like the symbol of the Static Feminine. Only now we add a line pushing out from those circles, led by the arrows of conquest, as armies of warriors set forth to conquer others. Put together, the arrow and the circle represent the modern symbol for the male (as well that used for the planet Mars, a planet associated with fiery aggression). This new order rises in opposition—*in every way possible*—to the Static Feminine, from whose base it had sprung. It moves outward from the protective circle of the mother and forges in an opposite direction.

As we walled ourselves off from Nature and became pitted against each other, the original harmonic unity was divided. This turmoil would create fluctuations in the balance between humans and Nature, affecting weather, illness, and social harmony. As a result, we see an increased emphasis on order and control through stronger human rule, along with ritual sacrifices of animals and occasionally humans to appease the anger of the old gods.

MARDUK AND TIAMAT

One myth in particular seems to indicate a turning point in the changing of the divine guard: the myth of Marduk and Tiamat, as told in the Babylonian epic, the *Enuma Elish*. This myth, whose name means "from on high," was known throughout the ancient world. It was celebrated at the new year for close to a millennium, from the late Bronze Age well into the Iron Age. [9] It tells the story of how the archetypal Mother is finally and totally vanquished, and a new order established upon the foundation of her slain body. Its archetypal symbolism is so significant for the points we are exploring, I present it here in detail, italicizing certain passages in order to emphasize their importance.

Tiamat, whose name means *salt waters* or *primeval ocean,* represents all that we have mentioned as our archaic beginnings: original chaos, undifferentiated consciousness, and the primal ocean from which we all came. Though the myth begins when Heaven and Earth had not yet been named or separated, the goddess Tiamat nevertheless has a husband, the Great Father Apsu, (sweet waters) and even a son, Mummu, who represents the mist on the waters. This represents a pre-differentiated time, where all the waters of awareness mingle as one. The *Enuma Elish* was recited at the springtime, when the annual flood of the Tigris and Euphrates rivers would cover the land with fresh water and mingle with the sea, shrouded with mists. It also represents the undivided unity of the Static Feminine.

As the sweet waters of pleasure mix with the salt waters of creation, Apsu and Tiamat give birth to a series of children, grandchildren, and great-great-great grandchildren, who grow into an entire order of gods and goddesses, each with their place in the cosmos. (Sumerians were said to have worshipped some 3,000 localized deities, certainly a large family.) Apsu, as irritable fathers are wont to do, complained that his children were noisy and disruptive, and that he could not rest or sleep.

We have already stated that in a culture that worships birth, there will be children—boy children and girl children. The polytheism that follows creates a number of contentious pantheons, each pocket of culture having its own theology. It is not surprising that this would create a "household" of squabbles, upsetting the peaceful order of things. Do we not, as parents, know this to be true of young children? Do we not get annoyed at their messy and noisy childishness, much as we love them? That Apsu wanted to sleep indicates that he was tired, perhaps because his role as father was complete. Yet he would not pass the mantle gracefully on to his children.

Apsu takes counsel with his son, Mummu, and suggests that the noisy children should simply be destroyed. Mummu, who thinks that he alone would be immune from this tyranny, agrees. Together, Apsu and Mummu, father and son, take their plans to Tiamat. She protests, as mothers are wont to do. "Why destroy what we ourselves have brought into being?" she cried. "Their way may be painful, but let us take it good naturedly."[10] Yet Mummu and Apsu persist in their plan, ignoring Tiamat's cries.

We can see how the struggle begins with an archetypal rivalry between the older and younger generations—an old story indeed. This struggle is fed by a prodigal son who separates his parents and plots against his siblings. Notice how the conflict first dances in the spheres of father and son, with the mother initially refusing to play. Though she, too, was disturbed by the turmoil, she maintains her static feminine nature—at least for a time.

The children get word of their father's plan and put a circle around themselves, much like the walled fortifications that appeared around cities. A younger son, Ea, then chants an incantation that brings the sleep his father had been longing for, whereupon Ea steals his father's crown, robe, and godly radiance, adopting it for himself. Ea is now imbued with the power of a god. (Once we have found our own divinity, the godlike stature of our parents is greatly reduced. Their rule holds less power in our psyche and is easier to overcome.) With the child as a god and the father now asleep, the father is easily slain. Ea then captures the traitorous Mummu and takes him prisoner. Ea takes his father's place in the sweet waters of Apsu, from where he produces, with his wife, Damkina, the god Marduk.

Now Marduk was a symbol of the third chakra, if ever there was one. "His figure was enticing,... manly his going forth. He was a leader from the start. He had four eyes and as many ears, and when his lips moved, *fire* blazed forth. He was... clothed with the radiance of ten gods, with a majesty to inspire fear."[11]

Such a god is not born without creating waves. Tiamat's waters were agitated, no doubt by the loss of her husband and the disturbing course of unsettling events. Some of her children became concerned. They claimed that they could not rest until she avenged the death of Apsu, that it was her duty to do so. Now the static element of the Good Mother turns into its opposite. The Terrible Mother awakens, saying: "Let us make storm. Let us make war against the gods."

Her children then rally to her side, furious and vengeful in their plotting and scheming,. Harkening back to the son-lover motif, Tiamat takes her eldest child, Kingu, and mates with him, putting him in charge of the battle. Tiamat herself creates "a monster brood of serpents, 'sharp of tooth and merciless of fang' whose bodies are filled with poison instead of blood." (All of the children in this brood were her *sons,* we might note.) What are the results of war but an inheritance of toxically angry children, "armed to the teeth" with animal nature aroused?

She affixes the tablet of destinies to Kingu's breast and says to her sons, "May the opening of your mouths quiet the *fire* god." Thus water and fire, elements of second and third chakra respectively, engage in a battle for supremacy. As the battle ensues, fear and trembling erupt. Ea and Anu refuse to confront the monsters, at which point they set Marduk to the task, for he is the most powerful. Marduk agrees—on the condition *that he is given supreme power.* Anxious to be bailed out, the sibling gods readily agree, and empower Marduk with magical weaponry guaranteed to crush any enemy and *never lose its power.* Marduk establishes his weapons of mace, spear, and thunderbolt and "set lightning before him, and with burning flame filled his body." He mounted a chariot and with his thunderbolt summoned the seven winds.

> "Then joined issue Tiamat and Marduk, wisest of gods,
> They strove in single combat, locked in battle,
> The lord spread out his net to enfold her,
> The Evil Wind, which followed behind, he let loose in her face.
> When Tiamat opened her mouth to consume him,
> He drove in the Evil Wind that she close not her lips.

As the fierce winds charged her belly,
Her body was distended and her mouth was wide open.
He released the arrow, it tore her belly,
It cut through her insides, *splitting the heart.*
Having thus subdued her, he extinguished her life.
He cast down her carcass to stand upon it."[12]

The terrible mother has often been referred to as a consuming force. Is it not compulsive, unconscious consumption that distends our belly? But moving through the belly (third chakra area) he "splits her heart." Marduk then captures all the gods who fought with Tiamat in a great net, and takes the tablet of destinies for himself.

We see here how the father was killed when his power was stolen, but the mother is defeated by a loss of the heart. For when the mother's love is no longer available, her influence wanes in the psyche. The central integrating principle of the archaic unity destroyed, her carcass now becomes the bloody ground of the new order.

"With his unsparing mace he crushed her skull,
When the arteries of her blood he had severed,
The North Wind bore it to places undisclosed.
On seeing this, his *fathers* were joyful and jubilant,
They brought gifts of homage, they to him.
Then the lord paused to view her dead body,
That he might divide the monster and do artful works.
He split her like a shellfish into two parts:
Half of her he set up and sealed it as sky."[13]

Marduk then assigns the gods to their new cosmic order, such as the signs of the zodiac, the cycle of the moon, the counting of time, and the gates of the rivers, marking the beginnings of intellectual thinking. When this is done and the gods are assembled, they want to know who instigated Tiamat's anger. Marduk answers that it was Kingu (the son-lover who avenges this mother). The gods, wanting a race to "free them from compulsory service" then ask for Kingu to bear the guilt of the struggle and be sacrificed. Thus Kingu, bearing the guilt for the slaughter, becomes a sacrificial scapegoat, much like the later Jesus of Nazareth who dies for the sins of others. *From this sacrifice, the gods create the race of man.*

> "They imposed on him his guilt and severed his blood vessels.
> Out of his blood, they fashioned mankind.
> He imposed the service and set free the gods."[14]

The gods, liberated from their duties, are now free to be served by a lesser class of beings: the humans. It is by our labors that the gods continue to exist. Just as the kings of these times were served by slaves, our role was defined as servants or slaves to the gods.

THE BALANCE OF BIRTH AND DEATH

This myth attempts to grapple with many polarities of existence: Heaven and Earth, Mother and Father, birth and death, by creating a primal separation between previously undifferentiated archetypal realms. Human consciousness exists between these realms, struggling to find understanding and create some sense of order. From the proliferation of children to the murder of their mother, this myth struggles to reconcile the forces of creation and destruction. It also defines the role of humans in the cosmos—here defined as slaves to the gods.

Birth and death are primary cosmic forces which must be kept in balance for existence to continue. While they occur constantly in Nature's creation and destruction, both sides of this equation must be fully understood to approach any kind of spiritual maturity. From the early cave dweller who did not understand the process of conception, but merely observed that creation happened, to the uprisings of war that bring massive death tolls, humans have been struggling to make sense these primary forces as long as we've walked on hind legs.

In our current world, the exponential curve of human birth

has created a population that seriously threatens the biosphere. Simultaneously, we have built nuclear arsenals capable of destroying all higher life forms many times over. The reins over life and death, creation and destruction, now rest in our hands. How do we bring them into the balance characteristic of the fourth chakra?

To answer that question, we must move from myth to historical reality and look more deeply into the events of the *Dynamic Masculine* era and the militarization of society. Here we find the challenges of the fiery initiation that forged individual wills into the blunt instrument of military power.

ESSENTIAL POINTS

• Rising populations created new challenges for food and land, and required a new means of social organization, including division of labor.

• Temple bureaucracies managed the distribution of goods and maintained social order. They evolved into hierarchical centers of power.

• This period is typified by the Dynamic Masculine overthrow of the Great Mother cultures, turning most previous values to their opposites. Developmentally, it corresponds to the childhood stage of awakening will and rebelling against the mother.

• Myths of separation between the God and Goddess as World Parents, or between the Goddess and her son or daughter, emerged during this time.

• The Babylonian myth of Marduk and Tiamat graphically illustrates the violent overthrow of the old order, the establishment of a masculine dominance, and the role of humans as slaves to the gods.

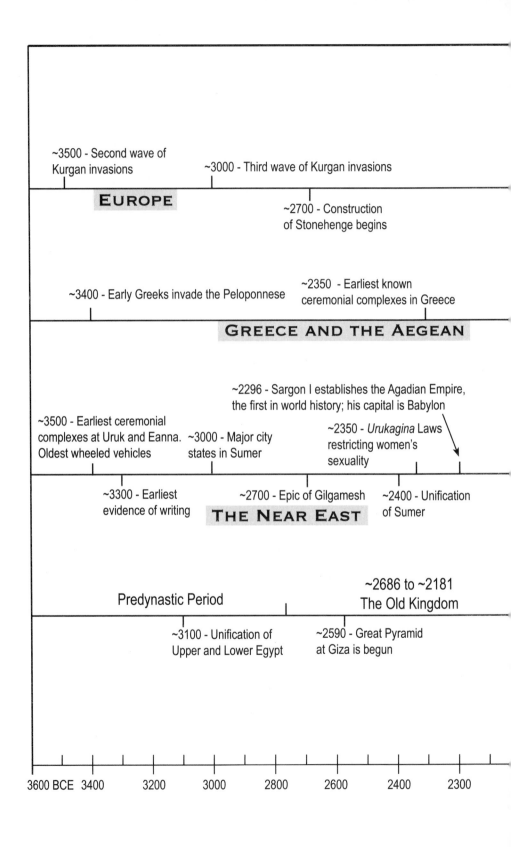

EUROPE

~3500 - Second wave of
Kurgan invasions

~3000 - Third wave of Kurgan invasions

~2700 - Construction
of Stonehenge begins

GREECE AND THE AEGEAN

~3400 - Early Greeks invade the Peloponnese

~2350 - Earliest known
ceremonial complexes in Greece

THE NEAR EAST

~2296 - Sargon I establishes the Agadian Empire,
the first in world history; his capital is Babylon

~3500 - Earliest ceremonial
complexes at Uruk and Eanna.
Oldest wheeled vehicles

~3000 - Major city
states in Sumer

~2350 - *Urukagina* Laws
restricting women's
sexuality

~3300 - Earliest
evidence of writing

~2700 - Epic of Gilgamesh

~2400 - Unification
of Sumer

Predynastic Period

~2686 to ~2181
The Old Kingdom

~3100 - Unification of
Upper and Lower Egypt

~2590 - Great Pyramid
at Giza is begun

3600 BCE   3400   3200   3000   2800   2600   2400   2300

TIME CHART 3 - THE FIRST EMPIRES

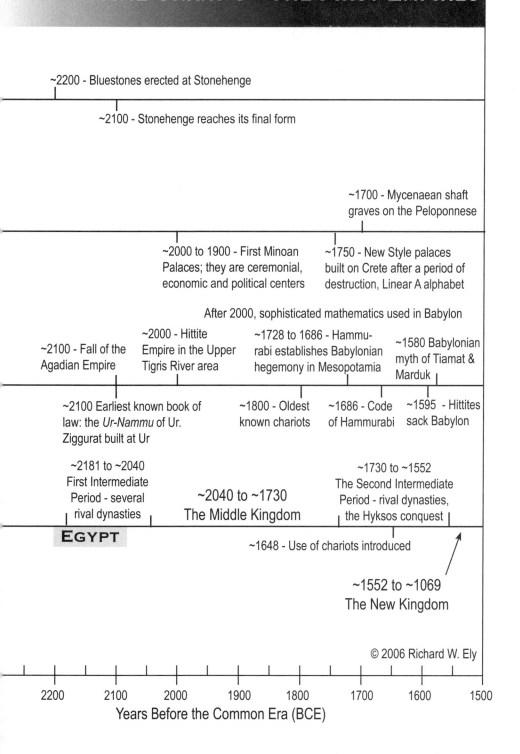

~2200 - Bluestones erected at Stonehenge

~2100 - Stonehenge reaches its final form

~1700 - Mycenaean shaft graves on the Peloponnese

~2000 to 1900 - First Minoan Palaces; they are ceremonial, economic and political centers

~1750 - New Style palaces built on Crete after a period of destruction, Linear A alphabet

After 2000, sophisticated mathematics used in Babylon

~2100 - Fall of the Agadian Empire

~2000 - Hittite Empire in the Upper Tigris River area

~1728 to 1686 - Hammurabi establishes Babylonian hegemony in Mesopotamia

~1580 Babylonian myth of Tiamat & Marduk

~2100 Earliest known book of law: the *Ur-Nammu* of Ur. Ziggurat built at Ur

~1800 - Oldest known chariots

~1686 - Code of Hammurabi

~1595 - Hittites sack Babylon

~2181 to ~2040 First Intermediate Period - several rival dynasties

~2040 to ~1730 The Middle Kingdom

~1730 to ~1552 The Second Intermediate Period - rival dynasties, the Hyksos conquest

EGYPT

~1648 - Use of chariots introduced

~1552 to ~1069 The New Kingdom

© 2006 Richard W. Ely

2200   2100   2000   1900   1800   1700   1600   1500

Years Before the Common Era (BCE)

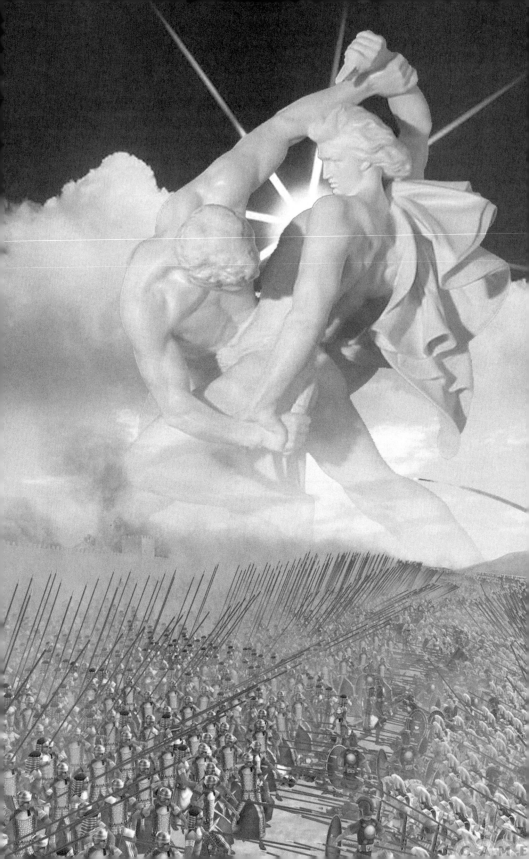

CHAPTER 7

THE BIRTH OF THE HERO

From Bronze to Iron

The need for many to act as one required the one to control the many.

—Andrew Bard Shmookler

S ince civilization began, the leading edge of culture has always been found at the meeting point of land and water. It is no surprise, then, that the third chakra era first arose on the dusty plains between the rivers of the Tigris and Euphrates. Alluvial valleys fertilized by annual spring floods were natural places for agriculture to prosper, while the coastline offered fishing and safe harbors for trade. With such ideal conditions for an abundant food supply, humanity grew like cells in a petrie dish. With a growing population, our ancestors found themselves in a new and different world, one that challenged every facet of their lives.

In 8500 B.C.E., the valley between these rivers was a dry, dusty plain, sparsely dotted by a few humble villages. By 3000 B.C.E., bustling cities sparkled along the riverbanks like glittering white jewels set among miles of green, irrigated fields, spotted with groves of date palms. Massive temples towered the plains, while people thronged in the streets. It was here, in what we would later call the cradle of civilization, that Mother Earth rocked her exploding population of toddlers into their early childhood.

As the Sumerian civilization spread across the fertile crescent,

Egyptian culture flourished across the desert to the West. While the Nile River rose and fell with its seasonal fluctuations, so did the many dynasties of the Egyptian Empire, with an overall continuity that spanned 2,500 years. Further to the East, along the Indus River, village settlements grew into sophisticated cities, such as Harappa and Mohenjo-Daro, around 2500 B.C.E., and by 1500 B.C.E. there were complex cities along the Yellow River in China.

These cultures rose up more or less concurrently, yet independent of each other. With successful farming and trading, their populations grew rapidly. However, the fertile valleys of the Tigris-Euphrates, Nile, and Indus rivers are all areas of circumscribed land, bordered by desert, sea, or mountains, which created natural barriers to growth. Within this limitation, expanding populations converged upon each other relentlessly, creating inevitable conflict.

From 10,000 to 3000 B.C.E., as population grew larger, the small cities of Mesopotamia were plagued by fights between neighbors over their sources of survival: land and water (elements of the first two chakras). What began as local skirmishes escalated into larger and bloodier forays until, centuries later, whole armies of men were waging all-out wars in a relentless compulsion to expand and conquer the territory around them. As these wars escalated, the archaic instinct toward survival, once oriented to the challenges of Nature, became directed instead into defense against other humans. Survival became militarized, forging divergent personal wills into singular collective entities of power and might.

WALLING OUT NATURE

The escalation of military skirmishes was coupled with the construction of strategic defenses. Villages that had been embedded in the natural world began surrounding themselves with fortified walls, something that was very rare prior to 3000 B.C.E. The city walls were like a cell membrane that sheltered its people within and defended them from invasion without. The administrative intelligence of each city emanated from its temple complex, which served as the cell's nucleus. Within the boundaries of these fortifications, cities grew large and dense. In Mesopotamia, for example, the city of Uruk crowded a population of 50,000 people into a mere 1,000 acres. They lived along narrow streets, in simple mud brick houses piled on top of each other.

Gilgamesh, a legendary hero of his time, was the King of Uruk. Many are the tales told of his conquests, and great was his reign. In one tale, Gilgamesh grows arrogant in his power, and restless within the walls of his city. The people of Uruk complain that no women are left as virgins, no son left to follow his father. Instead of responding to these complaints, the king seeks even more power. Gilgamesh says:

> "O Shamash, hear me, Shamash, let my voice be heard. Here in this city man dies oppressed at heart. I have looked over the wall and seen the bodies floating on the river and that will be my lot also. . . .Therefore I would enter the forest; because I have not established my name stamped in brick as my destiny decreed, I will go to the country where the cedar is cut. I will set up my name where the names of famous men are written and where no man's name is written I will raise a monument to the gods."[1]

His comrade in crime, the wild man Enkidu, dies along the way, teaching Gilgamesh the lesson of mortality. Gilgamesh grieves deeply, and tries to petition the gods for eternal life, but despite many trials, he remains unsuccessful. At last he returns to Uruk, to seek his immortality in the mud brick walls that surround the city.

> When the journey was accomplished, they arrived at Uruk, the strong-walled city. Gilgamesh spoke to Urshanabi, the ferryman, "Urshanabi, climb up onto the wall of Uruk. Inspect its foundation terrace, and examine well the brickwork; see if it is not made of burnt brick, and did not the

seven wise men lay these foundations? One third of the whole is city, one third is garden, and one third is field. . . . These parts and precinct are all Uruk. [2]

The erection of a wall represents an accompishment as well as a defense. The accomplishment is the triumph over Nature. Symbolically, it represents the ability to make distinctions, something commonly associated with the masculine psyche. As a defense, however, it cuts two ways, just as defenses do in our psyches: while they protect, they also deny. To be walled away from potential enemies was to be separated from Nature as well, and here lies an important and often overlooked shift, one that I believe is equally as significant as pushing seeds into the ground.

With walls around us, we were no longer immersed in Nature as an everyday experience. Our minds were no longer filled with the images of fields and forests, birds and beasts. Though there were still many who worked in the fields to provide food, the focus of human activity took place within the city walls. Consciousness within these cities became focused then—*as it still is now*—more upon a social order created amongst humans than upon the organic order that exists in Nature.

This human departure from Nature's limits brought us instead to the nature of human limits. Young and naïve as we were, those limits were many. We were still children, who knew little about the larger world. Still ruled by an instinctual distrust of the unfamiliar, we entered the uncharted territory of large-scale, cooperative living, where people with different gods, languages, or traditions converged upon each other. Like a child whose world shifts from family to school, we moved from the *intimately personal village* to the *vastly impersonal city*.

The worship of life brought with it the necessity to deal with life's abundance. Without the most basic technology we take for granted today, the feeding and governing of 50,000 people in a limited space, walled off from Nature, posed an enormous challenge of coordination—far beyond anything the human race had yet encountered. This period initially had no myths for this kind of living. Having mastered the maternal challenge of producing enough food, the next set of problems–housing, the distribution of goods, and defense–did not find their solutions in the natural world.

The realm of the Great Mother was rapidly losing relevance. Though she would remain strong in the ancestral unconscious for millennia to come, her ways were fading with each successive generation born and raised within city walls. When the mother is overthrown, her children are thrown into anarchy–at least until the father appears. While anarchy may have worked well for the smaller villages of the previous era, it was unworkable in cities of 50,000 or more people. Andrew Bard Shmookler, describes this as tempestuous at best:

> "Anarchy creates an environment in which each actor, group or individual must be the guarantor of his own security... In such an environment, survival as an autonomous entity requires a readiness to fight in defense of one's honor."[3]

It was into this vacuum of social governance that the age of power rallied. A new force was rising–that of the prodigal son–whose young feet stepped decisively into the footprints of the disappearing Mother. His awakened will could amass enough power over others to provide effective leadership and coordinate large numbers of people into coherent and obedient groups. Under his rule grew city-states and empires.

We know that group coordination–largely through slavery–made possible vast architectural and irrigation projects. More food could be produced with less labor. With a greater percentage of the population freed from farming to develop other pursuits, labor began to specialize. Some people made pottery, others wove cloth, while still others made jewelry, built houses, worked as scribes, or conducted the distribution of grain.

We might think that such a flowering and prosperous period would be an idyllic golden age. In many ways it was. The invention of writing and mathematics, the development of crafts and architecture, all mark this time as expansive in every way. Yet every light has its shadow. Along with the quantum leap in intellectual horizons grew the dark powers of warfare and slavery, ruled by tyrannical young kings, drunk on their power. For even though leaders were rising up to meet the challenges of a populous civilization, they were nonetheless young and naïve. (Alexander the Great, for example, was only nineteen when he started his career.) Their conquests were often fueled by ego. At Abu Simbel in Egypt, Ramses built statues thirty feet tall, cut 180 feet into a cliff. The Mesopotamian ruler, Ur-Nammu, built the largest ziggurat of his time, and made sure every brick was inscribed with his name. The fuel for feeding the imperial ego was the sweat of slaves and the blood of conquered people. As my mythologist friend, Hari Meyers states, "Empire is the collective expression of personal aggrandizement."[4]

A leader's job was to maintain order, coordinate the group's production of resources, and provide protection. This fell to people who had both the passion and the ability to wield that kind of power. As women were biologically destined to bear and suckle their many children, it would fall more naturally to the men to defend their village when attacked. This only needed to occur once, with its attendant slaughter, to engender a system whereby the men trained each other as soldiers in preparation for the next time. Such training, deemed essential to survival, diverted time and resources into developing weapons and strategies for defense.

Since women had been representatives of the previous *natural* order, it was men who became rulers of the new *social* order. This new order had to coordinate individual wills into a cohesive and powerful group force. In the early childhood of our civilization, this occurred through dictatorial parental rule, handed down through a pyramidal hierarchy of one man's might over another. Such a power dynamic fed the awakening young ego like gasoline on a fire. The social anarchy of an earlier time became hierarchically stratified, with the few ruling the many. If Nature had been a harsh taskmistress in the past, the ever-growing presence of violence and warfare were harsher still.

As tribes and city-states invaded each other, seeking to expand their power and prosperity, an unholy choice was forced upon any cluster of humanity that wanted to maintain its ways: *adapt to militarism or disappear into oblivion.* In his insightful book, *The Parable of the Tribes,* Andrew Bard Schmookler describes four possible outcomes for a society invaded by militant marauders, paraphrased below: [5]

1. They can be destroyed completely, with the invaders taking over their city.
2. They can surrender peacefully and be absorbed into the ways of the invading culture.
3. They can run for their lives, with many dying in the process, leaving their homeland behind to be taken over by the invaders.
4. They can develop a militaristic society and become just like their attackers.

Each possibility leads to the same outcome. Whether by destruction (1), absorption (2), withdrawal (3), or imitation (4), the area invaded becomes militarized.

To survive, civilized life had no choice but to develop along military lines. This is not to proclaim that war is inevitable, but that it is self-propagating. Aggression creates defense, and war begets war.

Those who failed to do develop militarily were simply killed, leaving the aggressive victors to mate with the women and dominate the gene pool. Throughout history, the big guy has always dominated the little guy. The horseman dominated the farmers; the chariots beat the foot soldiers; the iron replaced the bronze, and the guns and cannons wiped out those with arrows and spears. Its grisly culmination in the atomic bombs of Hiroshima and Nagasaki provides an enormous imperative to avoid what happens next. In applying this reasoning to our future, Schmookler states:

"Doubtless, part of our present problem is that the nuclear arms race is an atavistic attachment to a strategy that is no longer adaptive.... Our means of self-protection have long also been a source of our own endangerment."[6]

Those who survived these attacks, and lived long enough to become our ancestors, were the ones with the best weapons, the biggest armies, and most importantly, the organizational ability to wield them with single-minded purpose. For an army would fail if its actions were disorganized. These actions needed to be meticulously coordinated, even while adapting to new and dangerous situations. Smaller bands could be democratic, but larger armies required absolute obedience. Larger groups had more power and were capable of greater domination. They became the victors who called the shots, wrote the history, and shaped the world from which we came.

The old adage of divide and conquer shows the importance of a unified front. Dissenters were dangerous. They could undermine the group's resolve, and were therefore branded as traitors, ostracized, or executed—which gives us some insight into why pacifists meet such hostility during times of war. If a soldier argued for peace, or rebelled against his commander, he could undermine their army's ability to act as a single-minded force. Emotions such as fear and doubt were liabilities, as they could spread contagiously among the troops. In the face of battle, men were forced to deny their fear, as well as any sentimentality for the wives or children they left behind. To deny fear, love, longing, and need is to deny feelings in general, a habit which still plagues many men today as they struggle to recover their authentic inner life. This denial of feeling made it possible to commit heinous acts of brutality and oppression without sensitivity or compassion. The softer emotions were ridiculed, and associated with the "weaker" sex.

To repress emotion, then, would have been a requirement in the militarized male world. Emotional repression also requires a denial of the body in which feelings and sensations occur. Feelings, according to Jung, are the underlying source of our values. To suppress feelings is to create a culture without values—where nothing is sacred and everything is treated the same. Ken Wilber has called this lack of values, "flatland," a state where the interior world is denied and everything is equal to everything else.[7]

To live among violence, one has to suppress feelings of fear and disgust. Yet to suppress these feelings is to allow violence to continue unabated. Internal repression creates a wall around the heart—a psychological parallel to the physical wall that surrounded and protected the growing community of people.

The challenges and ordeals of battle have been a male initiation rite for a very long time. Living far from home and community, relying on strength and endurance, facing death on a daily basis, and encountering new worlds—these were all experiences that were believed to turn a boy into a man. For the chosen few who were best at killing others while escaping that fate themselves—it was the most common path chosen for a man to become a hero.

THE HERO'S QUEST

From the birth of the many, and the need to control them effectively, came the power of the one. This one became the Hero—a single male whose fantastic and often fanatic deeds shaped the fate of his people and the course of human history.

If a society could only survive by the maintenance of large, cohesive power structures, then this cohesion needed to be forged by some kind of singular purpose. Such privilege and responsibility fell best to a single individual whose personal power was potent enough to command huge numbers of men to leave their homes, wives and children, and face hunger, discomfort, and death on a daily basis. This required enormous charisma and organizational abilities. In addition, this ruler needed to be able to round up enough resources to support his armies on the campaign, feeding, clothing, and protecting tens of thousands of men, while constantly on the move in unfamiliar enemy territory. Alexander the Great had to procure 52,000 tons of provisions to feed 87,000 infantry, 18,000 cavalry, and 52,000 followers—for a mere *four month* interval out of his thirteen year campaign.[8]

All this to be accomplished with the meager technology of the 4th century B.C.E.!

Because fights over land and water were intricately tied up with the seasonal shifts in flooding and drought, the priests, who held this knowledge, were assumed to have a favored audience with the gods. Hence they were invested with political power. With this power, they built temples to house themselves and store excess grain, with their palaces serving as elaborate centers of administration—the nucleus of theocractic rule.

As the shape of the Egyptian pyramids or the Mesopotamian ziggurats might imply, power was seen as emanating from a single source on high that ruled in hierarchical fashion: from God to sacred king, then successively to the ruling bureaucrats, then merchants, then peasants and finally slaves. As fighting escalated and civilizations became embroiled in hostilities, war forced a change in the ruling theocracies. In early Sumer, for example, prior to 2800 B.C.E., decisions were made by councils of elders. However, in times of crisis, such as a war, the council appointed a single leader, called a *lugal,* which literally meant "big man." Eventually, as he retained his Hero status during peacetime and ruled over community life, this word came to mean "king."

So we see here how the institution of kingship grew out of a military structure superimposed upon an older religio-political system. The absolute authority of a commander over his army served as the prototype for the king's authority over the city. And king he remained, passing his rule to his male heirs and assembling all others into his kingdom. From his subjects, he took tributes, increasing his wealth. With slaves captured in conquest, he built palaces and temples.

As consciousness shifted from the world of Nature to the world of humans, the locus of power shifted from the Great Mother to the absolute rule of a single man whose status was elevated to that of a god. The protection and survival of his people depended upon his sole power and wisdom. Through his rule, the disparate elements of a culture were homogenized into something that could at least live in peace with itself, if not with its neighbors. But this peace was bought at the price of dictatorial rule. It was to the king's will that his subjects surrendered their own.

The first forays into power, then, were wildly unequal, as suggested in the last chapter. If we think there is a great gap between rich and poor in today's society, we need only look back at the ancient kings who lived in luxurious, palatial estates with tens of thousands of slaves to know that this economic gap is a vestige of a very old story. The Egyptian pharoah Amenhotep had as many as 90,000 slaves. In ancient Rome, emperors could have 20,000, while the wealthy might have only 4,000, and the merely comfortable, as many as 500.[9] The complete disregard for basic human rights in these social underclasses is utterly appalling. Assyrian King Shalmaneser (1274-1245 B.C.E.), for example, once took 14,000 slaves in battle, and forced them into submission by blinding them all.[10] Often slaves were castrated to become eunuchs. Even in the more rational periods in Greece and Rome, slaves were tortured, crucified, or forced to wear "gulp preventers" to keep them from eating food that they handled. Human life was abundant, bought and sold as a commodity, with little regard for the tragic experience of others. With the realm of feeling denied, how could there be compassion?

A narrowing hierarchy of power dominated the greater masses, which means that most people were power-*less*. To those lower down the pyramid, the only way to achieve freedom was to emulate those who had power. They might become a Hero themselves, striving to evolve their own will and strength to dominate others as a way of overcoming their own oppression. The more brutal the leader, the more brutality would be seen as the way to overcome their own violation and achieve freedom. It was the model of the time.

Thus the Age of the Hero brought forth its archetypal theme of the Hero's Quest—the initiatory journey to find inner power and exaltation through heroic deeds. Most of the myths along this theme were allegories of how the light of male consciousness triumphed over the dark, unconscious feminine. The positive side of this quest was that it often forced an awakening of individuation within the people that embarked upon it. A Hero was one whose third chakra had been ignited—with its attributes of power and autonomy, assertiveness and confidence.

Yet the Hero's quest is *inherently based on conflict*. Heroes are created by their *triumph* in conflict, whether internal or external. It may be a conflict between old and new ways of being, between reason and instinct, or between one country and another, but a man only becomes a Hero by engaging in some kind of battle and emerging victorious. Is it any wonder that when the big man at the top needs to appear heroic, he does so by creating a conflict he thinks he can win?

Much has been written about the glory of the Hero's Quest. It has become one of the dominant myths of our time. Stripped of its initiatory elements, it shows up far too often as the passion to become rich, famous, or powerful—purely for the sake of the ego. Rather than evolving consciousness, it arrests it. Without the feminine balance of rest, safety, feeling, and connection, this shadow side of the fiery third chakra is burning our resources and consuming our world.

At its deepest level, the Hero's Quest follows all the steps of an intiatory journey: separation, loss, confinement, revelation, transformation and finally, return. It is an archetypal journey for the evolution of consciousness—both individually and collectively. Joseph Campbell, in his classic book, *The Hero with a Thousand Faces,* describes both its light and dark side in a way all too familiar in our present world. On the positive side, he states:

> "The effect of the successful adventure of the hero is the unlocking and release again of the flow of life into the body of the world. The miracle of this flow may be represented in physical terms as a circulation of food substance, dynamically as a streaming of energy, or spiritually as a manifestation of grace."[11]

Campbell also points out the shadow side: the overextension of the quest, its dissociation from everyday life, and the abuse of the powers gained. Campbell's discussion of King Minos, one of many mythic heroes of the past, is a description that is all too reminiscent of economic heroes today:

> "The figure of the tyrant-monster is.... the hoarder of general benefit. He is the monster avid for the greedy rights of 'my and mine.' The havoc wrought by him is described in mythology and fairy tale as being universal throughout his domain.... The inflated ego of the tyrant is a curse to himself and his world—no matter how his affairs may seem to prosper."[12]

The wielding of power clearly relates to the issues of the third chakra, sometimes called the navel chakra because of its location. Campbell goes on to state:

> "The World Navel, then is ubiquitous. And since it is the source of all existence, it yields the world's plenitude of both good and evil."[13]

Thus the Hero has both a light and dark side. As he amasses power, the choice to act in the service of good or evil is equally open. To act wisely on that choice requires integration of the shadow and strength of character. To realize we are capable of both good *and* evil is necessary in order to awaken the responsibility we desperately need to see accompanying our heroic power.

EVOLVING THE THIRD CHAKRA

The social development of power brought tremendous gifts, yet it came at a price. The conquest of tribes and city-states forged vast empires, capable of great wealth and great works. But the constant warfare and strife robbed its people of a safe ground, separated men and women, and suppressed the feeling function that kept us in touch with ourselves, each other. With the Great Mother slain, defensive

walls shut us out of the garden. This era coordinated greater numbers of people and spread common languages, customs, and crafts,
spawning developments in writing and mathematics. Yet this power
became increasingly impersonal, too often brutal, with an economy
built on conquest and slavery. The construction of great monuments
and palatial estates were triumphs of the ancient world, but they
served to edify the ego of transient rulers, who were subject, like any
other mortal, to being slain by a sword.

Schmookler points out that our reality now "selects" for power.
This means that our choices are based on the maximization of power,
rather than on the increase of love, peace, or freedom. Because survival is at stake, and power is equated with survival, the only choice
in this myth is to choose paths that lead to more power. We "choose"
to support the military at the cost of social programs. We get passionate about the patriotism of war, rallying to support the troops, right
or wrong, sublimating our own sense of powerless with a militant
nationalism. Avenging deaths becomes more important than solving
the problems that caused them. In a further twist, many believe the
myth that this kind of power will bring us the very peace, love, and
freedom that it denies, and that fighting wars will bring peace.

As the Dynamic Masculine forces expanded outward, conquering
new territories and cultures, everything was toppled on its head–the
new order differentiating from the previous one in every way possible. Values shifted from the feminine to the masculine, from Earth
to sky, body to spirit, and the natural order to social hierarchy. This
reflects a basic dialectical process common in childhood, as well
as history, and evolving systems: reacting against what is, creating
something new, and then normalizing that novelty until the cycle
repeats again, or a new integration is reached.

Thus the culture of the Dynamic Masculine emancipated itself
from the Great Mother and established new ground. In order to
maintain that ground–and its separation from all that preceded it–
the Dynamic Masculine became the *Static Masculine,* instituting a set
of values, customs, and beliefs that have carried culture from the
early Greek philosophers to the present day. If we are to outgrow the

rigidity that holds our culture in its destructive patterns, we need to understand the dominant masculine valence of our most recent era, which we will explore in the next four chapters.

ESSENTIAL POINTS

• Hostilities between settlements created the need for defense. Men were the likely gender to be called to that task.

• Aggression spread militarism, whether by conquest, defense, surrender, or flight. Early civilizations had little choice but to form around militaristic principles.

• Walls were built around cities as protection, but they simultaneously crowded people together in a man-made environment, walling out Nature.

• War coopted the heroic impulse. It was a central initiation for men, and a way to become a Hero. The glory of war forced a repression of other more sensitive emotions.

• The Hero's Quest has both a light and a dark side. Power, once attained, enables both good and evil.

• The creation of a militaristic society that selects for power has contributed to our current civilization's obsessive love of power.

After 1600, Phoenician traders
reach the tin mines of Cornwall

EUROPE

~1450 - Fall of Crete to the
Mycenaeans; all palaces
save Knossos are burned;
Earliest Mycenaean citadels
on the mainland; Greek
Linear B alphabet in Crete

1250 - Widespread
use of iron

~1475 - The eruption of Thera volcano
in the Aegean Sea and the ensuing
tsunami had a devastating effect on the
Minoan civilization

~1200 - Trojan War; fall of
the Mycenaean civilization;
demographic collapse

~1200 and later - Devastating attacks
by the Sea People, possibly including
the Philistines and/or the Mycenaeans,
sweep across the Mediterranean region

THE NEAR EAST

~1500 - Hittites
destroy Babylon

~1400 - The Hittites
obtain iron weapons

~1200 - Collapse of the Hittite Empire.
Rise of Zoroastrianism in Persia

~1379 to ~1358 - Reign of
Akhenaten; he unsuccessfully
attempted to impose solar
monotheism on Egypt

~1345 to ~1335 -
Reign of Tutankhamun

~1184 to ~1152 - Reign of Ramses III,
the last great Pharaoh of Egypt; he
repels an invasion by the Sea Peoples

~1552 to ~1069 The New Kingdom

~1460 to ~1482 - Reign
of Queen Hatshepsut

~1200 - The great temple of Abu Simbel
~1200 - Traditional date of Exodus

EGYPT

After 1200, the secret of making
iron weapons was widely known

1500 BCE 1450   1400   1350   1300   1250   1200   1150

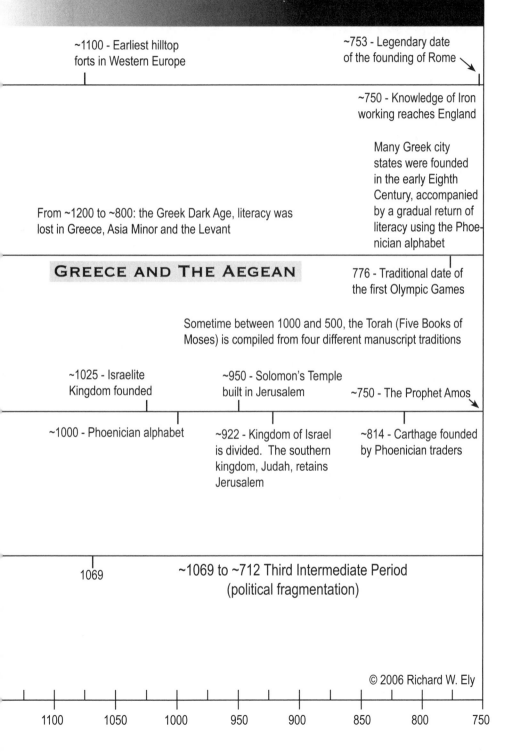

TIME CHART 4 - THE IRON AGE

~1100 - Earliest hilltop
forts in Western Europe

~753 - Legendary date
of the founding of Rome

~750 - Knowledge of Iron
working reaches England

Many Greek city
states were founded
in the early Eighth
Century, accompanied
by a gradual return of
literacy using the Phoe-
nician alphabet

From ~1200 to ~800: the Greek Dark Age, literacy was
lost in Greece, Asia Minor and the Levant

GREECE AND THE AEGEAN

776 - Traditional date of
the first Olympic Games

Sometime between 1000 and 500, the Torah (Five Books of
Moses) is compiled from four different manuscript traditions

~1025 - Israelite
Kingdom founded

~950 - Solomon's Temple
built in Jerusalem

~750 - The Prophet Amos

~1000 - Phoenician alphabet

~922 - Kingdom of Israel
is divided. The southern
kingdom, Judah, retains
Jerusalem

~814 - Carthage founded
by Phoenician traders

1069

~1069 to ~712 Third Intermediate Period
(political fragmentation)

| 1100 | 1050 | 1000 | 950 | 900 | 850 | 800 | 750 |

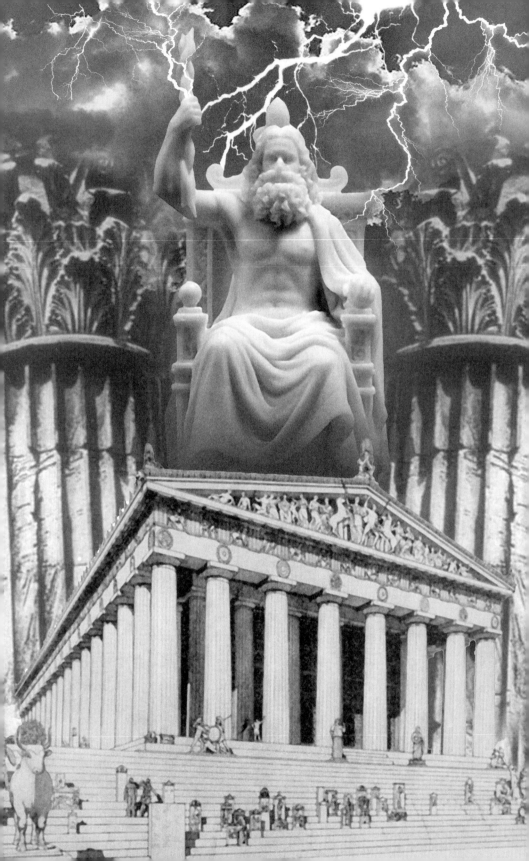

FROM ARCHETYPES TO IDEAS

The Dawn of the Static Masculine

> *What lies in our power to do, lies in our power not to do.*

—Aristotle

As population grew within the walled cities of ancient times, the organic roots of our past were paved over with cobblestone streets. Daily activities took place within a dense array of dwellings, civic plazas, and temples. Merchants of all kinds traded goods in bustling markets, exchanging news and ideas with strangers from distant lands. City populations expanded from tens of thousands to hundreds of thousands. It was a social world of diverse peoples, carrying on the complex business of living together in close quarters.

The Greek settlements in Asia Minor led the way for a new social organization—the *polis*—an independent, self-governing city-state, ruled by the collective will of an awakening citizenry. Each polis had its own dialect, religious traditions, and customs. Class distinctions still ranged from tyrants to slaves, but there was an emerging middle class of merchants rising from the profits of seafaring trade. People took pride in their city, and gathered in large public squares for assemblies, events, and conversation. They had a sense of collectively influencing their world. Ideas were explored and debated with passion. Participation was considered vital. Councils of elected citizens gradually replaced the monopoly on power of hereditary kings, giving birth to the first democracy in Athens. Only males could become citizens, and at first this was limited by heredity to an elite class. Over time, citizenship expanded to include some commoners and foreigners, even emancipated slaves–but never women.

Freed from the rudimentary chores of survival by the labors of women and slaves, the masculine elite had more leisure to contemplate the nature of the world. Superstition and rationality flowed into a heady brew of philosophical ambrosia that awakened a new kind of thinking. Human civilization was becoming more ordered. Men turned their attention to the gods and attempted to find order there as well. Homer penned his famous epics, *The Iliad* and *The Odyssey*, where the gods intervened in the lives of men. Hesiod's *Theogony* ordered the entire pantheon of divine archetypes into a kind of family geneology. Here we see the birth of Eros, god of desire that draws things together, born from the separation between Gaia, the Earth Mother, and Cronos, chaos or time. In the entire geneology, there is never any intermarriage between offspring of the separated parents. Later, the powers of Eros would give way to Logos, as word or logic, focused more on making distinctions than drawing things together. With a detachment that allowed for a more objective contemplation, the golden age of Greece burst forth with the intellectual foundations of Western civilization: medicine, history, geometry, science, rhetoric, and philosophy.

The focus of consciousness shifted upward, becoming more cerebral than earthy, transcending the instincts and urges of the lower chakras for a "higher" rationality. This rationality was not the logic of material attainment, oriented toward survival or sensory results, but a thinking focused on abstract ideas. Though one might argue that our core instincts, honed from millions of years of evolution, might actually be quite rational, the triumph of consciousness at this time was the capacity for reason and detachment–the ability to step back and ask questions about the underlying forces of creation. In a world of colliding ideas, what were the common denominators? Of what was the world made and how was it ordered? What was real and what was ephemeral?

Human civilization was maturing. The personal ties of family and clan were absorbed and expanded by an increasingly impersonal urban life. Though the gods and goddesses still bound the psyche to mythic archetypes, they were beginning to lose their power and influence. Just as it is with maturing children, mother and father's influence was still present, but less immediate. Instead, acceptance of laws regulated human behavior; impersonal codes that could be written, preserved, and applied to all.

THE EMERGENCE OF LAW AND ORDER

The rebellious will of the petulant child was maturing from the stage of moral development that psychologist Lawrence Kohlberg calls the *good boy/nice girl* to the morality dictated by *law and order*. In Kohlberg's theory, this takes us from the post-toddler stage to middle childhood, the time when a child goes to school and becomes socialized into a system outside the family. This is also a time of childhood when boys and girls ignore each other and play in separate worlds, a condition that lasts until adolescence—when the first blush of puberty draws the sexes toward each other again.

Where the Dynamic Masculine seized power in the previous era by overthrowing the Great Mother, the next task of the ruling paradigim was to keep that power. Such power was, by definition, everything opposite to the ground that preceded it, so the original wholeness had to be resisted—walled off, both literally and psychologically. In this way, the Dynamic Masculine forces that had established their dominion matured into the *Static Masculine*—a force that held power through the organizing principles of *reason and logic, laws and conformity*. Conquered lands required governing to maintain order and economic flow. Laws could reach across distances and establish universal social prinicples. Laws were propagated by the written word and enforced by the elite members of society who could read. In contrast to the oral tradition that preceded it, written words are static, unchanging. Literal truth was, quite literally, a *written* truth, frozen into stasis at the time of its writing.

The Static Masculine holds things in place. Its purpose is stability, but rather than the stability of the Static Feminine, which is cyclic and grounded in instincts, the Static Masculine is linear and grounded in logic. Its focuses on distinctions: it divides, rules, and regulates. The rigidity of its laws forges the chaos of converging populations into a homogenized cultural soup. They provided a common ethic for the social world which was slowly finding stability in the hum of urban life. Static forms do stabilize, but they also create rigidity.

As always, new ways of thinking clashed with the old. Myths and legends increasingly clashed with logical discourse. The gods and goddesses of Nature were now worshipped in man-made temples. Their stories reflected irrational antics that played whimsically with human fate. Sacrifice became a means to appease their whims, with many thousands of bulls, goats, and pigs slaughtered as offerings to increasingly distant and angry gods. Were the gods angry because we had turned away from their natural realms? Or was it just our projection resulting, perhaps, from the constant aggression of the time? Beneath the excitement of civilized life, cities were still rife with poverty and disease. Traumatized by the proximity of war, people looked for more rational explanations for the forces that generated reality, hesitant to leave the old gods behind. A philosophical tension ensued, as the mythic and the rational began to diverge.

Logical discourse began with the Pre-Socratic philosophers, to whom we owe the first division of the cosmos into the essential elements of earth, water, fire, and air, elements which happen to correspond to the first four chakras. (Not that chakras were known or had ever been mentioned by the Greeks. However, they had long been part of an oral tradition in India and it is possible there was undocumented cross-cultural influence.) Within these elements the Greeks looked at binary distinctions, such as hot and cold, moist and dry, light and dark. Curiously, as the fourth and fifth centuries B.C.E. mark the earliest glimmerings of the heart chakra—the Milesian philosopher, Anaximenes, posited that the first principle, from which all others were derived, was air, corresponding to the element classically associated with the heart chakra. Thales had proposed that the gods and all things came from water (chakra two), while Heraclitus associated Logos with the element fire (chakra three). Meanwhile, Heraclitus focused on the eternal nature of *being*—a step beyond the constant *doing* of third chakra consciousness.

Socrates, who was revered as the wisest man of his day, believed that the key to happiness was the development of a rational, moral character. He introduced the idea of *ethical rationalism*—an ethics based on logical sense rather than the antics of the gods or the authority of the state. He felt that to know the good was to do the good—that humans, when given educated choices, would naturally choose moral behavior. Socrates was a prominent supporter of gender equality, and held fast to the passion of personal dialog, eschewing the written word. Unfortunately, his habit of deep questioning and independent thinking marked him as a troublemaker, resulting in his public trial and forced suicide in 399 B.C.E. In his final act of passionate dedication to the truth, he chose to drink the poison hemlock rather than recant his views. He was remembered as saying: "I was really too honest a man to be a politician and still live."[1]

Socrates' student, Plato, carried on the inquiry for an even deeper order. He believed that appearances were deceptive and that the senses couldn't be trusted. Using the analogy of firelight casting shadows on the wall of a cave, he saw the known world as but a shadow of a hidden, divine flame, which emanated from a world of perfection, beauty, and abstract forms. These ideal forms led the mind upward, toward transcendence. The material realm, which had once been the only ground of our being, took a step backward in Plato's philosophy. Non-material ideal forms generated the changeable, physical world. These ideals were eternal, while matter was temporal. Human instincts were seen as base, compared to the awakening rational mind.

To Plato's student, Aristotle, the reverse was true: ideas rose out of existing physical forms. Both Plato and Aristotle were addressing the relationship between spirit and matter, recognizing that they influenced each other—the question was how. Later, a famous

Rennaissance painting by Rafael, called "The School of Athens" depicted Plato pointing upwards and Aristotle pointing downward, highlighting their philosophical differences. Thus mind and matter began their separation, along with myth and reason. The value previously attributed to the material world, shifted to the mental world of ideas. In this separation begins an inherently dueling dualism that plays out in the cosmic battle between good and evil.

Nowhere does this split make itself more apparent than in the philosophy of Manichaeism, where we see the irrevocable division of the cosmos into Good and Evil, emanating from a Zoroastrian myth circa 1200 B.C.E. As the story goes, Father Time (Zurvan) sacrifices for a thousand years to give birth to a son, and comes to doubt whether his actions will ever bear fruit. At last, two brothers are born, Ahura Mazda (Ohrmazd), representing light, is born from the merit of his sacrifices. Ahriman, representing darkness, is born from his doubt. Ahriman, knowing that the privileges of kingship will go to the first born, rips through the womb to be born ahead of his brother. To keep his sacrificial vow, Zurvan had to grant the dark brother kingship for nine thousand years, when it will at last be his brother's turn to reign. From this myth, we see how evil, or darkness, is derived as the first condition, but with the intervention of time, good can prevail in the end. Thus evil is born from doubt, the negation of a first emanation or impulse. (Notice the absence of any feminine figure in this myth concerning womb and birth.)

Manichaeism was spread by the Persian prophet, Mani, in the third century C.E. Mani taught that spirit carries the good, while matter blocks out the light of spirit and becomes its evil enemy. Of course, if matter is evil, then so is the entire earthly creation, humans as well, and especially our physical bodies. Good then becomes the *prisoner* of evil, and the only way out of this trap is through a series of savior-messengers. Manichaeists believed that even the institution of marriage was evil, not only because they abhorred the sexual act, but because having children brought the continual imprisonment of light in physical bodies. In the next chapter, we will see how this idea influenced the development of Christianity.

The dialectical battle between good and evil is an underlying theme of the Static Masculine era. It still rules our culture today, as the "axis of evil" is projected onto foreign lands and cultures, while our own shadow is denied. While we could argue that this ethical dualism invites us to rise above evil and evolve our actions toward the good, evidence that this inducement is working seems patently thin. Such atrocities as the Inquisition, the Holocaust, two World Wars, countless other genocidal events, as well as racism, poverty, and the destruction of the environment—all these are testaments to the failure of this philosophy to achieve its goal. In order to understand why, we must return to our story and see how these ideas spread throughout the ancient world.

FROM MACEDONIA TO ROME

Alexander the Great was Aristotle's student. With a direct lineage to Plato and Socrates, Alexander was well schooled in Greek ideals. His father was Philip of Macedon, a powerful ruler who united Greece in 338 B.C.E. Upon his father's murder, two years later, the nineteen year old Alexander, seeing the unity that his father had created, set out to conquer the rest of the known world. In a mere thirteen years, he conquered the Persian Empire and united the lands from Greece to India. Though fierce as a fighter and mighty as a general, he was humane to his enemies, allowing them to keep their ways, while infusing his own. As a result of this respect, he was able to spread the rationality of Greek ideals, language, and customs across the con-quered lands. Even though his death at age thirty-three fragmented his huge empire, the flavor of Greek culture had been infused into the immense cross-cultural maelstrom that he had ruled. Alexander's Hellenic world provided the foundation of Western civilization: a way of life that was masculine, logical, and imperial.

Alexander had also met Jewish tribes on his forays through Persia, where Cyrus the Great had freed them from captivity in Babylon two hundred years earlier. These were yet another people organized by

Static Masculine principles. They lived by a strict moral code, keeping a sacred covenant with a single, all-powerful male deity. By accepting the divine commandments of Moses, they allied themselves with a fierce and terrible god who could punish or reward, save or damn. As the Chosen People, they believed that they were divinely summoned to bring the spiritual light of peace and prosperity to the promised land. This would come about through a future Messiah, who would demonstrate divine powers and lead his people to the realization of Heaven on Earth. After centuries of brutal existence, wandering the desert in search of a homeland, one can imagine how important it would have been to the Hebrews to obey the commandments of their powerful god, Yahweh, to the letter of the law.

With Alexander's death, his empire fell to the quarrels of his survivors. The pinnacle of Greek society—along with its democratic organization—quickly declined. Culture reached out for a new center of stabilization. The Roman sense of *carpe diem* seized the day and took on the massive task of social coordination that brought civilization to a new level of organization.

At its height in the second century C.E., the Roman Empire ruled over sixty million people, spreading across two million square miles of territory. To feed, clothe, and govern a diverse population of this magnitude without the transportation and communication devices we take for granted today was a remarkable feat. It was achieved through a combination of third chakra political ambition and ruthless militarism with fourth chakra acceptance of diversity. This acceptance engendered a sense of belonging for those males willing to acknowledge Roman authority—and crushing domination to those who weren't. As Roman conquests expanded the empire's borders, the Roman world became wealthy, bringing back booty for imperial palaces, and slaves by the thousands.

Rome was a sizzling cultural stew: a city of wealth and squalor, terror and grandeur, sophistication and savagery. It was ruled by a Republican oligarchy that owned most of the land. Its large public buildings allowed huge numbers to gather—the Circus Maximus could seat 250,000 people. One Roman bath could accommodate three thousand people.[2] Despite the Roman talent for law and order, killing and enslavement were commonplace throughout Roman society, even for sport or entertainment. The famed Colisseum could seat 50,000 spectators, where on a single day thousands of animals might be slaughtered, or hundreds of gladiators might slice each other accompanied by cheers and jeers from the audience. Members of the Senate murdered each other with little attempt to hide their actions. This led to more killings—as avenging murder was a duty whose avoidance led to humiliation. Unwanted babies were thrown on the village dung heap, where the poor might rescue them to raise as slaves. No room for childishness here—life was brutal and dictatorial.

However, the Romans cared greatly for art and beauty, with palatial homes for the rich and elaborate ritual customs for all occasions. Their genius for laws and social contracts created consistent standards for conducting business among wildly diverse peoples. Extensive roadways enabled people to travel more easily. They spread far from their homelands, no longer supported by their native social customs. Platonic ideals sought reconciliation with Greek polytheism and the Jewish monotheism that was emerging from the East.

Men and women led separate lives in the Greek and Roman world. Even though the divine feminine was still worshipped through various goddesses, they were much reduced in stature. The Great Mother figure of Hera or Juno (her Greek and Roman names) was now a jealous bitch, whining about her husband's antics. The romantic passions associated with the goddess of love, known as Aphrodite or Venus, were seen as a wicked curse that induced madness. Mistress of the animals and wild places, Artemis or Diana, became a murdering maiden protecting her nakedness. Medusa's head full of snakes turned men to stone with a mere glance. Hardly an appealing sense of the divine for any of them! Even the legendary founding of Rome was pointedly devoid of a mother, as the abandoned twin boys Romulus and Remus, had to be suckled by a she-wolf instead.

In the mortal realm, women, in both Roman and Greek societies, held the legal status of slaves. Women were largely confined to their houses, regarded as property, and expected to be obedient. In

Roman law, the *Pater familias,* or eldest male, held the powers of life and death over his wife and the rest of the family. Daughters lived by the absolute rule of their father; wives subjected to their husbands. The society of men set the tone for the civilized world.

Along the edges of the Roman Empire, border wars were constant. The Romans relentlessly conquered and looted their neighbors, bringing back continuous supplies of slaves to build their extensive palaces, streets, and aqueducts. Sometimes ten thousand slaves would come through the gates of Rome in a single day.[3] In the city of Rome itself, up to 40 percent of its one million inhabitants were slaves.

Yet the Roman Empire maintained an internal peace, known as the *Pax Romana,* for more than six centuries. This allowed Greek, Jewish, and Christian ideas to weave their disparate fibers into a single myth that would eventually become central to all. Rome's inner stability, wealth, and extensive road system gave it the power to amplify new ideas throughout its vast empire. Members of this massive cross-cultural world were crying for a new story that would give them stability, social cohesion, and peace. It was into this fertile soil that the seed of Christianity was cast.

ESSENTIAL POINTS

• After seizing power by ovethrowing the original Static Feminine natural order, the Dyamic Masculine holds that power through the establishment of social order. This occurs, in part, through the creation of laws that act as ethical codes for a growing population of diverse people. The Dynamic Masculine matures into the Static Masculine, whose attributes are reason and logic, law and order.

• Philosophically, the intellect turned toward perceiving the order inherent in creation itself, with many differing views about the relationship between ideas and forms, spirit and matter. This period gave birth to many of the intellectual foundations of Western civilization.

• Alexander the Great spread Greek ideals throughout the Persian Empire and the lands to the East. After his death, the center of Static Masculine culture fell to the Roman Empire.

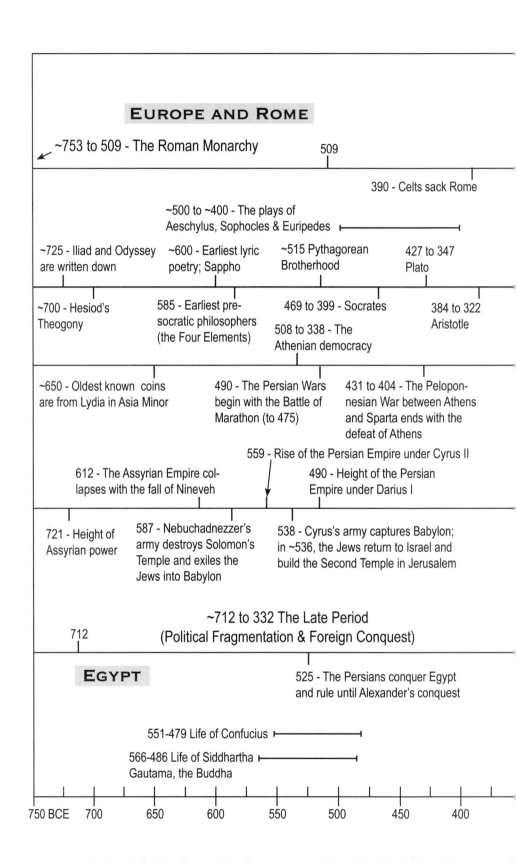

EUROPE AND ROME

~753 to 509 - The Roman Monarchy 509

390 - Celts sack Rome

~500 to ~400 - The plays of
Aeschylus, Sophocles & Euripedes

~725 - Iliad and Odyssey
are written down

~600 - Earliest lyric
poetry; Sappho

~515 Pythagorean
Brotherhood

427 to 347
Plato

~700 - Hesiod's
Theogony

585 - Earliest pre-
socratic philosophers
(the Four Elements)

469 to 399 - Socrates

508 to 338 - The
Athenian democracy

384 to 322
Aristotle

~650 - Oldest known coins
are from Lydia in Asia Minor

490 - The Persian Wars
begin with the Battle of
Marathon (to 475)

431 to 404 - The Pelopon-
nesian War between Athens
and Sparta ends with the
defeat of Athens

559 - Rise of the Persian Empire under Cyrus II

612 - The Assyrian Empire collapses with the fall of Nineveh

490 - Height of the Persian
Empire under Darius I

721 - Height of
Assyrian power

587 - Nebuchadnezzer's
army destroys Solomon's
Temple and exiles the
Jews into Babylon

538 - Cyrus's army captures Babylon;
in ~536, the Jews return to Israel and
build the Second Temple in Jerusalem

~712 to 332 The Late Period
(Political Fragmentation & Foreign Conquest)

712

EGYPT

525 - The Persians conquer Egypt
and rule until Alexander's conquest

551-479 Life of Confucius

566-486 Life of Siddhartha
Gautama, the Buddha

750 BCE   700   650   600   550   500   450   400

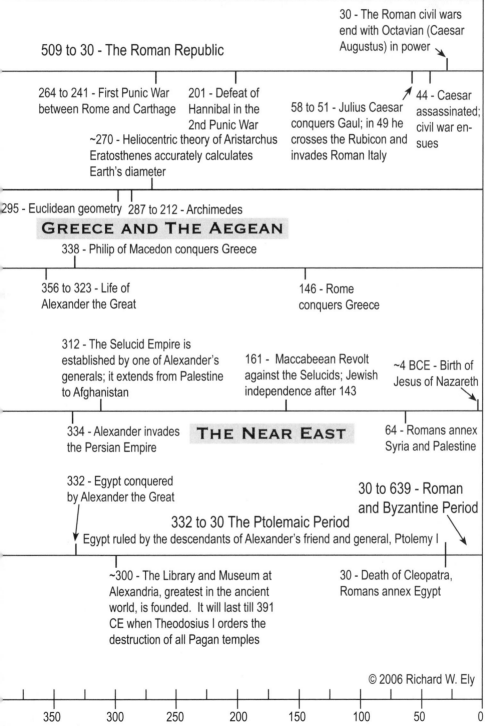

509 to 30 - The Roman Republic

30 - The Roman civil wars end with Octavian (Caesar Augustus) in power

264 to 241 - First Punic War between Rome and Carthage

201 - Defeat of Hannibal in the 2nd Punic War

58 to 51 - Julius Caesar conquers Gaul; in 49 he crosses the Rubicon and invades Roman Italy

44 - Caesar assassinated; civil war ensues

~270 - Heliocentric theory of Aristarchus Eratosthenes accurately calculates Earth's diameter

295 - Euclidean geometry   287 to 212 - Archimedes

GREECE AND THE AEGEAN

338 - Philip of Macedon conquers Greece

356 to 323 - Life of Alexander the Great

146 - Rome conquers Greece

312 - The Selucid Empire is established by one of Alexander's generals; it extends from Palestine to Afghanistan

161 - Maccabeean Revolt against the Selucids; Jewish independence after 143

~4 BCE - Birth of Jesus of Nazareth

334 - Alexander invades the Persian Empire

THE NEAR EAST

64 - Romans annex Syria and Palestine

332 - Egypt conquered by Alexander the Great

30 to 639 - Roman and Byzantine Period

332 to 30 The Ptolemaic Period
Egypt ruled by the descendants of Alexander's friend and general, Ptolemy I

~300 - The Library and Museum at Alexandria, greatest in the ancient world, is founded. It will last till 391 CE when Theodosius I orders the destruction of all Pagan temples

30 - Death of Cleopatra, Romans annex Egypt

350   300   250   200   150   100   50   0

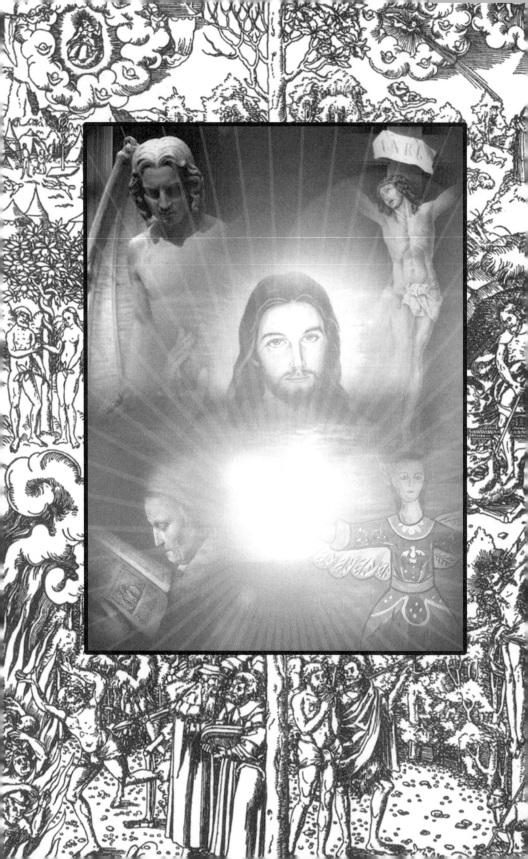

LIKE FATHER, LIKE SON
Early Christianity and The Biblical Myth

> *The images of myth are reflections of the spiritual potentialities of every one of us. Through contemplating these, we evoke their power in our own lives.*

—Joseph Campbell

When Jesus was born, Galilee was an idyllic place: a self-sufficient land of natural beauty, dotted with small villages, hot springs, a rolling river, and plenty of food. Though politically ruled by Rome, it was a land set apart from the whirlwind of political intrigue. Its population was of mixed race, sophisticated in Greek culture and faithful to Jewish law. They had a spirit of independence and a way of life worth protecting. Today, we might even call them *progressives,* free thinkers who lived peacefully with their environment and each other. Only when Herod the Great's successor, Archelaus, failed to command the independent spirit of Judaea, did Rome direct its attention toward controlling and subduing the region. In a world of empires ruled more by force than wisdom, this was the land—and the political climate—that gave birth to what has become the central myth of the Static Masculine era.

The Christian myth of the life, death, and resurrection of Jesus has had a greater effect on the shaping of Western civilization than any myth in our collective history. One third of the global population today–2.1 billion people as of 2005–define themselves as Christian, with estimates as high as 86 percent of the population in the United States.[2] Regardless of how you feel about this religion–whether you're a true believer or an atheist, a Buddhist, a Jew, a Muslim, or a Pagan–Christianity dominates the spiritual airwaves throughout much of the world. In the West, it holds the collective consciousness in a set of aspirations and fears, assumptions and beliefs that influence every facet of our civilization: education, health care, population control, environment, economics, sexual mores, women's rights, and political elections.

Like any religion, Christianity's development has had its twists and turns, with many events and contributors shaping its doctrines, and numerous interpretations of that doctrine. Countless volumes have been written about Christianity's history and beliefs, and bloody wars have been fought over its interpretation. What I attempt to tell here is a broad sweep of its salient points, comparing its original heart chakra vision of a loving social community to the way that vision played out in a third chakra paradigm of power. My purpose is neither to defend nor denigrate Christianity, but to illustrate–within the limits of a these few pages–both its brilliant light and its equally dark shadow. Only by bringing both polarities to consciousness can we come to the integrative wholeness necessary for an opening of the heart.

Christianity is based on the story of a simple man whose gentle presence taught His followers a new way to think about life and community. Jesus of Nazareth[3] was a radical visionary, an avatar of the heart chakra. His central message of love stood in radical contrast to the aggressive and dominating third chakra values of the time. He taught his followers to love their enemies, to turn the other cheek, and to practice forgiveness against trespassers–ideas that were revolutionary at the time, and hence controversial. Where ancient kings had been distant and authoritarian rulers, whose power was forged in conquest and whose wealth was built with the sweat of slaves, here was a prophet with a different kind of story, ripe with new hope and meaning. Like the Buddha five centuries before him, (whose wisdom had not yet migrated to the Western world) Jesus modeled compassion over judgment. He collapsed the stratifications of a classist and sexist society into a new community of social equality.

In the myth that grew out of His brief existence, Jesus was the product of an immaculate conception between a divine father and a virgin, human mother. As a result, He was regarded as both human and divine, an issue to be hotly debated in the centuries that followed. He even claimed his own divinity with the statement that "I and the father are one," and told his followers that they too were gods.[4] The archetypal son was maturing; the boy-become-man was now merging with the Father archetype, a symbol of divine consciousness.

Women had already been reduced to the status of a daughter–submissive, invisible, and obedient to husband and father. Jesus' father was God, his mother was mortal–certainly not a relationship of equals in the literal sense. (A deeper reading of the Virgin Mother who mates with God suggests a symbol of the virgin Earth who brings forth life as a result of penetration by the radiant sun.) But in the view that grew out of the Christian myth, Mother Mary was a passive recipient, stripped of sexuality and free will, a mere vessel, whose worship would later be forbidden. If she represented a reduced form of the Great Mother, her counterpart in Mary Magdalene, sunk to the status of prostitute. With the mother reduced to a maiden, and the maiden seen as a whore, the natural trinity of Mother, Father, and Child was replaced by a masculine duality–Father and Son–with the Holy Ghost to be added later–a ghost in place of what was once a living mother.

Masculine and feminine archetypal dynamics had now turned completely about. With women subdued to the status of powerless young girls, the Mother-Son motif of the Static Feminine era was now replaced by a dynamic of Father-Daughter. To reach the maturity required for egalitarian relationships, each gender must eventually outgrow its parents. For women, this wouldn't happen for nearly two thousand years, during which time conditions would get far worse before they started getting better.

REVOLUTIONARY SPIRITUALITY

Jesus was a rebel. He flouted Jewish law and customs—working on the Sabbath, associating with tax collectors, lepers, and whores, and advocating equal treatment of women. He preached that spiritual salvation was available to anyone, Jew or gentile, rich or poor, slave or master. Even women were welcome to participate. In a hierarchical world of haves and have nots, where social status was absolute, he leveled the playing field with equal opportunity spirituality. His philosophy did not require abstract questioning, detachment, or logic. Nor did it require wealth or status. By contrast the poor were actively invited to participate, and to share meals with those of higher classes, a practice that broke strong social taboos.

Jesus only required faith and love—faith that the individual would find salvation in the kingdom of God, and love as God's divine gift, to be shared unconditionally. His followers believed that He performed miracles as a demonstration of His love and His divine powers. Scarcity turned to plenty; water turned into wine. Diseases were healed; eyesight restored; [5] even the dead could be raised! It's easy to see the appeal that this egalitarian, spiritual utopia had on the ancient world. It was an exhilarating social experiment: a tantalizing belief in a world free of suffering; the promise of a sane society.

From the Gnostic perspective, (a view that was heavily suppressed in the centuries that followed) the Jesus story is an allegory for the process of initiation. Its elements combine the myths of the Greek mystery cults with the Jewish prophecy of the savior-king, creating a natural fusion of the two cultures. His baptism or purification, followed by His period of isolation in the desert, then crucifixion and resurrection, reflect the stages of initiation through which a deeper, divine reality is revealed.

If evolution is the gods' way of making more gods, Jesus was an example of evolution's next iteration, a living ideal of what could be possible for a human with advanced consciousness. His teachings were mystical clues about how to evolve our own consciousness and wake up to the miraculous power of the divine within. However,

His evolutionary vision was not limited to individual consciousness, but was centered around a radical social vision of community that broke down the barriers of racial and hierarchical status, redeemed the poor and dispossessed, and sought to harmonise the tensions between Jews and Romans.

A central vision of Jesus' teachings was that the kingdom of God was accessible right here on Earth, available to anyone. This radical idea addressed the previous separation of the World Parents, restoring the archetypal split between Heaven and Earth, and seeing humanity as one expanded family. Early Christian communities transcended the old boundaries of clan, tribe, and race by calling each other brother, sister, reverend mother. Priests were called fathers. Even Christ was called Lord, as in lord of the manor. Later the word Pope would come from the word for Papa. It was a radically adventurous movement that created, through love, the unity that the great empires had tried to forge through warfare. Unity—of the archetypal realms of Heaven and Earth, Father and Son, masculine and feminine, and one tribe to another—was the social message of Christ's new story. It carried a grand synthesis into a fragmented world.

These were rich ideas and they infused the early communities with a spiritual passion that spread across the land. As the gospel spread westward, through the Roman Empire, the teachings of Jesus were taken as literal fact to be believed, rather than clues to an initiatory experience. Christianity's fourth chakra focus on love and community entered a world ruled by third chakra dynamics. Though originally formed in reaction to Roman dominance, the early Christian communities quickly became coopted by the very system they were trying to transcend.

The Roman world was ruled by power, not love, by forced obedience, not cooperative inspiration. To keep the downtrodden masses from revolting, the Romans maintained a strict reign of terror. Crucifixion was one of the many ways in which they displayed their power. The Jews, believing their covenant was with the land they lived upon, rather than Rome, resisted Rome's taxation. In 4 B.C.E., the historian Josephus tells of a field of two thousand Jews crucified near Galilee for this rebellion, their corpses left on the crosses as an example to others.[6]

By contrast, Jesus did not force or manipulate. Unlike the kings of his day, He was not born of wealth or political privilege, as his humble birth in a manger implies. He didn't rule a physical kingdom but a spiritual one, fusing the roles of priest and king into a single figure once again. His followers were inspired by love, not power; by the reward of spiritual understanding, not material wealth. He preached a simple but radical gospel: experience God's love; love your neighbor; share what you have; miracles are possible.

> "As the Father has loved me, so have I loved you; abide in my love…. This is my commandment, that you love one another as I have loved you."　　　　　—John 15: 10-12

The early Jesus movement was a grand experiment carried out by social revolutionaries high on the energy of a new vision. Like the flower children of the sixties, they recognized each other as members of a new society, united by their vision of the possible. They overcame the boundaries of race and class, and gathered together for meals, sharing their hopes, dreams, and prayers. They were brothers and sisters in a common cause, inspired and held together by their love for each other and for Jesus as their teacher. He was the intermediary to a spiritual realm that could be shared by all.

When, just 33 years after His birth, and only three years or less after he began teaching, the prophet was brutally murdered, the blow to His followers would have been monumental. With such an untimely death, Jesus's message of hope and love risked becoming obscured for eternity. The movement was young and still unformed. Very little had been written down. Many still doubted his authority. But death followed by a story of resurrection made His life miraculous. His teachings were preserved and revered as the word of God. No longer a simple prophet with a progressive vision, Jesus became a figure of immortality, the Christos or Messiah. (Whether this was a real or symbolic resurrection was a subject of controversy between the Gnostics, who saw His life as an allegory for spiritual initiation, and the orthodox Christians, who interpreted the events literally.)

As birth was the numinous mystery of the Great Mother, it had been death that was the powerful shaper of reality in the third chakra era, perhaps the ultimate male mystery. It was death through war, and the fight against death through immortalized tombs and palaces, that propelled human behavior into the obedience of the Static Masculine paradigm. And where the ancient mystery religions had commonly celebrated the cycle of life, death, and rebirth in their rituals, the death and rebirth of Jesus made this mystery into a concrete reality, one that could be shared by all, symbolically ritualized again and again. While the sacred king of ancient times was, on occasion, sacrificed for the good of the land, the sacrifice of Jesus was for all time and all people, a sacrifice more fitting for the values of the day. The death and resurrection of the Christ echoes an older cycle of the Pagan god of the harvest, such as Dionysius or Osiris, who is cut down annually to arise again each springtime.

Death being the powerful motivator that it is, the horror of the crucifixion inspired an extraordinary zeal in His disciples to redeem Christ's death by propagating His message far and wide. Unfortunately, the macabre image of His body dying on the cross replaced the image of the fish that had preceded it as His symbol. The cross then became the dominant religious icon for spreading His message, an image ubiquitous to the present day. It's as if the entire philosophy of love and egalitarian community were frozen in arrested development from that point onward.

CHRISTIANITY AFTER JESUS

Most of what has come down to us about the life and death of Jesus was written after He died. Those who followed Jesus when He was alive did not need scripture—they had a living experience. Many were poor and illiterate. But as Christianity became Romanized, it became a religion of the book.

The prolific first century apostle Paul shaped much of Christian theology through his writings. A product of his times, Paul was a Jew, a Roman citizen, and a Greek by education. He never met Jesus alive, but was converted by a vision he received on the road to Damascus—a journey that had begun with a firm intention to put a stop the growing Christian cult! As the Greek mentality was already grounded in the mystery cults celebrating death and rebirth, the Greek Corinthians saw the resurrection of Christ as cause for celebration to be accompanied by ecstatic rites. Based on letters written at the time (which may have been forged), it seemed that Paul felt uncomfortable with the spirit of celebration. Reflecting instead the notion of the Greek noble death and the ideal of martyrdom, he stressed the need for seriousness. According to Paul, Christ's obedience unto death exemplified the proper spiritual attitude for the Christian community.[7] This death was the ultimate sacrifice for the love of God. Thus the religious zeal of the early Christians became infused with the idea that *willingness to suffer* demonstrated moral character. The cross was the perfect symbol to remind them of Christ's suffering.

Gareth Hill sees the cross as the central symbol for the Static Masculine archetype, representing "opposites held in the differentiated tension of an order state."[8] The lines of the cross create distinctions, boundaries, and walls. The horizontal line of the cross draws a division between above and below, Heaven and Earth, mind and body. The vertical line of the cross divides left from right, rational thinking from intuitive, male from female, good from evil. In this sense, the separation that had already been created by the Dynamic Masculine—the separation of the World Parents, the separation of Heaven and Earth, masculine and feminine, mind and body—was now given a symbol that expressed, maintained, and rigidified that separation.

If we place a human body against a cross, the lines intersect at the heart. Though Jesus was a prophet of the heart, who preached a message of love and unity for all people, the cross upon which He was crucified was firmly planted in the soil of a paradigm that was anything but loving. The ground of Roman soil did *not* unify men and women, spirit and body, or civilization and Nature.

Yet the divine kingdom that Jesus prophesied was not another dominant empire, but a promise of human redemption in a world of blinding paradoxes and acute spiritual hunger. Unfortunately, an empire ruled by force and obedience was the social structure of the time. It's no surprise then, that, as Christianity spread through the Roman Empire, it was coopted by the imperial values that ruled that empire. The divine and timely message of love, no longer renewed and updated by its living founder, was instead spread by messengers whose cultural milieu was institutional, authoritarian, and enormously efficient. As Joseph Campbell said to Bill Moyers in *The Power of Myth:* "The power impulse is the fundamental impulse in European history. And it got into our religious traditions."[9] As Christianity became Romanized, it became a servant of imperial values rather than mystical enlightenment.

CHRISTIAN MARTYRS

Early Christians were not immediately accepted in the Roman Empire, but remained fringe members of society in the first centuries of the common era. As a result, they kept largely to themselves in those early years. Their unwillingness to sacrifice to the emperor's divine cult was seen as politically contemptuous, and their refusal to honor the old gods earned them the term *atheists*. Such refusal threatened social stability. What if the gods got angry, and sought retribution by sending pestilence or drought? Before the gods could act, Roman officials took the upper hand, and persecuted some of the Christians instead. Brought before tribunals, they were asked to renounce their faith—or face public execution. Many chose martyrdom, finding more freedom in death than in life. Even in the face of tortuous deaths, the martyrs believed that their acts demonstrated the strength of the faith, and were the highest calling they could aspire to. Though not intentional, this proved to be an effective marketing tool—for what kind of God could inspire such zeal?

A decisive turning point came in 312 C.E., when the originally Pagan and immensely influential emperor, Constantine, received a vision in which he saw a large cross in the sky, emblazoned with the words, "In this sign, thou shalt conquer." As if in answer, he won his next battle miraculously. Ostensibly, he knew little about the Christian religion at the time, and struggled with how to align his victory with the fact that the God of Christ was not a God of war. Yet with this omen he saw an opportunity to solidify his power and unite the multi-ethnic Roman Empire under a single set of beliefs. He reversed his predecessors' persecution of Christians, and instead began rewarding them with money, tax exemptions, and prestigious positions. By this act, he cleared the way for all church dignitaries to serve his imperial rule. In the century that followed, the number of Christians grew from 5 million to 30 million.[10]

With this unification of church and state, political rulers were allowed to influence church doctrine. Constantine presided over the first ecumenical council at Nicea, in 325 C.E., where the issue of Jesus' divinity was debated. Was Jesus mortal or divine, a man or a God? The council eliminated any possibility of a logical trinity composed of father, mother, and child, and replaced it with the Father, Son and the Holy Ghost—a non-living, sexless spirit. All forms of Christianity, other than the form we now know as Orthodox, were banned.

After Julian, the last Pagan emperor of Rome, died in 363 C.E., the entire pantheon of the old gods and goddesses dissappeared—along with all their diversity and messy passions—into a wholly masculine monotheism. In 388 the Emperor Theodosius had the Pagan temples destroyed, which resulted in the loss of the famed temple and library in Alexandria in 389 and the Altar of Victory in the Roman Senate in 391.[11] Any traces of the initiatory tradition of the Gnostics were destroyed.[12] Orthodox Christianity became the official state religion, a means of bringing spiritual unification to the Roman Empire.

What was brought under the umbrella of unity was all that was above ground: the social world, religious dogma, behavioral codes, and the values of the Static Masculine. What was left out of this unity were all aspects of the first two chakras: the sacredness of the Earth, the body, sexuality, and pleasure. Class distinctions remained extreme, as did the lower-class status of women.

The heroic impulse of the power-oriented third chakra was projected outward, onto the figure of Jesus. He was the new hero, and the common man was relieved of the journey, at least in the outward sense. The heroic impulse now took place on the inner planes, as reason and logic battled with passion and instinct.

Though this was an attempt to rise to the level of the heart chakra, it denied or distorted the previous levels, which were oriented to survival, sexuality, and power. Women were left out of the divine picture, and continued to be repressed. The new social order wasn't playing with a full deck, and true unity could not be achieved. Where the mystery religions such as the Eleusinian rites of Demeter, or the rites of Orpheus, were about finding wisdom through a personal descent, Christians believed only in ascension, with the high being mightier than the low. The gap between Heaven and Earth—to which Jesus had proposed a synthesis—grew wider.

THE ROLE OF SIN

Having turned away from our biological roots and the laws of Nature, with millennia of warfare and domination, the world was far from a utopian dream of exalted splendor. Most people were still poor, with disease and violence as a constant presence. Christ had promised that the divine kingdom would be manifest as Heaven on Earth, yet the mundane world was still full of suffering. This awkward contradiction had to be addressed. What could explain this? What was the difference between those who were exalted and those who suffered, those who had plenty, and those who had little or nothing?

Wealth, status, and power, long equated with temple bureaucracies, were seen as God's gifts, proof of God's grace. Those who were dealt short hands in these matters must be sinners, their sins the reason for their unfortunate state. If they had done nothing wrong, then they must be the victims of original sin—a sin they had nothing to do with, yet still had to overcome. Only with deeper attempts at purification, sacrifice, and self-denial (more suffering) could one hope for redemption. Rather than question the *source* of that suffering, Christianity gave it a moral value: by enduring it, you earned credit toward your eventual salvation. With the attitude of no pain, no gain, suffering and hardship became the mark a true orthodox Christian's life. It was a means of purification, a viable road to God. And that suffering, like the suffering of Christ, was to purge us of our sins. This was a convenient philosophy for those who imposed a brutal social order. By giving suffering a moral value, one need not question its causes.

It is interesting to note that the word *sin* occurs in early Jewish texts in reference to behavior that is out of accord with the rules of the Torah.[13] The early Jesus movement was grounded in Jewish law, yet it sought to include gentiles as equal members of the community—a major focus of Paul's ministry. That gentiles had a different set of social customs, including not being circumcized, posed a critical problem in the early communities. These differences, according to Christ's message, were to be "forgiven" in the service of forming a larger community, hence forgiveness of sins.[14] (I imagine that aspiring Christian males breathed a sigh of relief at the time.)

Since the promised kingdom had not yet arrived, it was pushed toward the end of time *(eschaton),* where all people would meet a judgment that would recognize the worthy and damn the rest. The presence or absence of "sin" determined that outcome, and it became incumbent upon the good Christian to curtail certain behaviors in favor of others so as to fare better on that fateful day. Which behaviors to curtail changed over time, but what is clear is that the physical body, pleasure, and sexuality were considered the most incriminating. Therefore, the gulf widened further between men and women, Eros and Logos, mind and body. Guilt, over the inner forces that were indeed natural pervaded one's very being and deepened the believer's need for strict control.

THE TWISTING OF SEX AND POWER

If sexuality had not received enough of a blow from the ascetic attitudes of the first century, its final throttle came from one of Christianity's most influential writers: St. Augustine, Bishop of Hippo. Born under the sign of Scorpio (Nov. 13, 354 C.E.) in Thagaste, North Africa, he was the son of a Pagan father and a Christian mother—a splendid setup for wrestling with the contradictions of his time. His father, Patricius, was known for his frequent affairs and, as fathers are wont to do, encouraged his son to pursue his passions. As a young man, Augustine lived well, fathering a child out of wedlock, and living with his concubine, whom he apparently loved for many years. He was also drawn toward the dualistic teachings of Manichaeism, with its eternal battle between good and evil, where the human body, like all matter, was considered evil. Despite nine years of study, he never officially joined that faith, yet it is clear it influenced his thinking and teachings throughout his life.

Augustine's mother, Monica, was emotionally enmeshed with her son, apparently suffering greatly when he did not live according to her expectations. Deploring her husband's infidelity, she begged Augustine to curb his desires, and pressured him to leave his concubine for a woman of higher status. To further that goal, she saw to his education. He developed a talent for rhetoric that would make him one of the most prolific writers of his time—including the first deeply introspective autobiography, *Confessions,* which is how we know so much about his inner process.

Monica prayed fervently that Augustine would see the error of his Pagan ways and convert to Christianity. Her prayers were answered when at thirty years of age, Augustine encountered the teachings of Plato, and experienced the preaching of St. Ambrose. During a meditation, he heard a child's voice inside his head that said repeatedly, "Take it and read, take it and read." He randomly opened the Bible to the following passage in Paul's epistle to the Romans:

"Not in revelling and drunkenness, not in lust and wantonness, not in quarrels and rivalries. Rather arm yourselves with the Lord Jesus Christ; spend no more thought on nature and nature's appetites."

(Romans 13:13-14)

This passage spoke directly to his inner struggles. Here he found integration of his Manichaen roots, his Platonic aspirations, and his spiritual longing. He could at last make peace with his suffering mother, who promptly found him a suitable marriage and sent his concubine back to Carthage. He chose to follow Christ and lead a celibate life—or at least he tried.

Old habits die hard; his sexual passions did not succumb to his will. He was unable to control his desire, a major subject of his *Confessions*. Because he could not *will* his desire away (his member rose and fell without his conscious control) he concluded that free will was not something that he possessed. Nor did he believe that anyone else possessed such a thing, or even that it was *possible* to have free will, lashing out at those who professed otherwise.

Through long and tortuous reasoning, he came to believe that the original Adam himself was void of free will, and that Adam's sin of copulation with Eve was passed down through the generations in the substance of semen. Therefore all descendents of Adam— meaning everyone: Pagans, Christians, and Jews alike—were guilty of original sin from the moment of conception, having been con- taminated by this vicious substance for the whole of their lives. Beginning life in sin, and stripped of the free will to do anything about it, humans couldn't do anything *but* sin. Elaine Pagels, in *Adam, Eve, and the Serpent* states:

"Augustine believed that by defining spontaneous sexual desire as the proof and penalty of original sin he has suc- ceeded in implicating the whole human race, except, of course, for Christ. Christ alone of all humankind, Augustine explains, was born without *libido*—being born, he believes, without the intervention of semen that transmits its effects.

But the rest of humankind issues from a procreative process that, ever since Adam, has sprung wildly out of control, marring the whole of human nature." [15]

Augustine further declared that Adam and Eve's sexual desire—and all the trouble it caused—was the result of their disobedience to God. Therefore, obedience to church and imperial authority alike was a way to counter this sin. It was a sign of obedience to God Himself. He believed that the dictatorial authority of the church was the only force that could liberate men from their evil nature, and was therefore necessary for governing a peaceful state. This belief amplified his conflicts with a rival church, the Donatists, who were known to be violently rebellious to authority in general. As time passed, Augustine became increasingly authoritarian. He supported the institution of fines and penalties, the denial of free discussion, the exile of Donatist bishops, and the use of physical coercion to maintain order. It seems that renouncing his sexuality made Augustine a very rigid man.

The idea of free will might have been saved by Pelagius, a popular Irish monk, whose more positive attitude professed that humans *did* possess their own will and could use it to work good deeds. Augustine, however, believed that Pelagian ideas would undermine church authority. With a bribe of eighty Numidian stallions, he induced the Pope to excommunicate Pelagius in 418 C.E.[16] From that point onward, church doctrine upheld the hereditary transmission of original sin.

One might wonder why the people of the fourth and fifth centuries would accept such convoluted reasoning when there were other voices arguing against it. The answer, Pagels argues, lies in the value to an imperial authority of the belief that their citizens were sinners who were incapable of self-control and therefore of self-government. This was a convenient philosophy for the few who wanted to rule the many. Augustine's beliefs made it a religious duty to submit to imperial rule. Church and state, utterly intertwined, need not separate their authority. Pagels explains:

> "It is Augustine's theology of the fall that made the uneasy alliance between the Catholic church and the imperial power palatable—not only justifiable but necessary—for the majority of Catholic Christians.... Augustine's theological legacy made sense out of a situation in which church and state had become inextricably interdependent."[17]

Free will—the contentiously complex element of the third chakra—was now culturally and scripturally suppressed. Without free will, there was no spark, no fire, and no evolution. Sexuality, passion, and the pageantry of the old rituals were now defined as sins. Innate sexual desire, and even the emotions of longing for connection with another, were to be chastized or made chaste. Intimacy between men and women went into further decline, though it had been eroding for centuries. With this loss of passion came a loss of heart. The center of the Roman Empire could no longer hold.

Despite six centuries of peace, power and prosperity—as well as its assertion of holding the high moral ground—the Roman Empire fell into political and moral corruption and collapsed. The factors deemed responsible, we might note, are all present today: an oppressive government, rapacious expansion, ambitious generals, barbarian incursions (read terrorism), power struggles between church and state, sustained inflation, moral decay, and epidemic disease. With the fall of the western empire at the end of the fourth century, its people were plunged into turmoil. Like traumatized children, desperately trying to survive difficult times by pleasing an authoritarian father, humankind entered the ensuing Dark Ages wearing a straight-jacket of moral restrictions lashed to the psyche with fear. The period that followed was a dark and depressive spiritual wasteland.

ESSENTIAL POINTS

• Christ's original vision of love and community was a revolutionary experiment in social equality that challenged both Jewish law and Roman authority.

• Christ's early death arrested the development of his message before it had matured throughout the movement.

• The death and resurrection of the Christ story reflects Greek mystery cults of the dying and reborn god.

• When Christianity spread through the Roman Empire, it became imperialized as a tool of political power.

• Augustine, a noted fourth century Christian writer, solidified the doctrine of original sin and the absence of free will.

• Stripped of its heart, rigid in its beliefs, the church-state theocracy of the Roman Empire collapsed.

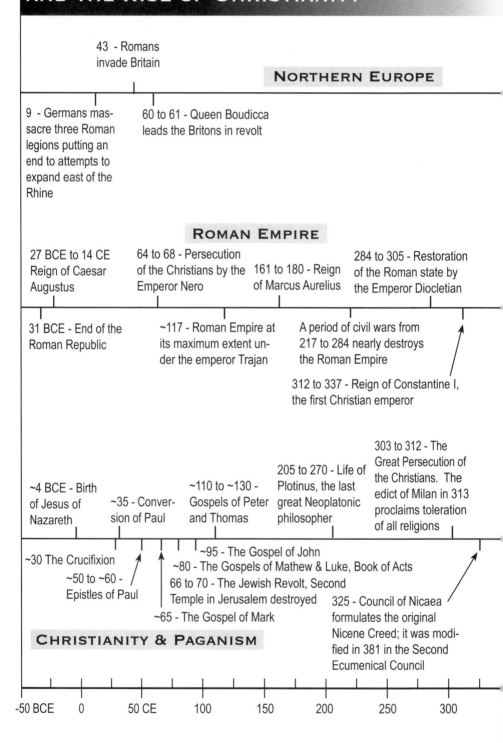

43 - Romans invade Britain

NORTHERN EUROPE

9 - Germans massacre three Roman legions putting an end to attempts to expand east of the Rhine

60 to 61 - Queen Boudicca leads the Britons in revolt

ROMAN EMPIRE

27 BCE to 14 CE Reign of Caesar Augustus

64 to 68 - Persecution of the Christians by the Emperor Nero

161 to 180 - Reign of Marcus Aurelius

284 to 305 - Restoration of the Roman state by the Emperor Diocletian

31 BCE - End of the Roman Republic

~117 - Roman Empire at its maximum extent under the emperor Trajan

A period of civil wars from 217 to 284 nearly destroys the Roman Empire

312 to 337 - Reign of Constantine I, the first Christian emperor

303 to 312 - The Great Persecution of the Christians. The edict of Milan in 313 proclaims toleration of all religions

~4 BCE - Birth of Jesus of Nazareth

~35 - Conversion of Paul

~110 to ~130 - Gospels of Peter and Thomas

205 to 270 - Life of Plotinus, the last great Neoplatonic philosopher

~30 The Crucifixion

~50 to ~60 - Epistles of Paul

~95 - The Gospel of John

~80 - The Gospels of Mathew & Luke, Book of Acts

66 to 70 - The Jewish Revolt, Second Temple in Jerusalem destroyed

~65 - The Gospel of Mark

325 - Council of Nicaea formulates the original Nicene Creed; it was modified in 381 in the Second Ecumenical Council

CHRISTIANITY & PAGANISM

-50 BCE   0   50 CE   100   150   200   250   300

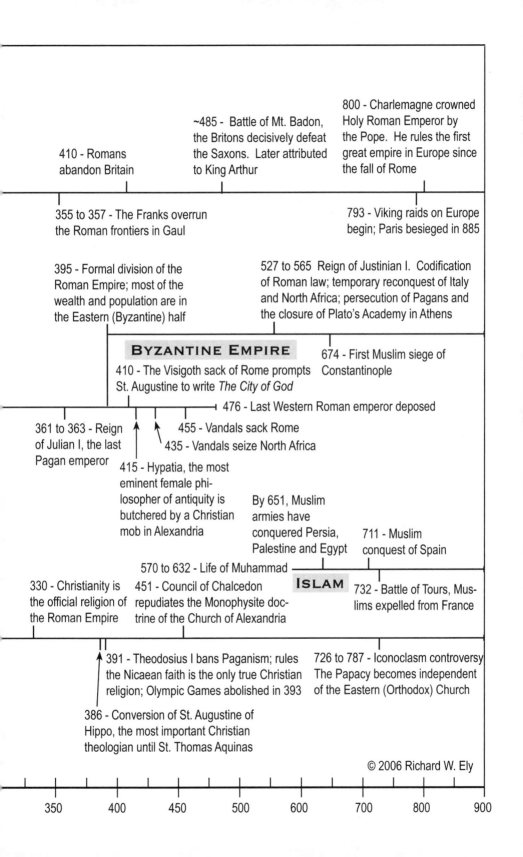

800 - Charlemagne crowned Holy Roman Emperor by the Pope. He rules the first great empire in Europe since the fall of Rome

~485 - Battle of Mt. Badon, the Britons decisively defeat the Saxons. Later attributed to King Arthur

410 - Romans abandon Britain

355 to 357 - The Franks overrun the Roman frontiers in Gaul

793 - Viking raids on Europe begin; Paris besieged in 885

395 - Formal division of the Roman Empire; most of the wealth and population are in the Eastern (Byzantine) half

527 to 565 Reign of Justinian I. Codification of Roman law; temporary reconquest of Italy and North Africa; persecution of Pagans and the closure of Plato's Academy in Athens

BYZANTINE EMPIRE

674 - First Muslim siege of Constantinople

410 - The Visigoth sack of Rome prompts St. Augustine to write *The City of God*

476 - Last Western Roman emperor deposed

361 to 363 - Reign of Julian I, the last Pagan emperor

455 - Vandals sack Rome
435 - Vandals seize North Africa

415 - Hypatia, the most eminent female philosopher of antiquity is butchered by a Christian mob in Alexandria

By 651, Muslim armies have conquered Persia, Palestine and Egypt

711 - Muslim conquest of Spain

570 to 632 - Life of Muhammad

330 - Christianity is the official religion of the Roman Empire

451 - Council of Chalcedon repudiates the Monophysite doctrine of the Church of Alexandria

ISLAM

732 - Battle of Tours, Muslims expelled from France

391 - Theodosius I bans Paganism; rules the Nicaean faith is the only true Christian religion; Olympic Games abolished in 393

726 to 787 - Iconoclasm controversy The Papacy becomes independent of the Eastern (Orthodox) Church

386 - Conversion of St. Augustine of Hippo, the most important Christian theologian until St. Thomas Aquinas

© 2006 Richard W. Ely

350   400   450   500   600   700   800   900

SHEDDING LIGHT
ON THE SHADOW

The Dark Ages and Beyond

> *One does not become enlightened by imagining figures of light,*
> *but by making the darkness conscious.*

—C. G. Jung

The promising pinnacle of Christ's vision of God's love, stripped of the passion and free will to sustain it, entered a dark time. Without a mother to help maintain natural order in the home, this need fell to a stern father, whose countenance grew ever more strict as he single parented humanity through its formative centuries of childhood. Social order was based on unquestioning obedience, with error punishable by damnation, pain, or death. Death, as a means of control, grew ever more menacing. Clement, Bishop of Rome, as early as the first century C.E. stated that whoever disobeys the divinely ordained authorities has disobeyed God Himself, and should "receive the death penalty."[1] By 435 this sentiment had grown to an established law that threatened any heretic in the entire Roman Empire with death. A Christian woman could even be executed for marrying a Jew.[2]

Under this kind of severity, the European world was greatly subdued; the ecstatic experience of the divine far removed from daily life. (The word *ecstasy* comes from "ex-static," meaning "beyond the static.") Religious experience was no longer direct, but needed to occur through mediating priests, who doled out blessings in exchange for supporting their massive hierarchy. Father's rules were written in books that became law, but only the elite had access to these books. Truth was literally and figuratively the letter of the law, static and unchanging. Morals and ethics were dictated by those who lived celibate lives in stone churches, removed from daily life and familial love. These codes had less to do with the establishment of a sane and egalitarian society than with strict adherence to the dominant masculine values that allowed such an unbalanced system to continue unopposed. Indignation over suffering was muted by the belief that it was just punishment for sins. Fear was rampant. In other works, I have named fear as the demon that appears when the first chakra's connection to ground is distorted.[3] When this happens to an entire culture, that fear can be used as a means of control. *Scared is what happens when the sacred gets scrambled.*

St. John Chrysostom, who initially opposed Augustine, saw fear as an organizing principle, essential to maintaining order: He writes:

> "If you were to deprive the world of magistrates and the fear that comes from them, houses, cities and nations would fall upon one another in unrestrained confusion, there being no one to repress, or repel, or persuade them to be peaceful through the fear of punishment."[4]

All that was rejected in the Great Reversal that overthrew the Static Feminine—the body, sexuality, passion, pleasure—became relegated to the shadow. It was denied, outlawed, policed, and punished. The divine Earth was seen as a material trap for spirit. Sin became equated with any behaviors that were contrary to the values of the masculine dominator structure. The Great Mother and her wide pantheon of Nature deities were obliterated from memory. Statues were beheaded, temples and artwork destroyed. Christian churches were erected on Pagan holy sites. Rituals or prayers to the Goddess were made a sin, punishable by death. The Divine Feminine archetype was sent to the Underworld, along with emotions, free will, and ecstatic spirituality. If one's unconscious objected and momentarily broke free from this repression, the offender would be labeled as crazy and summarily locked up or tortured. The unconscious repository in which humankind stored these feelings would not be discovered until the early twentieth century when they began to resurface on the psychoanalytic couches of Sigmund Freud and Carl Jung.

The mythology of a divine order based on Nature was replaced with the myth that Christianity had not only lifted society from an archaic primitivism, but that warfare, hierarchy, and male domination had always existed and were therefore natural. Where the old gods had held properties of dark and light within a single archetype, the Christian God was completely pure, while shadow aspects were projected outward, onto Nature, women, and heretics—and inward against one's instinctual human drives. The physical world, once a divine, magical creation, was now the province of the devil, an archetypal repository for all that was rejected.

A righteous spiritual path was to be marked by disengagement from the physical world—an impossible task, since we are, in fact, mortal creatures. With a dangerous dissociation that still persists today, all sense of the divine was removed from ordinary life, much as daily life had been removed from Nature millennia before. The divine realm was "other worldly," accessed only by disengagement from life, or by death itself, which would hopefully lead to a heavenly afterlife. In a period of cultural introversion, civilization drew inward toward the daunting task of managing the inner world, and shaping it according to the morality dictated by priests and the certainty of scripture. The exultant Christian spirit became mired in judgment, dogmatism, and resignation.

Yet we were willing to sell our souls for this stability, and its promise of salvation. It even carried a sense of grandeur, as we learned to build taller and higher, with elaborately arched cathedrals drawing our attention upwards. Their contrast to the humble, dirt-floor hovels in which the common people lived was stark. Religious services provided comfort in dark times, with angelic choral singing, and the most elaborate works of art to be found. Christianity continued to spread, offering a mixture of oppression and inspiration.

THE MIDDLE AGES AND THE CRUSADES

As the exquisite cathedrals rose from the ground of the Middle Ages, so did their cost. The church had to continue to amass wealth in order to maintain its elaborate hegemony. Church properties were free of taxes, and comprised up to a third of the land mass of Western Europe, with vast estates that produced abundant income.[5] The Church made money in a variety of ways. Imperial rulers made contributions, much as special interest groups do today. Through the selling of "indulgences," people could buy off their sins. The wealthy could buy eclesiastical offices (called "simony"), and the church confiscated the property of "heretics." (The word comes from the Greek *haeresis*, meaning "choice.")

When worship of the Virgin Mary swelled in the Middle Ages, the Church responded by strengthening its authoritarian structure. The Pope created a council of papal legates, called the curia, who could override the authority of any local bishops and archbishops, giving the Church a more centralized and dictatorial leadership. The Pope's power was now unlimited. He could proffer land deals with entire countries, even rule over kings. Pope Gregory VII, for example, excommunicated and deposed the Emperor Henry IV in 1076, forcing him to perform public penance–then promptly allying with his enemies. [6] The imperial powers of Europe were greatly subdued by the totalitarian rule of the Pope.

The Pope could even declare war, as did Pope Urban II, who launched the first Crusade in 1095. Word had come to Rome that infidels to the East were preventing pilgrimages to Jerusalem, a practice that had been peaceful for hundreds of years. With a common enemy to rally against, the dispirited imperial powers came together with religious zeal. In a wide appeal to all of Christendom, Pope Urban II promised complete remission of sin to any who would join the cause and make the long and treacherous journey to the East.

The initial response was a passionate cry of *Deus lo volt!* ("God wills it!") Crusaders took a public vow of military service, with resulting grants of indulgences and even land should they be lucky enough to return. Ostensibly to defend the Holy Land, the Crusades became a war against anyone who was not Christian, namely Muslims and Jews. Those who were attacked were astonished at the ferocity of the invaders. Entire villages of men, women and children were slaughtered. The chronicler, Raymond of Aguilers, illustrates how death became glorified in this description of a scene in Jerusalem, as it fell in 1099:

> "Wonderful things were to be seen. Numbers of the Saracens were beheaded. . . . Others were shot with arrows, or forced to jump from the towers; others were tortured for several days, then burned with flames. In the streets were seen piles of heads and hands and feet. One rode about everywhere amid the corpses of men and horses. In the temple of Solomon, the horses waded in blood up to their knees, nay, up to the bridle. It was a just and marvelous judgment of God, that this place should be filled with the blood of unbelievers." [7]

The Albigensian Crusades targeted the Cathars in Southern France—a powerful group of mystics that combined Christianity, Moslem Sufism, Jewish Kabbalah and Nature worship. Cathars allowed women to be priests and administer important rites. Under protection from the upper class, they grew immensely popular. In 1139 the Church began calling councils to condemn them, to little avail. In 1208, however, when their lands were promised away, the thirty year Albigensian Crusade against Southern France was launched. When asked how to tell Catholic from Cathar, the commanding legate replied, "Kill them all, for God knows his own!" [8]

What a strange twist to Christ's original message to believe that a man could be completely absolved of his sins by engaging in brutal genocide! Had the world gone mad? Had we lost all moral ground? The Crusades, in various bursts, lasted approximately two hundred years, killing hundreds of thousands of women and children, all in the name of a supposedly moral God. What was the lasting value from this killing spree? Though it did increase the wealth of Italy, lands that were invaded were not permanently gained; nor was the rise of Islam deterred. Rather, the permanent effects were to heighten the animosity between Christians and Muslims, breed increased anti-Semitism, and harden the schism between the Latin Christians of the West and the Greek Christians of the East.

Still, the people in the Middle Ages were restless. Through increased literacy and sophistication, they were waking up and questioning the absolute authority of the Catholic Church. Yet each heresy or revolt only increased the punitive authoritarianism of the papal hierarchy.

In 1231, this exceeded all previous limits with the establishment of the Papal Inquisition, formed by Pope Gregory IX. Formed as a separate tribunal, independent of bishops and prelates, it was a totalitarian regime. From village to village the inquisitors roamed, with their black robes and cowls, their stern faces, and their terrifying power. Unsuspecting peasants, mostly women, were captured without notice, removed from their homes, and confined in rat-infested prisons whose cost was exacted from their families. Those who were accused had no recourse to defend themselves. Often they never even knew the identity of their accusers or the nature of their crime. Yet they were brutally tortured until they confessed to heresy or condemned another. Most inquisitors came from the Dominican order, and all had a zealous hatred for heresy. Those who defended friends or family were labeled heretics as well, and could receive the same treatment as the accused. It was a miserable choice: humiliating public penance and possible life imprisonment for those who repented, or death by hanging or burning for those who would not. (This was an uncanny parallel to the early persecutions of Christians where the martyrs chose death rather than recant their faith.) Though the Crusades had massacred whole villages, the Inquisition was pointedly focused on cruelty. It was not a movement of conquest, but one of pure sadism.

It was also lucrative. The Church amassed wealth as it systematically confiscated the property of the victims. Inquisitors required local communities to pay for their trials, and took bribes from the upper classes in exchange for protection. The result was a *culturally instilled terror* that repressed the urge to speak or even think creatively. This created a fearful mistrust of one's own community. It also had a devastating impact on the European economy.

Why would anyone agree to participate in such atrocities? In the dualistic view of the times, anyone not joining the vengeance of the righteous was guilty of heresy. Even secular authorities could themselves be tied to the stake if they refused to exact these punishments. No one was safe to think or speak freely. Neighbor was pitted against neighbor, child against parent.

As fear prevailed, resentment toward the church went underground, silent and festering, while religiosity dominated all facets of society. Many intelligent people retreated into monasteries, withdrawing from everyday life. As if this were not enough to subdue the human spirit, the spread of the Black Death in 1348 cut across all classes, striking the pious as well as the commoner. The Church seized upon the plague as a demonstration of God's punishment for people's sin (not its own, of course) and used it as further proof of the need to obey Church authority. As medicines proved useless to stop the plague, the practice of medicine became suspect as well, including herbcraft and midwifery. Instead, the evil within was believed to be purged through bleeding, a barbaric practice that killed tens of thousands each year.[9]

A BREAK IN THE CLOUDS: THE ITALIAN RENAISSANCE

It is amazing that out of this cultural depravity, with all its suppression of wisdom, compassion, and creativity, there could even be a Renaissance, yet the human spirit continually proves to be more powerful than its circumstances. Out of a time riddled with pestilence, economic depression, and intellectual ignorance, there arose a new dawn, a rebirth of intellectual inquiry and creative expression.

In the late fourteenth century, in Northern Italy, the most urbanized and prosperous part of Europe, a movement burst forth to recover the glories of antiquity. It was certainly a dark time. Europe was at an all-time low. "Where have we gone wrong?" asked intellectuals of the time. Perhaps the wisdom of the ancients, long suppressed as Pagan writings, could provide some answers. Francesco Petrarch, a pre-Renaissance Italian with a passionate love for classical Greco-Roman texts, commenced a grand project for the reeducation of Europe. Voted the poet laureate of Europe, he seeded the Renaissance with a revival of romantic poetry and classic language, heralding the ideal of an autonomous individual with an interior emotional life. This reawakened—at least for a time—the spirit of the lost feminine and the passion of the human soul. A new hunger for learning followed, and with it, a renewal of scholarship and a revival in the art of rhetoric. Ancient manuscripts were recovered. Those who had money invested in art and literature, spawning a revival of creativity. Guilds formed, and with them a politics of the people. In Florence, 30 percent of the population was eligible to serve in office—including any adult male who paid taxes, owned property and matriculated in a guild. The dawning of civic humanism fueled its citizens with a sense of special destiny, a pride and passion to create the most beautiful cities and sophisticated works of art.

The Renaissance was the first self-conscious period in history, meaning that writers of the time were articulating that something new and different was happening – while it was occurring! Giovanni Bocaccio, (d. 1375) claimed that his world was different from the period before it. Leonardo Bruni (d. 1444) named the previous period the "Middle Ages." Matteo Palmieri, (d. 1440) claimed that Europe was experiencing a "rebirth."

Within the span of one lifetime, there were enormous achievements in knowledge and culture. Music and poetry, literature and science, all leapt from the shadows of their previous darkness. Clothes became colorful, music joyful, and creativity flourished. Because the plague had freed up a great deal of wealth from the many deceased, both the rulers of Italian city-states and the Church had funds for art and architecture. Da Vinci, Michelangelo, and Raphael produced their astounding works. Columbus discovered the New World. Gutenberg received a patent on the printing press. Literacy was on the rise. It was a welcome interlude of sunshine during a long, dark storm, a new awakening of love and knowledge, enchantment and creativity.

Unfortunately, it was to be short-lived. Even while Christianity was lavishly exploding with great works of art, the Catholic Church played a dual role of benefactor and oppressor, brewing a collective resentment that was kindling itself into a smoldering fire. While the common folk were waking up, both intellectually and spiritually, the Roman papacy was reaching new depths of corruption. Italian states surrounding Rome became mired in political battles in which greed, murder, and duplicity exceeded all reason. Pope Sixtus IV, for example, appointed relatives with no religious training, even children, as bishops and cardinals, giving them huge sums of money which they spent on lavish lifestyles. As successive Popes squandered the Church's massive wealth, they exacted more and more funds from the peasants, through taxes and the sale of indulgences. It became such a racket that one could even pay ahead for sins not yet committed, or pay for the deeds of deceased relatives to release them from purgatory!

SOCIAL PROTEST: THE PROTESTANT REFORMATION

While the Catholic hierarchy in Rome was falling from grace, religiosity continued to grow in Northern Europe, and with it a spirit of independence. Piety and poverty lived in stark contrast to Roman opulence. The printing press made the Bible widely available. Parents sat in on their children's classes, learning to read. People were thinking and questioning.

When at high noon on October 31, 1517 a monk by the name of Martin Luther posted 95 refutations of papal indulgences on the door of a German church, the smoldering resentment toward Catholicism flared into the blazing fire of the Protestant Reformation. This "protest," after which the movement was named, broke the thousand-year rule of the Roman Catholic Church as the only religious authority.

This marked the beginning of the rebellion against the father–perhaps the first hint of budding adolescence.

Protestantism was a movement that shifted the locus of power from church to state and from priest to layman. It opened the way for new ideas, and empowered the individual. It sought to rectify the Christian mission, through a return to its original values as stated in scripture. Yet it painted over the colorful joy of the Renaissance with a very dark brush. Like many reactionary movements, it took on the severity of the very system it was resisting.

In contrast to the Catholic Church, with its ostentatious cathedrals and elaborate rituals, Protestantism was simple: it relied on faith, grace, and scripture alone. Luther believed that the individual should be able to connect directly to God, without having to deal with a priest or the Catholic Church, which he felt had strayed too far from Christ's original message. Therefore scripture was the way to restore sanctity to the Christian lifestyle. Like Augustine, Luther believed that humans lacked free will, and were doomed to sin. He did not believe that sins could be bought off, or even "worked off" by good behavior, but redeemed only through God's grace as revealed through the Bible. Sins were merely a symptom of a deeper malady, which only faith could cure. Initially, he deplored the acts of the Inquisition and the rampant racism against Jews, Turks, and Moors, but it wasn't long before the Protestants came to commit equally heartless crimes against humanity.

Since Luther's interpretation of scripture did not accord divinity to Mother Mary, he discouraged her worship, and banned mother-son images of Mary and Jesus. The status of women continued to decline. In the earliest Christian writings, the Roman apostle Paul had described woman as the "weaker vessel."[10] From the works of Paul, Augustine, Tertullian, and Luther, the blame for sexual desire landed squarely on women as the devil's gateway. In the second century, father Tertullian wrote that: "Women are the gate by which the demon enters... it is on your account that Jesus died."[11] In the sixth century, the Council of Macon took a vote as to whether women had souls.[12] Even Thomas Aquinas, whose thirteenth century philosophy valued Nature as the perfection of the divine, left women entirely out of the equation. He said: "Nothing defective should have been produced in the first establishment of things; so woman ought not to have been produced." [13] And in the very town of Wittenberg, where Luther first tacked up his 95 refutations, there was debate over whether women were even human beings. [14] While the Catholic church had forbidden priests to marry, (some say to keep property from descending to potential heirs), Luther reversed that practice and eventually married and raised six children, some of them girls. Nonetheless he said, "Take women from their housewifery and they are good for nothing. . . . If women get tired and die of childbearing, there is no harm in that; let them die as long as they bear; they are made for that."[15]

The Catholic Church held fast to the idea that virtuous actions could influence salvation. When Pope Leo X issued a papal bull for Luther to withdraw his protestations, Luther simply burned it. The Catholics responded in a variety of ways, some positive, some negative. The Jesuits, an elite priestly order, stepped up the education of the young, founding hundreds of educational institutions throughout Europe. Yet more bloody wars ensued. Civil wars between Catholics and Protestants took the lives of hundreds of thousands, as a religion divided against itself killed for the supremacy of interpretation and the source of spiritual authority. These battles were as bloody as the Crusades. In France, on St. Bartholamew's Day (August 24, 1572) as many as ten thousand Protestants were slain in a single day.[16] Seventeen years after Luther nailed his objections on the church door, the Catholic Church had lost England, Denmark, Scotland, Sweden, Switzerland, and half of Germany to Protestantism.

On the spiritual front, each side entered an ever more aggressive competition for religious certainty. The Protestants reacted by adhering even more strictly to scripture, with increased judgment for any deviant behavior. Protestant mobs destroyed images and statues of Christian saints, much as the Catholic Church had destroyed Pagan art throughout the Roman Empire twelve hundred years earlier. Protestant sects fragmented, and each argued that their interpretation of scripture was the right one.

As the shadow aspects of human consciousness descended even deeper into the unconscious, the belief that humans were inherently flawed hardened into the bedrock of assumptions. Jesus' message of love and glory on earth was obscured, while His suffering and sacrifice were augmented. Both Catholics and Protestants became even more severe in their rejection of the physical body and sexuality, to the point where in some cases, even bathing was regarded as a sin. A Sorbonne prior *and doctor* wrote:

> "You must regard every kind of touching of your own and others' bodies, every liberty, as the most serious of sins; although these lewd acts may indeed be secret, they are loathsome in God's sight, who sees them all, is offended by them, and never fails to punish them most severely." [17]

Skin itself was considered a spiritual liability. Clerics decreed the female body was to be covered in dark clothing at all times. Home furnishings became very austere. Pleasure of all types was frowned upon, even public celebrations, theatrical productions, and the simple activities of children, such as swimming or sledding.

The God of love that had fueled Christian passion in the early days of the Jesus movement had become a God of fear and hate. Luther proclaimed:

> "This is the acme of faith, to believe that God, Who saves so few and condemns so many, is merciful; that He is just Who has made us necessarily doomed to damnation, so that.... He seems to delight in the tortures of the wretched, and to be more deserving of hatred than of love. If by any effort of reason I could conceive how God, who shows so much anger and iniquity, could be merciful and just, there would be no need of faith," [18]

It didn't get any better with Luther's successor John Calvin, a Frenchman, whose mother had died during his infancy. Like Luther,

Calvin believed that humans were a sorry, sinful lot, with women at the bottom of the heap. He ordered church elders to spy on families and denounced all dancing, singing, playing cards, or boisterous behavior. Sex before marriage resulted in death, and his own stepson and daughter-in-law were executed, along with their lovers. Any single woman found pregnant was instantly drowned. Even a child was beheaded for striking his parents.[19] Since Luther had proved that print was such a powerful medium, Calvin's regime controlled the press, with any criticism punishable by death.

Meanwhile, as the Italian Renaissance came to an end, the Spanish Inquisition continued to torture and murder thousands of victims. By 1570 it had established independent tribunals as far away as Peru, Mexico, and Goa, India.[20] But punishment for mere heresy wasn't enough to demonstrate religious purity. In Spain, just as Columbus was discovering the New World, King Ferdinand and Queen Isabella launched a vicious campaign forcing first Jews and then Muslims into exile, killing those who resisted by the thousands. Pope Innocent VIII declared in 1484 that witchcraft was a central threat to the Christian world. While advancing the fortunes of his sixteen children, he commissioned the creation of a manual for eradicating witches, called the *Malleus Maleficarum*. Aided by the invention of the printing press, this heinous torture manual spread rapidly throughout Europe, fueling an epidemic of insanity whose cruelty knew no bounds. Hundreds of thousands of women—and many men—were tortured, hanged, or burned. Children could be flogged while being forced to watch their mothers go up in flames. Though the worship of Mary had risen and fallen over the centuries, Protestants entirely dismissed her. In one of the torture devices invented by the inquisitors, was a statue of Mary from which protruded sharp knives and nails.[21]

If this was not enough to turn the Great Mother into a wild beast, Christianity changed the ancient, goat-footed god, Pan, into an image of the devil. Just as Pan's life-giving meaning was distorted to represent something contrary to life, the devil was equated with everything that was opposite to Christianity. He was believed to work his evil by reversing all values. Thus the devil could be summoned by saying the Lord's Prayer backwards: worshippers of the devil were said to fly, or stand on their heads. Women, in particular, were accused of cavorting with the devil. Under pain of torture, they even fabricated confessions to that effect. All that was magical, mythical, or connected with Nature was associated with witchcraft, until it became a heresy *not* to believe in the evil deeds and presence of witches.

As religion took on the exacting task of subjecting divine spirit to the rigor of the written word, the scientific community was making provable discoveries that contradicted those very words. Christianity and science diverged. Monotheistic religion, initially born of Static Masculine rationality, stuck fast to its irrational behavior, claiming sole jurisdiction over the realm of spirit. Science found its viability in logic and rationality, and claimed jurisdiction over the realm of matter. They could only get along if they each stuck to their own territory, and left the other alone.

And so the material world, once the divine realm of the Great Mother, having been denigrated as evil and separated from spirit, was now completely inanimate, a lifeless demonstration of laws and principles to be inspected and dissected, used and abused, by the rational but dissociated intellect. The gap between Nature and the spirit of "mankind," that began to diverge when we first walled our cities, had grown to a complete separation. Into this abyss stepped the rational world of science.

ESSENTIAL POINTS

• Christianity entered a dark time in which heresy was punishable by death.

• Spirituality was expressed through obedience to authority.

• The Middle Ages had very little innovation and few intellectual breakthroughs. The Renaissance was the first period to name its own awakening.

• The Reformation began as a protest against the Catholic Church but became ever more authoritarian in its interpretation of doctrine.

• Hundreds of thousands, if not millions, died in the name of the Christian God through the combined results of the Crusades, and the Papal and Spanish Inquisitions. This frightening irrationality set the stage for science to claim the next period of awakening.

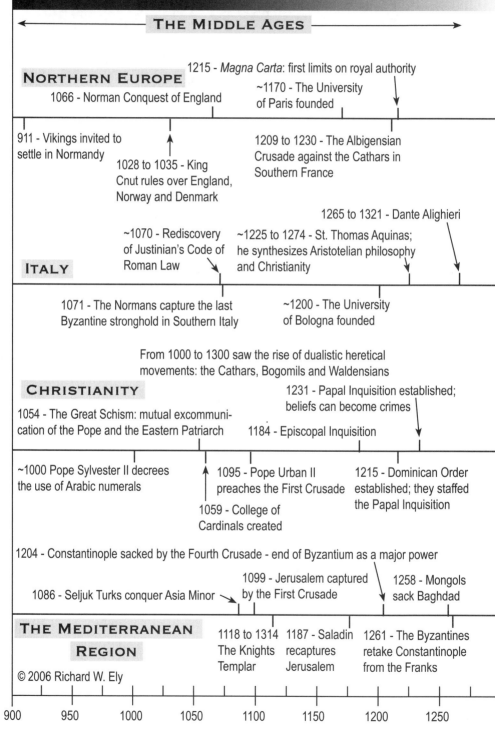

TIME CHART 7 - THE MIDDLE AGES
TO THE PROTESTANT REFORMATION

THE MIDDLE AGES

NORTHERN EUROPE

1215 - *Magna Carta*: first limits on royal authority

~1170 - The University of Paris founded

1066 - Norman Conquest of England

911 - Vikings invited to settle in Normandy

1028 to 1035 - King Cnut rules over England, Norway and Denmark

1209 to 1230 - The Albigensian Crusade against the Cathars in Southern France

1265 to 1321 - Dante Alighieri

~1070 - Rediscovery of Justinian's Code of Roman Law

~1225 to 1274 - St. Thomas Aquinas; he synthesizes Aristotelian philosophy and Christianity

ITALY

1071 - The Normans capture the last Byzantine stronghold in Southern Italy

~1200 - The University of Bologna founded

From 1000 to 1300 saw the rise of dualistic heretical movements: the Cathars, Bogomils and Waldensians

CHRISTIANITY

1231 - Papal Inquisition established; beliefs can become crimes

1054 - The Great Schism: mutual excommunication of the Pope and the Eastern Patriarch

1184 - Episcopal Inquisition

~1000 Pope Sylvester II decrees the use of Arabic numerals

1095 - Pope Urban II preaches the First Crusade

1215 - Dominican Order established; they staffed the Papal Inquisition

1059 - College of Cardinals created

1204 - Constantinople sacked by the Fourth Crusade - end of Byzantium as a major power

1099 - Jerusalem captured by the First Crusade

1258 - Mongols sack Baghdad

1086 - Seljuk Turks conquer Asia Minor

THE MEDITERRANEAN
REGION

1118 to 1314 The Knights Templar

1187 - Saladin recaptures Jerusalem

1261 - The Byzantines retake Constantinople from the Franks

© 2006 Richard W. Ely

900   950   1000   1050   1100   1150   1200   1250

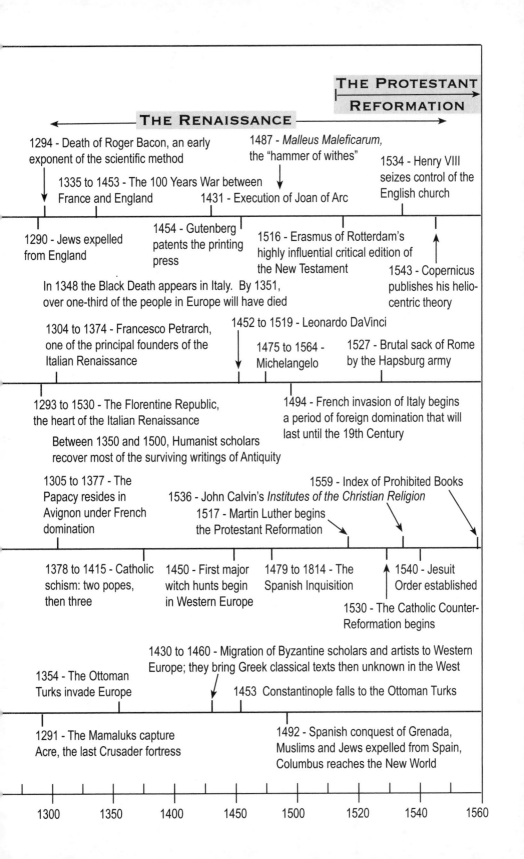

THE PROTESTANT REFORMATION

THE RENAISSANCE

1294 - Death of Roger Bacon, an early exponent of the scientific method

1487 - *Malleus Maleficarum,* the "hammer of withes"

1534 - Henry VIII seizes control of the English church

1335 to 1453 - The 100 Years War between France and England

1431 - Execution of Joan of Arc

1290 - Jews expelled from England

1454 - Gutenberg patents the printing press

1516 - Erasmus of Rotterdam's highly influential critical edition of the New Testament

1543 - Copernicus publishes his helio-centric theory

In 1348 the Black Death appears in Italy. By 1351, over one-third of the people in Europe will have died

1304 to 1374 - Francesco Petrarch, one of the principal founders of the Italian Renaissance

1452 to 1519 - Leonardo DaVinci

1475 to 1564 - Michelangelo

1527 - Brutal sack of Rome by the Hapsburg army

1293 to 1530 - The Florentine Republic, the heart of the Italian Renaissance

1494 - French invasion of Italy begins a period of foreign domination that will last until the 19th Century

Between 1350 and 1500, Humanist scholars recover most of the surviving writings of Antiquity

1305 to 1377 - The Papacy resides in Avignon under French domination

1559 - Index of Prohibited Books

1536 - John Calvin's *Institutes of the Christian Religion*

1517 - Martin Luther begins the Protestant Reformation

1378 to 1415 - Catholic schism: two popes, then three

1450 - First major witch hunts begin in Western Europe

1479 to 1814 - The Spanish Inquisition

1540 - Jesuit Order established

1530 - The Catholic Counter-Reformation begins

1430 to 1460 - Migration of Byzantine scholars and artists to Western Europe; they bring Greek classical texts then unknown in the West

1354 - The Ottoman Turks invade Europe

1453 Constantinople falls to the Ottoman Turks

1291 - The Mamaluks capture Acre, the last Crusader fortress

1492 - Spanish conquest of Grenada, Muslims and Jews expelled from Spain, Columbus reaches the New World

1300   1350   1400   1450   1500   1520   1540   1560

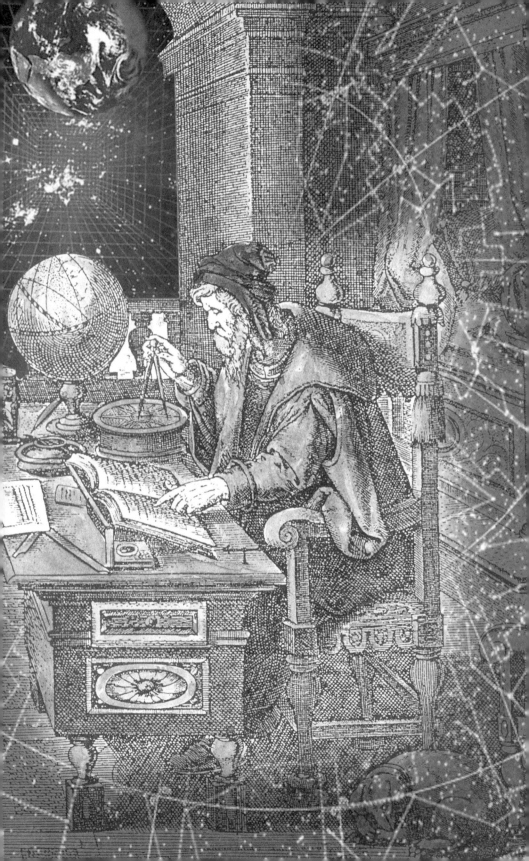

FROM FAITH TO REASON

The Enlightenment

> *I admit nothing as true of them that is not deduced, with the clarity of a mathematical demonstration, from common notions whose truth we cannot doubt. Because all the phenomena of nature can be explained in this way, I think that no other principles of physics need be admitted, nor are to be desired.*

—Rene Descartes

New ideas, by necessity, emerge from the ground of their particular era. Like flowers in a garden, each one blossoms with a different face, yet they sprout from a common soil, washed down by the streams of time. Each idea grows from the foundation of knowledge composted by the life of earlier ideas. And like flowers, ideas need the appropriate season and climate in order to blossom.

We have seen how Christianity was a heart-based idea born in the soil of a "power over" paradigm. The imperialism of the Roman Empire and the internal wars against our own nature thoroughly trampled the mythic ground of preceding eras. Christ's seeds of love and acceptance were carried on the winds of a patriarchal mindset that demonized Nature, sexuality, the body, and women. The brief awakening of the Renaissance was crushed, though not without considerably warming the intellectual climate through the rise of literacy and the recovery of ancient texts. The spiritual climate, however, fell into a restless darkness, waiting for a new dawn.

The insanity of the Inquisition and the Catholic-Protestant wars left a cold chill on the world. People were fearful and subdued, terrorized into docile obedience. At a time that would correspond to our cultural pre-pubescence, rebelliousness was thoroughly quelled. Questioning was dangerous. Students learned their lessons well: work hard; keep in line; believe what you're told. Women were especially subdued. They knew their place—obeying their husbands, raising their children, keeping quiet—with eyes downturned and bodies well covered. Men were dissociated from their feelings, and dared not express their individuality.

Yet, there was a payoff. With the wildness of human passions somewhat tamed, life proceeded more predictably. As cultural children, we were growing up. We were well-behaved and properly socialized; we knew our roles and played them dutifully. We had mastered both the instincts of survival and the demands of procreation—the first two chakras. Power was slowly trickling down to the commoner but was still held firmly by those best adapted to maintaining the status quo.

It was out of this climate, deeply frozen in the feeling function, with a ground well weeded of feminine influence, that the shoots of the Scientific Revolution began to sprout. At the height of the witch burnings—an irrational collective psychosis if ever there was one—science offered a sane alternative: rational, empirical study, focused on predictable, inanimate objects. With Christianity monopolizing the realm of spirit, the world of matter lay rejected—evil at its roots, inconsequential at best. From this dissociated state the human mind was able to examine matter without reverence—as an inanimate thing, devoid of spirit. The Earth Mother had long been removed from the center of focus. This gave us enough separation from Nature to regard her objectively, and to see her components as a series of objects.

The Earth Mother had been replaced by the Sky Father. As if in parallel, Copernicus suggested that the Earth was not the center of the cosmos, but actually orbited the sun—a revolutionary idea in every sense of the word! From his first realization in 1514 at the height of the Renaissance, it would still be twenty years before he dared share it with the Pope (who initially approved of his research). Reluctant to publish his findings in a climate dangerous to heretical ideas, Copernicus waited until the end of his life to make public his research. He held his published manuscript in his hand for the first time just one day before he died in 1543.[1] His ideas, however, did not die, but continued to push against the vehement repression of reason. (Luther had called reason the greatest enemy to faith, the Devil's greatest whore.[2])

Copernicus was not alone in his belief, nor was he the only one to fear persecution. Half a century later, in 1600, Giordano Bruno was executed by the Inquisition. One of his crimes was daring to agree with Copernicus. But truth cannot be hidden forever. When Galileo saw the same thing through his telescope, ten years after that, it would seem that the proper order of the heavens was obvious. Yet even Galileo, who enjoyed great respect for his scientific observations and mathematical scholarship, faced persecution for his findings. At the ripe age of seventy, while in poor health, he was abducted from his home, taken to Rome, and forced to recant his views before a Catholic tribunal. In an attempt to keep his views quiet, he was confined to house arrest for the last eight years of his life. His book, *The Dialogue of the Two Chief Systems of the World (1632),* remained on the Church's Index of Prohibited Books as late as 1835.[3]

Still, there were many who had looked through Galileo's telescope. When Kepler published his laws of planetary motion in 1609, the idea of a mathematically sensible movement of heavenly bodies fell into place. The Catholic hierarchy, knowing the truth, chose to support scripture instead. In doing so, they froze the budding flower of heliocentric theory and seriously undermined their intellectual credibility. As time passed and the enlightened view of the solar system became more widely accepted, a dividing line was crossed. The church lost respect and science gained it. Faith and fact diverged.

Yet the precision with which the heavenly bodies moved through the cosmos was seen by most as proof of God's perfection. How else could something be so exquisitely designed? As explanation replaced mystery, God's role in influencing the present was diminished.

God was now seen as a distant father, a divine architect, who had designed the universe, then abandoned the kids to raise themselves. Divinity was no longer obtained through faith or deeds but, like a carrot dangling before our eyes, it just might be found through scientific discovery. By cracking the codes of creation, we, too, could approach godhood. Excitement grew with each mystery solved. The world became rational, explainable, and potentially controllable. Discovering the secrets of matter held a glimmering possibility of regaining our power. As science became the new religion, scientists became the new priests.

Among them was Francis Bacon, often touted as the founding father of modern science for his establishment of the "scientific method." In 1597, while the men of his time were torturing witches for their devilish secrets, Bacon suggested that the scientist needed to "torture nature's secrets from her."[4] Nature was a "she" who should be "constrained," made a "slave" and "forced out of her natural state" so that "human knowledge and human power meet as one."[5] In graphic sexual symbolism, Bacon wrote that Nature's "holes and corners were to be entered and penetrated."[6] He described this new method of inquiry as a "masculine birth," one that would bring forth a blessed race of heroes and supermen. Man's role was to have dominion over the natural world, and scientific knowledge was the means. He wrote of a technocratic utopia, ruled by a scientific priesthood who would make decisions for the good of the state.[7]

Prior to this, most philosophical inquiry had examined either the realms of spirit—an invisible force that could be known only through faith or subjective experience—or the realm of matter; the visible, inanimate world, understandable through rational inquiry and objective experience.[8] It wasn't until Rene Descartes' revelation of *cogito ergo sum,* "I think, therefore I am," that science began to consider the *source* of our questioning—*consciousness itself.* Though sages of the East had been talking about consciousness for thousands of years, Rene Descartes popularized the notion that a thinking "I" exists within each one of us.

Doubt, the Zoroastrian evil twin from two millennia earlier,[9] was now the gateway from which Descartes' thinking emerged. He alone seemed able to separate his belief systems from his cultural milieu. He realized that if he'd been raised Muslim or Jewish, he might not have believed as a Christian, raising doubt as to the ultimate truth of Christianity or any other worldview. Doubting everything he could possibly contemplate, he finally realized that the only thing of which he could be absolutely certain was that there existed within him an aware, thinking consciousness that was capable of doubting. Even the body could be an illusion, he thought. Only the fact of his thinking was indelible proof of his existence.

Descartes' ideas grew from the ground of a good Jesuit education, where he was renowned for his brilliance in mathematics. The flower of his thought was that the universe and the human body were devices that operated mechanically. Consciousness was the ghost in the machine, much like the driver in a car today. *Mind and body were completely separate.* He states: "there is nothing included in the concept of body that belongs to the mind; and nothing in that of mind that belongs to the body."[10] Like Bacon, Descartes believed that the aim of science was the domination and control of nature—plants and animals being simply machines without soul or spirit. He promoted the notion that Nature was a mechanical system whose language was mathematics, precise and logical.

Descartes considered this to be a divine revelation, one that could promise certainty in an uncertain world. Cartesian rationalism considerably cooled the fires of the witch burnings, for if spirit and matter were separate realms, then how could someone's thoughts make the crops fail? As rationalism slowly began to replace superstition (at least among the elite classes), the human experiment took a giant step forward. The sprouts of reason were growing into a sturdy tree.

By the time Sir Isaac Newton's apple had fallen into this mathematical garden, the gravitational force beneath the ground of science had congealed into a paradigm that concretized the static masculine separation of spirit and matter, Heaven and Earth, mind and body. Gravity was the force that moved the worlds. Newton's discoveries were hailed as the enlightened triumph of reason over medieval ignorance. Following Newton's publication of the *Principia* in 1687, the enlightened view was that the universe was made of material particles that moved according to mathematically predictable laws and principles. It was a purely mechancial system. That which could not be seen or measured was given little, if any importance. Though Newton had been a deeply religious man, his theories explained much that had been attributed to God and furthered the eventual separation of science and religion. This view dominated scientific inquiry for the ensuing three hundred years.

These ideas made fertile the garden of the eighteenth century Enlightenment. An explosion of understanding lifted us out of the Dark Ages of superstition, persecution, and church hegemony, and into a period bursting with information and understanding. It took power out of the heavens and brought it down to "man." Long-held mysteries were solved, with a promise of increasing freedom for all. We can imagine the relief and appeal that such rationalism would have, given the history that prededed it.

If Descartes was the person most remembered in the West for acknowledging consciousness as a viable entity, it was Charles Darwin who popularized the concept of evolutionary thinking. With *Origin of Species* (1859), he examined the way natural selection demonstrated an evolutionary process. To Darwin, evolution happened by chance and necessity, rather than by external design on the part of a divine architect. Such a view further undermined the belief in God as the noble creator. Simultaneously, the elite view of humans as the pinnacle of creation was deflated by the revelation that we were just another animal crawling our way up the food chain. The divine, within and without, took another step backward.

Darwin's theories of natural selection, however, were interpreted through the third chakra dynamics of struggle and competition, leaving us with a legacy of the idea of "survival of the fittest." A closer reading of his texts reveals that he spoke far more often of such things as love and cooperation as important evolutionary forces, and that it was actually Herbert Spencer who coined the term "survival of the fittest."[11] David Loye, a noted scientist and evolutionary theorist, actually did a word count on Darwin's 900 page original manuscript (*Descent of Man,* 1871) and discovered, to his amazement, that "survival of the fittest" only occurred twice in the entire text, and the second time was as an apology for exaggerating its importance! [12] "Competition" was only mentioned nine times, "selfishness," twelve times. By contrast, he spoke of love, mind, and brain nearly one hundred times each, with additional emphasis on consciousness, intellect, higher morality, and imagination. While Darwin's theories have been taught to school-age children the world round, his emphasis on love, conscience, and moral agency has been pointedly overlooked. The aggressive and dominating values of the time ignored these aspects of his theory for the ensuing century.

Darwin's theories had far-reaching implications for the shaping of society. On the one hand he dealt another blow to Biblical authority by suggesting (as geologists had done previously) that the Earth was indeed far older than had previously been imagined—far too old and complex to have been created in merely six days. He also demonstrated the paradox that dynamic change was the enduring principle of creation, challenging the previous view of a fixed and unchanging reality. Despite ample proof, his theories of evolution were still banned as late as 1951 by the Catholics and 1967 by some Protestants. [13] With the debate over Intelligent Design today, the battle to teach the science of evolution in our school systems is still being hotly challenged by some Christian conservatives.

Secondly, the idea of natural selection through competition contributed to an egocentricity that gave every man permission to serve himself above all others. Otto Amman, in 1911, said, "Bravery, cunning and competition are virtues. Darwin must become the new religion of Germany," [14] a view that contributed to the rise of Nazism. In the U.S., William Graham Sumner, a political and social science professor at Yale, taught that, "Millionaires are a product of natural selection. Let it be understood that we cannot go outside this alternative: liberty, inequality, survival of the fittest, not liberty, equality, survival of the unfittest." [15] This brick has been a building block in justifying corporate greed and neo-conservative politics.

But surely we run ahead of ourselves. For the fruits of the Enlightenment gave us not only a rational understanding of the world around us, but also a cascade of inventions and discoveries that liberated us from the rigors of survival. Life improved in essential ways. Through the microscope we discovered bacteria, and learned to use sanitation to prevent disease. Along with better nutrition, this increased life span. Machines extended the power of the human body and reduced our dependence on servants and slaves. With great reluctance, the captains of industry distributed more income to the average man, enlarging the middle class. Power was slowly trickling down to the masses.

By the time the steam engines of the Industrial Revolution began spewing carbon into the air, the mechanical worldview was mechanizing our lives, using machines to fertilize the fields, pave the roads, harvest the forests, and to make more machinery. Consumption of resources amplified exponentially, along with population. The relationship of man and machine surpassed our relationships with God, with Nature, and with each other. This was called progress.

And indeed it was. The standard of living rose dramatically for most of the Western world in the latter half of the nineteenth century. The promise of a better life made by religion was actually delivered by industrialism. No longer did the common people live in dirt hovels. Mass production distributed food and goods far and wide. We could travel by rail and see more of the world. We may have had to slave away in a factory to pay for our homes, but their privacy allowed insulation from the harsh world we were creating, and offered us more privacy from each other. We continually sought to improve our private world with furnishings. A previously missing, but essential element of the third chakra began to develop—*the sovereignty of the individual.*

CREEPING INDIVIDUALISM

Today, we take for granted the idea that each person is an individual, but this was not always so. If we backtrack to Hellenic Greece, we find that a person who kept to himself and did not particpate in the democracy of the *polis* was called an *idiotes,* from which we get our word for idiot. Jeremy Rifkin, in *Biosphere Politics,* describes how the idea of an individual self was not even well developed in the Middle Ages, where a man who wandered by himself was considered effeminate at best, or more often, insane and ridiculed. Communal living was the norm—among the better off, extended families, servants, even animals all shared a single dwelling with a great hall. Those with less means lived in one-room houses, where three generations might sleep in one bed. As the economics of communal living shifted towards a paycheck for individual workers, privacy became a privilege of wealth and a new ideal to attain. Though the gap between rich and poor has always been present, the rich were now able to withdraw further from society into their own enclaves, set apart from the masses. They became even more removed from the rest of society.

The walls that first defended our cities in ancient times, then enclosed us in great halls in the Middle Ages, by the nineteenth century surrounded each family unit, with further walls for individual bedrooms. Rifkin goes on to describe how the increasing privatization led to shame. The Protestants had put an end to public baths, and bodily functions were increasingly hidden from view. Sex, bathing, elimination, and sleeping became increasingly private affairs.

With an increasingly impersonal universe that resulted from a mechanical world view, an industrial lifestyle, and a social world walled off from Nature, each other, and our own natural instincts, it is no surprise that by 1888, Nietzsche, while singing praises to the power of individual will, could make the fateful proclamation that "God is dead." Faith in the church had waned; spirituality was at an all-time low; the world around us deemed lifeless and mechanical. The Goddess had long been forgotten. We had become spiritual orphans, lost from our mythic ground, abandoned by both Mother and Father, hungry for a new spiritual home.

MATTER AND SPIRIT

From the eighteenth to the twentieth century, materialism gradually took over as the new creed, back with a vengeance from its rejection by Christianity. Scientific materialism asserted that only matter and energy are real. Consciousness, spirit, soul, and all non-physical qualities were exiled from legitimate study because they could not be objectively measured. Objectivity became more important than subjectivity. The world was regarded as an "it" to be manipulated and used for our own purposes.

Materialism, however, hearkens back to our original thesis, of matter as the primal ground, the basic matrix, as the word itself derives from *mater* or mother. Similarly, the words *nature* and *physical* both come from words that connote birth. The Latin *natura* has the same root as natal, meaning birth. The Greek word *phusis* means nature and its root *phu* has a primary meaning connected with birth.[16] In veiled form, whispers of the divine feminine realm were returning. In 1854, the Catholic Church had decided that Mary, like her son Jesus, was a product of immaculate conception. Since original sin was passed through semen, she was declared free of sin, and could therefore be worshipped again.[17]

As the trauma of the Burning Times retreated into the past, women felt safer to express their opinions, and the first shoots of feminism began to sprout, even as those sprouts were often crushed. In 1848 the first women's convention was held at Seneca Falls, New York, inspired by the rejection of women delegates to an anti-slavery convention in London. With little promotion and only a few days planning, three hundred women and forty men drew up a "Declaration of Sentiments" in which eighteen "injuries and usurpations" were listed. In 1869, John Stuart Mill called upon men to end "the legal subordination of one sex by another."[18] Three years later, Susan B. Anthony pulled the lever in a voting booth, believing that she would survive her subsequent arrest and conviction on the grounds that she met the fourteenth amendment's qualification for "person." (She lost her case.) By 1920, when women finally won the right to vote, only one woman from the Seneca Falls conference (Charlotte Woodward, a worker in a glove factory) had lived long enough to do so. Feminist writers entered the public discourse: Mary Wollstonecraft, Elizabeth Cady Stanton, Phyllis Wheatley (an emancipated slave), and Judith Sargeant Murray.

The repressed pole of Nature, passion, creativity, and imagination sprang back to life. Masculine and feminine values began to dance with each other again. Thinkers of the time divided into two camps: those who modeled reality with objective masculine logic (e.g. Kant, Hume, and Locke), and the Romantics, who reveled in Nature and the more feminine aspects of beauty and subjectivity (such as Rousseau, Goethe, and the poets, Byron, Keats, Shelley, and Blake). Whereas the scientists saw the world of Nature as devoid of spirit, the Romantics experienced Nature as infused with spirit. While the scientists measured and recorded all aspects of the outer world, the Romantics turned their intention to the inner world. The scientists projected onto the future, with an unstoppable idealism; the Romantics resisted modernity, fearing its estrangement, hearkening back to simpler principles. Each stream had its own validity.

As energy oscillated between these two philosophical poles, the technological world harnessed polarity in the form of electricity. We had not yet resolved the heart, but we were developing the cultural fifth chakra by the first means of electronic communication. By 1844, we could send messages by telegraph, opening the field of fast, long-distance communication—the first major leap in communication since the printing press in 1454. By 1880, four years after its invention, there were 54,000 customers with telephones.[19] By 1901 we bridged the Atlantic by radio, and by 1920 we were playing records and going to the movies. Even as we were courting our individuality, the interconnected networks were weaving a collective web, giving birth to new possibilities. The curve of discoveries was accelerating.

In our modern world, it is hard to imagine—save for an occasional power failure—the monumental triumph of the light bulb. Though we had means of transcending distance through travel and the telegraph, it wasn't until New Year's Day, 1879, that Thomas Edison engineered the first commercially viable light bulb. (Interestingly, he was a man who didn't like to sleep at night, but only periodically catnapped.) The world was electrified and illuminated. Primordial darkness took a giant step backwards. The third chakra harnessing of electromagnetic forces had opened the realms of fifth and sixth chakras, (related to the elements sound and light) enabling telegraph, telephone, radio, and motion pictures.

It wasn't long before science moved from the examination of forces to the examination of relationships. After Einstein's theories of special relativity (1905), neither science nor the Bible could claim an absolute point of view. Energy was not separate from matter; they existed on a continuum, as aspects of the same thing, symbolized by Einstein's famous equation ($E = MC2$).

With discoveries in quantum mechanics, we looked into smaller and smaller increments of matter, and discovered that subatomic particles move backward and forward in time, joining space and time in yet another continuum. Certainty became ambiguous as we discovered that photons and electrons behaved both like particles and waves. Material substance started to look more like empty space. We discovered that the observer influenced the experiment. The collapsed dimension of spacetime appeared more relative than absolute. The Static Masculine paradigm was losing its rigidity, no longer able to rely on predictability and certainty.

Meanwhile, as the positive and negative poles of electricity illuminated homes and ran factories, the budding science of psychology discovered the rejected pole of our psyche. Freud and Jung turned a focused eye onto the unconscious and the realm of the shadow. While Freud wasn't the first to talk about the unconscious (Romantics such as Goethe and Schiller had named the unconscious as a source of creativity), he was the first to explore this mysterious realm with rational analysis. If we had become divided selves, Freud gave voice to these divisions and named them. The id and the superego represented the disparate worlds of our biological instincts and intellectual conscience. The ego, as mediator between the two, was seen as the triumph of awakening from the insatiable jaws of the Dark Mother. Only the aware ego could rescue the vital energy from the realms of the unconscious, and only the superego could balance its dangerous contents.

The discovery of the unconscious was the uncovering the elements of the lower chakras: bodily instincts, sexual urges, and emotional traumas. They were contained or repressed by intricate walls erected within our psyches, called defenses, much like the walls around cities had been erected for defensive purposes, so long ago. We found common patterns in these psychological defenses and began to name them: repression, denial, projection, reaction formation, sublimation, displacement, regression, and dissociation. All were patterns by which the ego kept unwelcome material out of awareness.

The ego became the leading element of the psyche. Like a young shoot, it needed much coddling and encouragement. Psychoanalysis gave it that attention. People began to examine themselves, and reflect on their behavior, motivations, dreams and fantasies–some would say to the point of excessive self-absorption. Most important, people were awakening to a deeply interior "I." It became socially acceptable, even laudable, to make the most of that "I," to better oneself, to become rich, beautiful, accomplished, recognized, or admired–a privilege that had previously been limited to the elite. The ego now awakened among the masses.

With this awakening of the interior "I" came a quest for individual rights. Workers joined unions to fight for their rights. Women fought for the right to vote. Native Americans were given citizenship. We began to see that all sorts of subclasses, previously ignored, needed protection of their rights. As we moved into the 1960s, this blossomed into civil rights, women's rights, children's rights, gay rights, animal rights, and environmental rights.

Could it be that one must awaken the "I" in order to have a "we"? Could it be that we need to be in touch with our own pain and inner defenses to understand the defenses of others and make compassionate contact? Could it be that we had to establish the ego, find our own will, autonomy, and power, before we could voluntarily surrender to another? I believe this is an essential step in development, the reason why the third chakra precedes the fourth: we must find our autonomy before we can truly love.

Yet the ego is its own trap. It, too, can be insatiable, inflating itself to godlike proportions in order to maintain its illusion of power and separateness. While we think it took prodigious effort to break the hold of the sleepy unconscious and escape the jaws of the primal Mother, we may find it takes even greater strength to escape the constant demands of the ego. These demands consume both the psyche and its environment in quests for larger houses, more clothing, more money, and more power. They keep us isolated, alienated, and exhausted.

It was necessary to develop an ego in order to transcend it. We needed to discover the interior self to know that such a self existed in others. We needed the power to determine our own lives before we could use that power in service of something larger. We needed to learn separation before we could fully create union. The ego leads us toward awakening, yet can also stand as a barrier. It is the vehicle that drives the journey, but if we never get out of the vehicle, we never truly arrive at our destination.

Like every age, the scientific revolution generated both blessings and curses. We put an end to the witch burnings, but later dropped the atom bomb. We solved many of nature's mysteries, yet plundered her resources. We extended life-span through medical advances, yet created carcinogenic environments and spread diseases around the globe. We studied and categorized every conceivable life-form, yet we rendered a good portion of them extinct. We raised the standard of living with electric lights, refrigerators, automobiles, telephones, stereos, radios, televisions, cameras, computers, and countless other devices. Yet the creation of these products pollutes the air, water, and earth, while enslaving those who build them to the drudgery of factory assembly lines. We have created transportation that allows us to see the wonders of the world, yet the burning of fossil fuels is altering the climate.

The advances have been staggering. A little over five hundred years ago, Europe had just discovered North America. Now we can fly to the moon and beyond, and see pictures of the Earth hanging in space. Prior to the printing press, few people could read or even had access to books; now we have the Internet. In the Middle Ages, thousands of people died from the practice of bleeding, now we can transplant hearts and reattach limbs. In the First World, at least, we've abolished slavery and instituted democracy. Ken Wilber refers to these aspects as the "dignity of modernity."[20]

The trouble is, we have lost our ground in the process–the ground of the Earth, our bodies and our souls. We have gained privacy but lost community. We have transcended the limits of Nature, yet lost the experience of her majesty. We have risen above superstition, but the Goddess is forgotten and God is proclaimed dead. Many live mechanical lives, out of touch with the inner world of feeling, devoid of meaning. Advertising fills that void, resulting in a consumerism that devours our resources faster than they can be replaced. Like adolescents, we have more power than wisdom. We live for the moment at the cost of the future. The ability to differentiate from Nature and our inner world has brought us to a cultural dissociation, or as Wilber puts it, the "disaster of modernity."[21]

It is possible that the excesses of modernity can be addressed, and the blessings still harvested. We can reclaim what we have lost without denying what we have gained–*if, and only if*, we face the adolescent challenge of stabilizing our adult size as a population, and learn to grow spiritually, instead of physically. The great thrust of physical progress must now explore the frontiers of consciousness, and find mature relationships through the heart.

We have experienced the organic stability of the Static Feminine, the dominating upheaval of the Dynamic Masculine, and the restabilizing rationality of the Static Masculine. The Great Mother with her son-lover has been matched by the Great Father and his daughter-wife. To reach adulthood and enter egalitarian relationships, each gender has had to emancipate itself from the parental projection that results in domination by the Sacred Other. The masculine overthrew the Great Mother long, long ago. But the liberation of the repressed feminine is still relatively new. There is one more archetypal pattern that needs to be embraced in order to embrace the full quaternity and reach the heart: the dance of the Dynamic Feminine.

ESSENTIAL POINTS

• The rational discoveries of science slowly broke the hold of the Christian church on the European mind.

• Science and religion each claimed separate territory: science took the realm of matter; religion, the realm of spirit.

• The industrial revolution brought a rise in the standard of living and a mechanization of society.

• Technologies of electromagnetism created communication possibilities that began to unite people across distances.

• The repressed realm of the unconscious was examined by the psychologies of Freud and Jung, giving rise to the interior world of the individual.

TIME CHART 8 - SCIENCE AND INDUSTRY

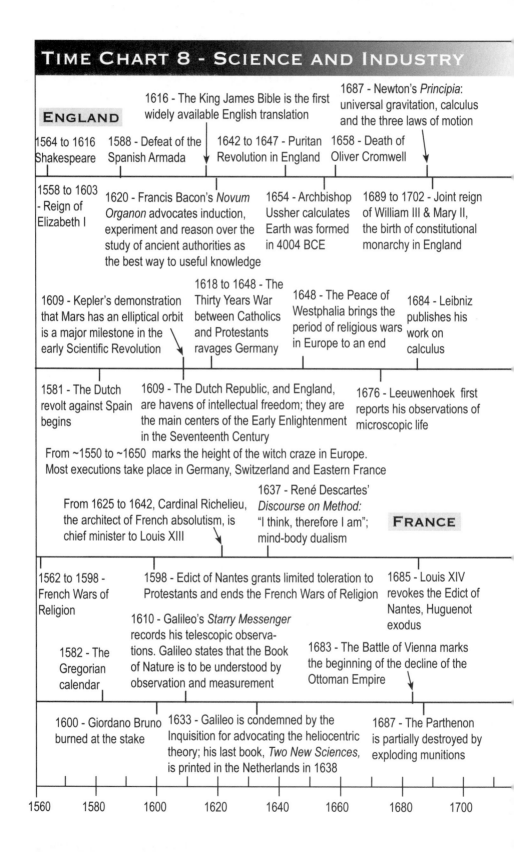

ENGLAND

1616 - The King James Bible is the first widely available English translation

1687 - Newton's *Principia*: universal gravitation, calculus and the three laws of motion

1564 to 1616 Shakespeare

1588 - Defeat of the Spanish Armada

1642 to 1647 - Puritan Revolution in England

1658 - Death of Oliver Cromwell

1558 to 1603 - Reign of Elizabeth I

1620 - Francis Bacon's *Novum Organon* advocates induction, experiment and reason over the study of ancient authorities as the best way to useful knowledge

1654 - Archbishop Ussher calculates Earth was formed in 4004 BCE

1689 to 1702 - Joint reign of William III & Mary II, the birth of constitutional monarchy in England

1609 - Kepler's demonstration that Mars has an elliptical orbit is a major milestone in the early Scientific Revolution

1618 to 1648 - The Thirty Years War between Catholics and Protestants ravages Germany

1648 - The Peace of Westphalia brings the period of religious wars in Europe to an end

1684 - Leibniz publishes his work on calculus

1581 - The Dutch revolt against Spain begins

1609 - The Dutch Republic, and England, are havens of intellectual freedom; they are the main centers of the Early Enlightenment in the Seventeenth Century

1676 - Leeuwenhoek first reports his observations of microscopic life

From ~1550 to ~1650 marks the height of the witch craze in Europe. Most executions take place in Germany, Switzerland and Eastern France

From 1625 to 1642, Cardinal Richelieu, the architect of French absolutism, is chief minister to Louis XIII

1637 - René Descartes' *Discourse on Method:* "I think, therefore I am"; mind-body dualism

FRANCE

1562 to 1598 - French Wars of Religion

1598 - Edict of Nantes grants limited toleration to Protestants and ends the French Wars of Religion

1685 - Louis XIV revokes the Edict of Nantes, Huguenot exodus

1582 - The Gregorian calendar

1610 - Galileo's *Starry Messenger* records his telescopic observations. Galileo states that the Book of Nature is to be understood by observation and measurement

1683 - The Battle of Vienna marks the beginning of the decline of the Ottoman Empire

1600 - Giordano Bruno burned at the stake

1633 - Galileo is condemned by the Inquisition for advocating the heliocentric theory; his last book, *Two New Sciences,* is printed in the Netherlands in 1638

1687 - The Parthenon is partially destroyed by exploding munitions

1560   1580   1600   1620   1640   1660   1680   1700

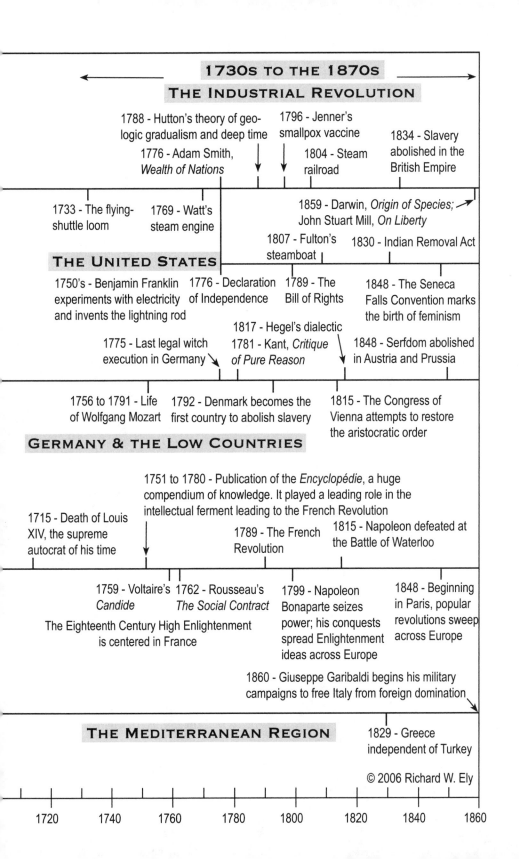

1730s TO THE 1870s

THE INDUSTRIAL REVOLUTION

1788 - Hutton's theory of geologic gradualism and deep time

1776 - Adam Smith,
Wealth of Nations

1796 - Jenner's
smallpox vaccine

1804 - Steam
railroad

1834 - Slavery
abolished in the
British Empire

1733 - The flying-
shuttle loom

1769 - Watt's
steam engine

1859 - Darwin, *Origin of Species;*
John Stuart Mill, *On Liberty*

1807 - Fulton's
steamboat

1830 - Indian Removal Act

THE UNITED STATES

1750's - Benjamin Franklin
experiments with electricity
and invents the lightning rod

1776 - Declaration
of Independence

1789 - The
Bill of Rights

1848 - The Seneca
Falls Convention marks
the birth of feminism

1775 - Last legal witch
execution in Germany

1817 - Hegel's dialectic

1781 - Kant, *Critique
of Pure Reason*

1848 - Serfdom abolished
in Austria and Prussia

1756 to 1791 - Life
of Wolfgang Mozart

1792 - Denmark becomes the
first country to abolish slavery

1815 - The Congress of
Vienna attempts to restore
the aristocratic order

GERMANY & THE LOW COUNTRIES

1751 to 1780 - Publication of the *Encyclopédie*, a huge
compendium of knowledge. It played a leading role in the
intellectual ferment leading to the French Revolution

1715 - Death of Louis
XIV, the supreme
autocrat of his time

1789 - The French
Revolution

1815 - Napoleon defeated at
the Battle of Waterloo

1759 - Voltaire's
Candide

1762 - Rousseau's
The Social Contract

The Eighteenth Century High Enlightenment
is centered in France

1799 - Napoleon
Bonaparte seizes
power; his conquests
spread Enlightenment
ideas across Europe

1848 - Beginning
in Paris, popular
revolutions sweep
across Europe

1860 - Giuseppe Garibaldi begins his military
campaigns to free Italy from foreign domination

THE MEDITERRANEAN REGION

1829 - Greece
independent of Turkey

© 2006 Richard W. Ely

| 1720 | 1740 | 1760 | 1780 | 1800 | 1820 | 1840 | 1860 |

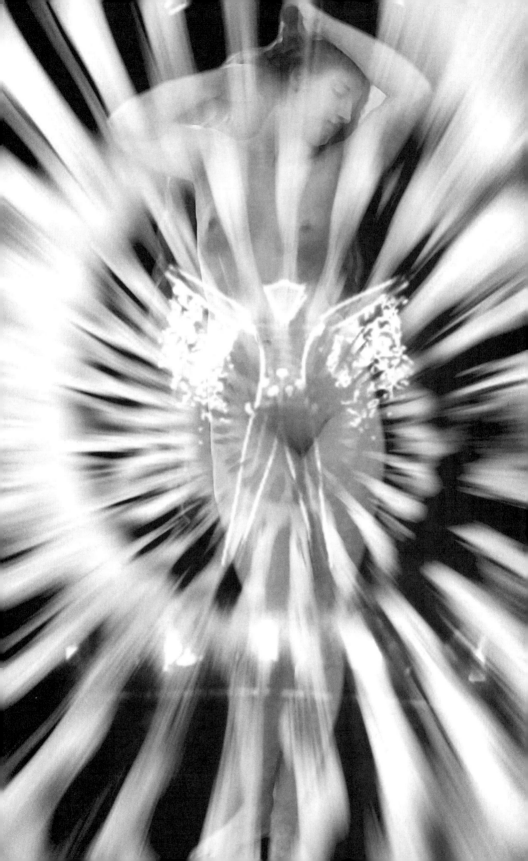

SPIRALING INTO ECSTASY

The Dynamic Feminine

> *In other words, it would appear, as far as the divine is concerned, that we are opening rather than closing, inventing rather than devolving, experimenting and thrusting and whispering new secrets to the moon rather than quivering in the corner, afraid of our own divine shadows, slouching toward death, unaware that our cosmic shoes are untied.*[1]

—Mark Morford

It's hot and dry in the Nevada desert during the last week of August. Like a huge snake, glistening in the sun, vehicles of every size and shape crawl northward from Reno for their annual pilgrimage to the middle of nowhere. They are heavily loaded with rolls of carpets, sofas, generators, people, costumes—and enough food and water for each passenger to survive for a week in extreme heat and cold, dust and wind – all to take part in a collective experiment in alternate reality.

For several days this procession pours its metallic sparkle into Black Rock City, a place that is nothing but empty land eleven months out of the year. Like the mythical story of Brigadoon, the Scottish village of the distant past that came to life once every hundred years, Black Rock City comes to life for *one week* each year, then vanishes into sand and dust immediately after. But where Brigadoon was a land preserved from the distant past, Black Rock City is a wave of the future. Or at least a future that tens of thousands of people believe is possible. And they are willing to put considerable time, money, and effort into proving it.

Black Rock City is a defiance of all probability and a testament to human possibility. That upwards of 35,000 people (as of 2005) can converge peacefully on a few square miles of land that has no roads, grass, trees, water, food, electricity, telephones, cell phone reception, shops, or buildings, and erect an entire city, over three miles wide, for a single week's habitation, is remarkable enough. That this city creates multiple newspapers and radio stations, a functioning postal system, high-tech nightclubs, and theme-based neighborhoods, with more art and entertainment than you could possibly experience in a week if you never slept a wink, is more remarkable still. That this occurs virtually outside the realm of monetary commerce proves that a peaceful, co-creative society that is not based on commercial enterprise can indeed exist–even if only for a week.[2]

Every aspect of this city is creative. Most attendees dress in outrageous costumes, or wear nothing at all, decorating their body with any combination of paint, sunscreen, tattoos, piercings, or scant bits of clothing. Tents, RVs, trucks, vans, and cars make up the neighborhoods, and are equally decorated or disguised. Art cars (sculptures of transportation) provide the only means of public transportation. Individuals walk, ride bicycles, or hitch rides on art cars. While everything that residents need must be transported to and from the site–even water and garbage–some camps have such unlikely features as hot tubs or swimming pools, available to anyone who might happen by with a need to get wet. Others have a dozen full-sized sofas, buildings that are several stories tall, revolving dance halls, geodesic domes, yurts, teepees, and pyramids, all with elaborate high-tech lighting, amplified music, and way-out-of-the-ordinary, interactive experiences.

The high point of the event occurs Saturday night, when a multi-story edifice topped with an eighty-foot wooden man loaded with fireworks is ceremonially burned to the ground. Circling the inferno are some 35,000 people in various states of attire and consciousness, who drum, dance, sing, pray, meditate, or gaze rapturously at the spectacle. Named for this conflagration, the festival is called *Burning Man*.

The express purpose of this event is Art, with a capital A. People come to see, share, and create Art together. Art installations can include huge temples several stories high, made of wooden dinosaur scraps; optical illusions of lakes; performance art; light sculptures; sound experiences; moving vehicles up to one hundred feet long; political statements; and unusual doorways to another world. One year, artist Zachary Coffin brought five eighteen-ton slabs of granite, and suspended them diagonally from a frame so that viewers could climb on them and view an aerial fireplace.[3] It took five trucks to haul them in from Alabama, just to be viewed for a week. Many artists work all year long on their installations for Burning Man, and most, like the wooden man himself, or the famed temples of David Best, are created for the sole purpose of temporary art—burned to ashes at the end of the week.

There are few rules at Burning Man. Exchange no money, be an active participant, and "leave no trace" of your presence after you leave, comprise the chief agreements. Burning Man runs on a "gift economy," which means that entertainment, rides, water, food, alcoholic drinks, massage, bike repair, yoga classes, newspapers, or any of other service or commodity, is freely given away. Even the barter system is frowned upon. If you need something, just ask. If you have something to share, offer it. If you think you have nothing, contribute your time: run errands, volunteer for the post office, deliver a singing or a stripping telegram. (If you know what a singing telegram is, you can guess what a stripping telegram might be.) Each participant is expected to contribute to the whole. If there is any kind of competition in Black Rock City, it is based on who can *give* the most, not on who *has* the most. The more people give of themselves, the more delightful the event becomes for everyone.

You cannot survive in the desert alone. Temperatures can range from 120 degrees in the day to near-freezing at night, with dust storms thick enough to obscure the face of the person sharing your

coffee cup. The entire event thrives on cooperative co-creation oriented toward community experience. My own cadre from Northern
California plans for most of the year to create its interdependent
neighborhood of over two hundred people. Bio-diesel generators provide electricity for all of its "citizens," with a large rented tent erected
as a common area for group gatherings, workshops, performances,
parties, meals, and daytime collapse from the night's escapades. A
bus transformed to look like a spaceship carries its people around.
Each neighborhood is a tribal entity, with its own distinct flavor that
adds to the whole.

Burning Man is a shining example of the Dynamic Feminine paradigm: erotic, creative, egalitarian. This is not to imply that it is ruled
by women, but rather that it's not ruled by much of anyone. It does,
however, imply that women are empowered, free, and respected
equally to men. It is highly communal, yet fiercely individualistic,
and wildly ecstatic.

A NEW RENAISSANCE

The Dynamic Feminine paradigm is the fourth archetypal pattern in
our historical progression—the missing piece to the four possibilities
of dynamic and static aspects of masculine and feminine principles.
This piece, *in conjunction with the other preceding pieces,* can take us the
rest of the way to the heart. It is the newest form dawning on the
social horizon, and it promises a much-needed balance to the eras
that have preceded it.

Where the cross was the symbol of the Static Masculine—rigid
and linear, logical and deterministic, Gareth Hill sees the Dynamic
Feminine as a spiral. Moving out from the center of the cross, the
spiral breaks down the rigidity and separation of the arms, and
moves toward a circular flowing expansion. But unlike the Static
Feminine circle of the ancient Great Mother, the spiral has no limits. It is not fixed, permanent, or repetitively cyclic, but non-linear
and ever expanding. It doesn't negate any of the other modalities

we have studied thus far. At its best, it incorporates them all. In the words of Gareth Hill:

> "The tendency of the dynamic feminine is undirected movement toward the new, the nonrational, the playful. It is the flow of experience, vital, spontaneous, open to the unexpected, yielding and responsive to being acted upon.... In its highest aspect, the dynamic feminine is the synthesizing creation of new possibilities and new combinations. It is the insight, awareness, gnosis, that comes only through actual experience. Its effects are the uplifting, ecstatic inspiration that comes from the experience of transformed awareness. Its central value is Eros, not in the image of the arrow shot from the bow of Amor, but that which is awakened by the arrow's piercing. Its attributes are participation and process."[4]

The Dynamic Feminine is simultaneously interior and exterior, collective and individual. By definition, the Dynamic Feminine seeks to move beyond the limitations of the Static Masculine. Its members seek ecstatic experience, and we might remember again that ecstatic means *ex-stasis,* or outside the realm of stasis. The focus on the inner world, however, is not private or removed, as in the contemplative traditions. It is instead a kind of group rapture, a shared witnessing of what individuals can create together in a communal happening that combines inner and outer experience as one.

The communities that form around these principles are far from conformist. Their members exhibit blatant individuality, if not eccentricity. Its central hallmark is creativity and connectedness, with a bold recovery of Eros, carried equally by both genders, neither preying upon the other, but both embodying the vitality of a sex-positive lifestyle. Its adherents tend to be fit and sexy, living embodied lives with flamboyant fashion statements.

The Dynamic Feminine does not come from a place of knowing, so much as from an openness based on the realization of how much we *don't know.* Process is more important than content, the means more important than the ends. (In systems terminology, homeorhesis (fluctuating around a dynamic process) is more important than homeostasis (fluctuating around a fixed point). A group meeting may spend more time, for example, on *how* the meeting is conducted than on the actual content of the agenda. (And yes, it does often take longer to get things done, but people are happier with the result.)

In science, the Dynamic Feminine can be seen in chaos theory, quantum physics, non-linear dynamics, and living systems theory. All are relatively indeterminate, fluctuating, and highly relational, speaking of a dynamic web of relationships more than things themselves. These forms transcend the static nature of science, calling us to still-deeper mysteries. In medicine, we find increased interest in alternative healing practices, herbology, energy healing, hypnotherapy, massage and bodywork, prayer, and meditation.

In the social realm, this movement is exhibited through nonviolent civil disobedience, participatory democracy, tribal events, country fairs, Rainbow Gatherings, Pagan festivals, multi-media concerts and raves, and religious ceremonies that are created spontaneously by small groups without leaders. These groups have women leaders more often than mainstream culture, yet men and men work together, sharing power equally.

The Dynamic Feminine movement is inherently tribal. The web-organized www.tribe.net, for example, boasts membership of 60,000 tribes. Though people still marry and raise children, the nuclear family is less important than the larger tribe, with children known and cared for by many. More people remain childless or have fewer children, giving more time and attention to helping other parents juggle the responsibilities of work and family.

Social interactions are both hi-tech and high-touch. Text messaging on cell phones, the Internet and e-mail, ipods, and digital communications in general are a native language to most. Displays of affection are removed from shame and privacy, and can be found in an easy sharing of love and touch. Hugs replace handshakes. Sexuality is not restricted to heterosexual dyads, and is more accepting of gays, bisexuals, and open relationships. There is general comfort with nudity and erotic costume. The body is exalted and kept fit; often decorated, pierced, and tattooed.

The Dynamic Feminine was largely born in the sixties through the psychedelic revolution that opened people's minds to the frontiers of consciousness and illuminated the tragedy of regimented lives. Just as the Apollo spacecraft circled the moon and relayed the first pictures of Earth from space, self-reflective consciousness awakened in the younger generation. As drug experiences dissolved the barriers of the ego, a higher order was revealed that transcended the rigid mechanics of corporate materialism. A new spirituality developed—one that harkened back to the practices of Eastern traditions, such as yoga and meditation, as people sought ways to achieve the same spiritual highs by natural means. There was a wide recognition of our collective potential, even if its achievement seemed to be a distant, idealized goal.

The exterior edges of the ego were not the only thing to dissolve, however. For the psychedelic experience made one more sensitive to the inner realm as well. Heightened awareness put people in touch. People discovered that the food they ate, the health of the body, and the degree to which personal issues were resolved had great bearing on the quality of their experience. Organic food, natural surroundings, and the practice of yoga, fasting, meditating, ecstatic dance, aerobic workouts, and wearing natural fibers; all these became valued as necessary ingredients to a clear psychological state – on or off drugs. Mind and body were no longer separate, but mutually influential. Mental health was no longer a quality of the mind alone, but now involved the body. Body-based therapies such as Bioenergetics, Rolfing, massage, yoga therapy, and breathwork emerged. There was a resurgence of Chinese medicine, chiropractic, herbology and homeopathy, to name but a few. Medicine began to recognize the influence of one's psychological state on health and disease. Consciousness was seen as a dimension worthy of deep study. People meditated, reflected, practiced yoga, and discovered that they had chakras.

The central vision of this movement is that life is an intricate, living web—all of it sacred. Its reverence is for Nature; its grief for its loss. Out of this realization rose the first Earth Day in 1970, with a back-to-the-land movement that spawned urban gardens, wilderness recreation, and the pursuit of deep ecology. If mind and body were no longer separate, neither were culture and planet. A new synthesis had begun, emerging from deep within. Deep polarities recognized each other as part of a larger unity.

Nonviolence is a fundamental value held by this movement. War and corporatism exhibit stark contrasts to the harmonic relatedness that individuals were experiencing—and therefore knew to be possible. The atrocities of the Vietnam war fueled moral outrage. The love children of the sixties, as they came to be called, gathered in hordes to march, to chant, to pray, and to hold candlelight vigils. The largest anti-war movement in the planet's history (at that time) took form across the nation, and pushed the stems of flowers into the barrels of rifles.

Leonard Shlain, based on his premise in *Alphabet vs. the Goddess,* might say that the ubiquity of the television, which allowed information to be conveyed in images rather than the written word, made possible a rebirth of feminine values. Certainly, Women's Liberation, as it was called at the time, played a huge role in making this movement possible. As women in the sixties went to consciousness-raising groups and compared stories, they discovered common themes. Many discovered that they were living someone else's life, with values that were alien to their own. They threw away the orange juice cans they tried to sleep on to curl (or straighten) their hair, kicked off their high heels and pantyhose, and began to dance barefoot on the grass. While their brothers burned draft cards, women burned their bras. A new kind of sisterhood began to emerge, with its own distinct flavors. Women were finding their own voice, their own style, and along with it, their righteous indignation over centuries of oppression.

In seeming coincidence, archaeological discoveries brought to light information about ancient goddesses that had long been buried and forgotten. We learned that God had not always been a man on a throne with a long, white beard, and that goddesses had many forms. We learned that there were once priestesses as well as priests, and that the divine feminine was not simply God in drag, but something equally holy—and wholly different. What first appeared as centuries of oppression stretched to several millennia.

As feminists fought for equal rights, women rebelled against their oppressors, be it their dictatorial fathers, college professors, bosses, or husbands, and set out to make their own way. They left the kitchen and entered the workplace. They set up rape crisis centers, child care agencies, and started their own businesses. Some decided they didn't need men anymore. Others transformed their relationships with men, patiently explaining *ad nauseum* the subtler aspects of sexism that still crept into most relationships. Women discovered the love of other women as they freed themselves from the romantic expectations of men. Women-only environments freed both gay and straight women from the expectation of dainty behavior, perfect hair-dos, uncomfortable clothing, and the mask of make-up. Men learned to make their own coffee. They, too, discovered the sacred in each other, and formed men's groups to redefine their identity as something other than oppressors of women. Same-sex love, both male and female, came out of the closet, and began the uphill journey for social acceptance.

RIGHTS FOR ALL

Gender issues were not the only battles fought by the Dynamic Feminine movement. The sixties also brought with it the civil rights movement, the environmental movement, the peace movement, and a heightened awareness of racism, ageism, child abuse, animal rights, gay rights, disabilities, and consumer rights. As the standard of living continued to grow for much of the population, it became increasingly obvious that it didn't improve for *all* of the population. The fight for rights of all kinds became part of the equalizing force of the spiral feminine, knocking down the arms of separation between left and right, above and below, formed from the masculine cross.

Self-reflection through psychotherapy entered the mainstream. People wanted to know more deeply who they really were beneath their gender-specified roles. Women wanted to find their power. And when their husbands and boyfriends were left behind in the dust, wondering what they'd done wrong and how they were going to survive, men began to enter therapy themselves. Self-help groups for alcoholism, drug abuse, gambling, sex, and the enabling of any of these addictions sprang up all over the country. The angry residue of five thousand years of a dominator paradigm flared into an energized awakening. Powerlessness became less tolerable.

Though there is still a very long way to go toward true equality, we are no longer surprised when women, blacks, or gays hold positions of power. Fewer people tell their daughters they can't become doctors, or tell their sons they have to go to war to be real men. Gay couples can walk down at least some streets holding hands. Now the fight is legislative: can gays marry and have the same privileges as other couples? Do black minorities have as much right to be rescued from the effects of a natural disaster? Can women find birth control as easily as men can find Viagra? In an overpopulated world, do women have the right to an abortion on demand? Do the more silent animals, forests, and oceans have any rights at all?

If the Static Feminine was our infancy, the Dynamic Masculine our terrible twos, and the Static Masculine our middle childhood, then the Dynamic Feminine can be said to be our adolescent awakening. It is the independent rebellion against the father, against fixed forms, institutions, rules and regulations. It is boldly embodied, passionately sexual, and highly individualistic. Women and men join together as equals – in relationships, in the workplace, even in politics. Sexuality is seen as a sacrament leading to a spiritual connection. Freedom and self-determination are essential, along with openness and flexibility, meaning and creativity.

In its negative aspect, the Dynamic Feminine valence can be so resistant to structure that it becomes ineffective. In extreme, it can be indulgently hedonistic, so fully in the moment that it goes nowhere, so bent on equality that no one can lead. New Age platitudes can replace grounded research. Altered states can take one so far into the cosmos that one loses touch with reality. This negative aspect results from denying the other archetypal patterns of the past–the steady grounding of the Static Feminine, the focused drive of the Dynamic Masculine, and the rigid structure of the Static Masculine.

The Dynamic Feminine seeks to redefine power by leveling the playing field. For those who are familiar with the Spiral Dynamic model of Don Beck, the Dynamic Feminine is inherently Green–with equal rights for all. At its worst it can become what Ken Wilber calls the "mean green meme," and fall to quarrelsome bickering and a valueless flatland, where everything is considered equal to everything else. It is highly resistant to imposed structure–to the Blue level of conformity and to the Orange level of capitalistic acquisition. It is not yet integral, but is an important step to getting there as it reclaims a wholeness within the self, and values equally both interior and exterior aspects of reality, both individual and collective. Its tribal values and behavior are fundamentally self-organizing through small, creative groups without outer leaders.

The bulk of progressive values reflect the Dynamic Feminine sentiment. In the words of Paul Ray, who coined the term, *Cultural Creatives*:

> "the new progressive values planetary rather than national interests, eco-sustainability rather than sentimental environmentalism, feminism rather than Heroic models, personal growth more than personal ambition, and condemns globalizing mega-corporations more than the religious right." [5]

The Dynamic Feminine emerges at a time when technology allows us to transcend the written word with multi-media downloads of high speed communication. Where reading is inherently static–a slow and linear mental process, building logically from one thought to another–information today is immediate and whole-brain. Rather than stare for hours at tiny text on a white page, (as you are doing right now) information is transferred instantaneously, through sound and images. Channel surfers can watch several programs at once. Cell phone users can access the Internet. Computers can talk and listen, remember and perform.

The Dynamic Feminine movement is still young. Scientifically, it began with Einstein's theory of relativity, socially with the feminist movement, technologically, with the advent of television and the Internet. Though it sports a steady increase, it is still outside of the mainstream, considered by many to be "fringe," and dismissed. We have yet to see the way it will mature, and how it will influence society as a whole. But if its early stages are any indication, it is delightfully creative, empowering, and embodied, with a strong focus on environmental sustainability and social justice.

The Dynamic Feminine alone is not the way of the future, but an essential shift in values, and a dissolution of past structure that is necessary to move forward into a truly holistic or integral paradigm. Because the Static Masculine is by nature rigid and unchanging, it becomes outdated in a dynamic and changing universe. Because the heart requires mutually fulfilling relationships and cooperative ventures, male domination must allow itself to be balanced by feminine values. But before we can dissolve the power paradigm that has controlled civilization for the last five thousand years, we must make an essential inquiry: What is the organizing principle that replaces it? And where are we now?

ESSENTIAL POINTS

• The Dynamic Feminine movement is typified by a reclamation of the body, sexuality, freedom, passion, community, and creativity.

• The social revolution of the sixties spawned a new awareness of the frontiers of consciousness.

• Major progress was made during this time in the realm of human rights and the claiming of personal freedom.

• This is a young movement that is still considered to be a fringe element to mainstream culture. We have not yet had time to see what its influence will be.

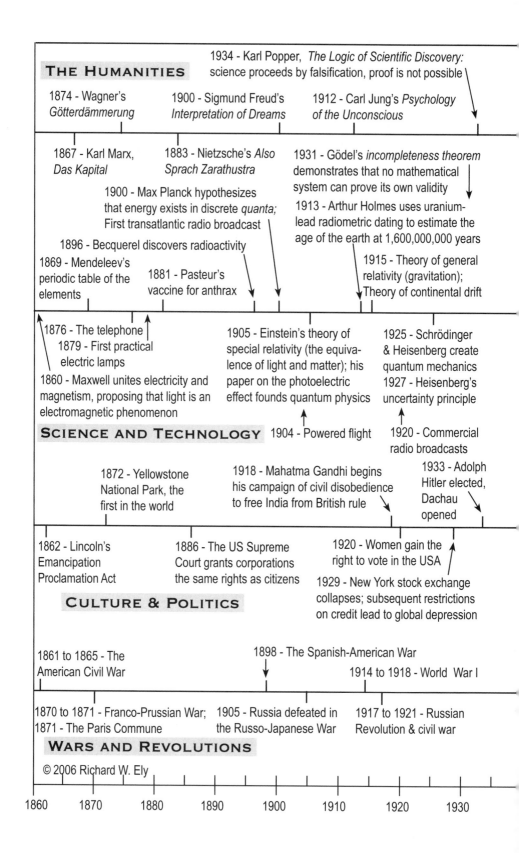

THE HUMANITIES

1934 - Karl Popper, *The Logic of Scientific Discovery:* science proceeds by falsification, proof is not possible

1874 - Wagner's *Götterdämmerung*

1900 - Sigmund Freud's *Interpretation of Dreams*

1912 - Carl Jung's *Psychology of the Unconscious*

1867 - Karl Marx, *Das Kapital*

1883 - Nietzsche's *Also Sprach Zarathustra*

1931 - Gödel's *incompleteness theorem* demonstrates that no mathematical system can prove its own validity

1900 - Max Planck hypothesizes that energy exists in discrete *quanta*; First transatlantic radio broadcast

1913 - Arthur Holmes uses uranium-lead radiometric dating to estimate the age of the earth at 1,600,000,000 years

1896 - Becquerel discovers radioactivity

1869 - Mendeleev's periodic table of the elements

1881 - Pasteur's vaccine for anthrax

1915 - Theory of general relativity (gravitation); Theory of continental drift

1876 - The telephone
1879 - First practical electric lamps

1905 - Einstein's theory of special relativity (the equivalence of light and matter); his paper on the photoelectric effect founds quantum physics

1925 - Schrödinger & Heisenberg create quantum mechanics

1927 - Heisenberg's uncertainty principle

1860 - Maxwell unites electricity and magnetism, proposing that light is an electromagnetic phenomenon

SCIENCE AND TECHNOLOGY

1904 - Powered flight

1920 - Commercial radio broadcasts

1872 - Yellowstone National Park, the first in the world

1918 - Mahatma Gandhi begins his campaign of civil disobedience to free India from British rule

1933 - Adolph Hitler elected, Dachau opened

1862 - Lincoln's Emancipation Proclamation Act

1886 - The US Supreme Court grants corporations the same rights as citizens

1920 - Women gain the right to vote in the USA

1929 - New York stock exchange collapses; subsequent restrictions on credit lead to global depression

CULTURE & POLITICS

1861 to 1865 - The American Civil War

1898 - The Spanish-American War

1914 to 1918 - World War I

1870 to 1871 - Franco-Prussian War; 1871 - The Paris Commune

1905 - Russia defeated in the Russo-Japanese War

1917 to 1921 - Russian Revolution & civil war

WARS AND REVOLUTIONS

© 2006 Richard W. Ely

| 1860 | 1870 | 1880 | 1890 | 1900 | 1910 | 1920 | 1930 |

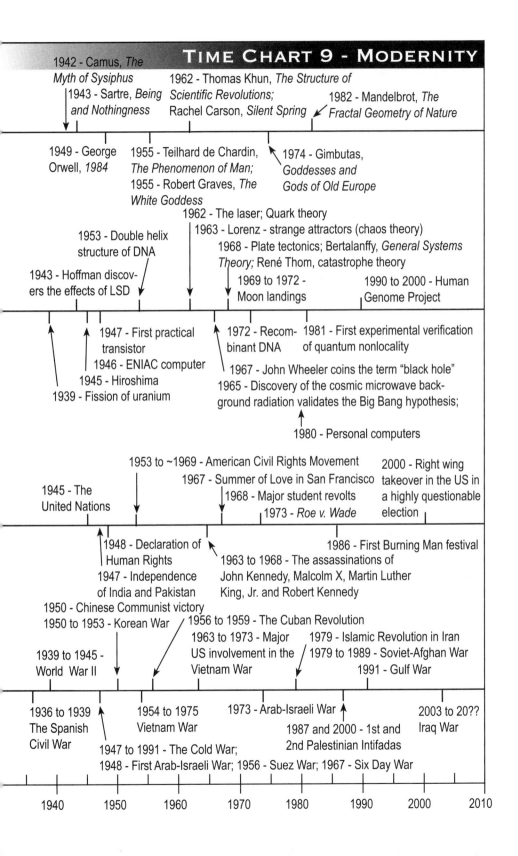

TIME CHART 9 - MODERNITY

1942 - Camus, *The Myth of Sysiphus*

1943 - Sartre, *Being and Nothingness*

1962 - Thomas Khun, *The Structure of Scientific Revolutions;*
Rachel Carson, *Silent Spring*

1982 - Mandelbrot, *The Fractal Geometry of Nature*

1949 - George Orwell, *1984*

1955 - Teilhard de Chardin, *The Phenomenon of Man;*
1955 - Robert Graves, *The White Goddess*

1974 - Gimbutas, *Goddesses and Gods of Old Europe*

1962 - The laser; Quark theory

1963 - Lorenz - strange attractors (chaos theory)

1968 - Plate tectonics; Bertalanffy, *General Systems Theory;* René Thom, catastrophe theory

1953 - Double helix structure of DNA

1943 - Hoffman discovers the effects of LSD

1969 to 1972 - Moon landings

1990 to 2000 - Human Genome Project

1947 - First practical transistor

1946 - ENIAC computer

1945 - Hiroshima

1939 - Fission of uranium

1972 - Recombinant DNA

1967 - John Wheeler coins the term "black hole"

1965 - Discovery of the cosmic microwave background radiation validates the Big Bang hypothesis;

1981 - First experimental verification of quantum nonlocality

1980 - Personal computers

1953 to ~1969 - American Civil Rights Movement

1967 - Summer of Love in San Francisco

1968 - Major student revolts

1973 - *Roe v. Wade*

2000 - Right wing takeover in the US in a highly questionable election

1945 - The United Nations

1948 - Declaration of Human Rights

1947 - Independence of India and Pakistan

1950 - Chinese Communist victory

1950 to 1953 - Korean War

1939 to 1945 - World War II

1986 - First Burning Man festival

1963 to 1968 - The assassinations of John Kennedy, Malcolm X, Martin Luther King, Jr. and Robert Kennedy

1956 to 1959 - The Cuban Revolution

1963 to 1973 - Major US involvement in the Vietnam War

1979 - Islamic Revolution in Iran

1979 to 1989 - Soviet-Afghan War

1991 - Gulf War

1936 to 1939 The Spanish Civil War

1954 to 1975 Vietnam War

1973 - Arab-Israeli War

2003 to 20?? Iraq War

1987 and 2000 - 1st and 2nd Palestinian Intifadas

1947 to 1991 - The Cold War;

1948 - First Arab-Israeli War; 1956 - Suez War; 1967 - Six Day War

1940   1950   1960   1970   1980   1990   2000   2010

CHAKRA	ONE	TWO	THREE
ELEMENT	Earth	Water	Fire
TASK	Survival	Procreation	Power
AGE	Infancy	Toddlerhood	Early childhood
TIME FRAME	Early humans to 10,000 BCE	10,000 BCE to 3000 BCE	3000 BCE to now
GENDER VALENCE	Static Feminine Mother only	Static Feminine Mother/Son	Dynamic Masculine Brother/sister
INITIATORY EXPERIENCE	Hunting	Procreation	War
CENTRAL BELIEFS	Nature is all	Magic influences Nature	Conquest is power
ORGANIZING PRINCIPLE	Nature	Seasonal cycles	Imperial authority
CHALLENGES	Survival	Population expansion	Coordination of labor
TECHNOLOGY	Hunting and gathering	Farming animal husbandry	Irrigation, metal-work
COLLECTIVE LIVING UNITS	Nomadic clans	Villages	City-states
POPULATION OF UNITS	Tens to Hundreds	Hundreds to Thousands	Tens of thousands
ACCOMPLISH-MENTS	Primitive art	Farming	Writing, mathematics, irrigation
SPIRAL DYNAMIC COLOR	Beige	Purple	Red

FOUR	FIVE	SIX	SEVEN
Air	Sound	Light	Thought
Love	Communication	Imagination	Realization
Middle childhood	Pre-adolescence	Adolescence	Maturity
Christian era to now	Renaissance to now	1900 to now	1960s to now
Static Masculine Father/Daughter	Static Masculine Father/daughter	Dynamic Feminine Erotic Partnership	Mystic Marriage Mature partnership
Asceticism	Scholarship	Mystical awakening	Union of Masculine and Feminine
The word is law	Knowledge is power	God/dess dwells within	Heaven on Earth
Written word	Commerce	Self-organizing	Global awakening
Cohesion of diversity	Mechanization, complexity	Environmental Sustainability	Integration
Weaponry, archictecture	Machines, movable type	Computers, Television	Consciousness
Cities	Nation States	Megapolis Urban sprawl	Eco-villages? space colonies?
Hundreds of thousands	Millions	Millions to tens of million	???
Law and order	Science, Education	Information network, human rights	World Peace
Blue	Orange	Green	Yellow/Turquoise

PART THREE

Where Are We Going?

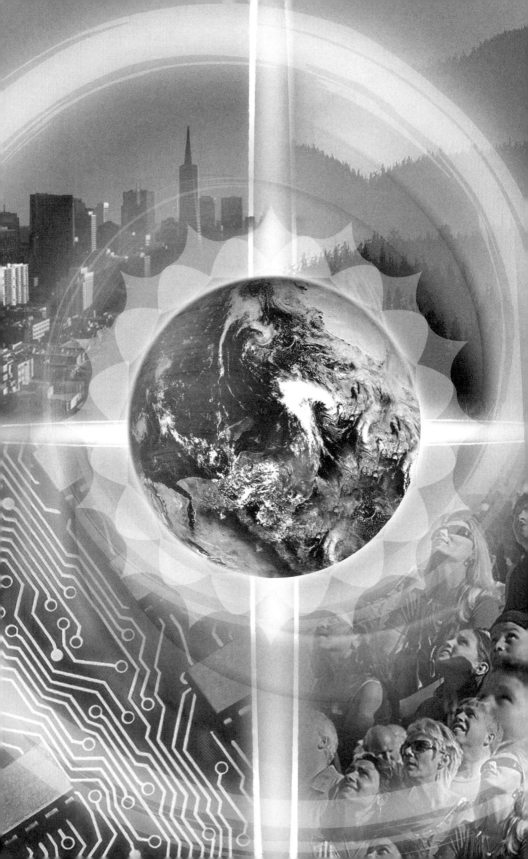

CHAPTER 13

NO TIME LIKE THE PRESENT

The Power of Now

> *When you act out of present-moment awareness, whatever you do becomes imbued with a sense of quality, care, and love — even the most simple action.*

—Eckhart Tolle

It is September 1, 2005. I begin my day by entering the present moment. My practice is to sit quietly, wherever I am, and simply listen to the sounds around me, extending my awareness even to the sounds I cannot hear but only imagine. I recently moved from my country home, where the predominant sound was birds and wind—and the cacophony of my own thoughts. There, I would quiet my mind and soften my breath, until I merged with the deeper rhythm of the surrounding woods beginning its day. I imagined that I heard the whispers of spirit urging me on.

Today, in my writing room on a hilltop in Marin County, California, I hear the encroaching sound of traffic, two barking dogs, an occasional siren, a helicopter, a plane, and a neighbor's radio. My own thoughts draw inward rather than out. To listen inside, I must retreat from the noise around me. I had forgotten how the din of civilization permeates every moment of urban life.

Permeating my own thoughts as I begin this chapter is news of the latest large-scale disaster: the levee breach in New Orleans that has destroyed the city. Though it will be old news by the time you read this, the debacle is just beginning as I write. My heart pounds with the implications. This is not a temporary loss or mild inconvenience. Most of the city will be underwater for weeks if not months and much of it will be utterly destroyed. Oils and chemicals, sofas and refrigerators, medicines and memories, along with unidentified corpses, are being washed indiscriminately out to the global sea. Over a million people are displaced, crowding together by the thousands in public facilities with no food, water, power, or sanitation. As relief efforts and humanitarian funds are assembled, and as looting runs rampant through the flooded city, I am reminded that crisis brings out both the best and worst in humanity. It is the bifurcation—the splitting in two—of a system on its way to a new order.

As hurricanes are one of Nature's cooling systems, one cannot help but consider the effects of global warming. Fueled from warmer oceans, such storms may become ever more violent. Like the Sumatra tsunami just a few months earlier, this is yet another event in the process of global initiation. I fear there will be more, but I also know that beneath the destruction, something greater is being born. Perhaps the city can be rebuilt with a more sensible plan in mind— ecological, artistic, humanitarian. But today, that is a long way off. There are more immediate concerns to deal with first.

If I listen deeper, I can imagine the buzz of millions of conversations, from breakfast mumblings to news commentaries, from schoolyard taunts to college lectures. How many people are talking about this very subject, headlined in every major newspaper? Such tragedies do focus our attention. They direct our consciousness toward the present moment.

Reaching deeper, there are many more sounds in this symphony of life. The sound of music and lovemaking, laughter and tears, old ones dying and babies being born. Somewhere in the world people are chanting or singing hymns, and somewhere else they are blowing each other up. The Burning Man festival is going on as I write; though I am not there this year I can hear the tribal beat entraining tens of thousands of people to a new rhythm of hope, even while military planes fly teenage soldiers to fight in Iraq.

I extend my consciousness to listen to the underlying heartbeat of civilization, coming together in a global awakening. I hear the cries inside people's hearts to continue the dance–to live, to love, and to thrive. I hear the cries of trees falling, the whispers of animals with nowhere to run. I hear the sound of a world converging upon itself, focusing our attention again and again, until we see through the illusions and recognize each other as aspects of the same being, sharing a living home together.

We cannot fail now. The best is yet to come. A sumptuous banquet awaits us–even while we fight over appetizers in the waiting room. The doors to the next realm will open when we humble ourselves enough to appreciate the beauty and majesty that surrounds us every day–in our environment, in the faces of our fellow beings, and in the unfolding of the mystery. For the global heart is awakening, calling us out of our complacent slumber and adolescent distractions, into the possibility of a world beyond our wildest dreams.

The rite of passage is beginning. The parent culture is dying. We who are here to experience this passage will be the hospice workers easing the last gasps of the old world while we simultaneously midwife the birth of the next era.[1] Like any birth, it can be painful and messy, but equally joyful. It requires the labors of all of us. For what we are birthing is far too large for any one person, organization, or country. Can we do it?

We have the tools and technology to paint a new picture, but we are floundering for lack of a guiding vision. It is clear to most that we need to end war, redistribute wealth, revise healthcare, support education. We need to overcome racism, agism, sexism, heterosexism, and all the other "isms" that place one group of people above or below another. We need to not only protect but restore our assaulted environment. We need to ease the stress of modern life. We need to feel peaceful and hopeful once again, able to move forward on the evolutionary trajectory that has brought us this far. These are the better-known issues that comprise the threads in the new tapestry we are weaving. What is the common denominator to these challenges?

Joanna Macy points out that future generations will look back and call our time the "Great Turning."[2] It is rare that such a thing can be named and consciously acted upon while it is actually happening. (The last time was the Renaissance.) It gives us a context in which to make sense of things, a way of putting it all in perspective. To turn the colossal Spaceship Earth away from five thousand years of linear momentum and point the arrow of evolution in a new direction takes incredible effort – all hands on deck, working together toward a new goal. Only a vision of what can be possible will aid our efforts in this turning. Is an awakening of the heart worth our efforts?

We tend to think of vision in terms of a fixed point in the future, but if the rate of change is continually accelerating, *there is no fixed point in the foreseeable future, there is only change*. Static systems will be outgrown by a rapidly changing society, much like the tight skin of the caterpillar rips open as its body expands. Our global, high-tech, overcrowded, post-modern, pre-dawn world is simply too complex to be ruled by the simplicity of an imperial system founded in the earliest phase of our written history – the era of young kings invading land masses to add to their egoic empires. Imperialism is a hold-over from our younger days. Imperial control is a liability now.

We are the children of the past and the parents of the future. But just where are we now? What has all this history wrought? What is its significance? In our long journey from the past to the future, now, as Eckhart Tolle is fond of pointing out, is the only thing that exists, and certainly the only thing we can change. The horses are breaking loose and the reins are falling into our own hands. What do we see as we look around? Where has all our progress taken us?

Once again we see both light and shadow, wealth and poverty, genius and lunacy. We live in a time that is both better and worse than ever before. At my local mini-mart, for example, a panhandler coming in from the street can buy wines and delicacies that previous generations could only dream of. Gregg Easterbrooke, in his book *The Progress Paradox,* points out that 99 percent of Americans and Europeans live better than most of the royalty of history.[3] The majority of Westerners, regardless of their economic status, have traveled on a plane at least once, while an increasing number travel the globe regularly. Ninety-eight percent of Westerners own a television, while in Third World countries, televisions are more common than indoor plumbing, giving a common window to us all.[4] One hundred years ago, only 8 percent of American homes had telephones. Today we walk down the street with cell phones that resemble small computers. In the developed world, the lower classes struggle less with whether they will die from starvation (with inner city violence being the worst survival threat) than whether they can afford the simple amenities that make for basic comfort—a safe and decent place to live, transportation, and clothing. (This is a movement from the struggle for survival (chakra one) to obtaining comfort (chakra two), while those with greater resources hold the positions of power (chakra three)). The average American has twice as much indoor space per person as he or she did even fifty years ago. Homes have far more amenities, such as central heating and air conditioning, and an array of electronic gadgets to make life easier.[5]

Yet this rosy outlook is a mere slice of the whole. While personal, indoor space may be expanding, our shared outdoor space is shrinking under the onslaught of freeways, shopping malls, and parking lots. At night, these are dotted with the sleeping bundles of homeless bodies who have no indoor space at all. Worldwide, *20 million people* live as internally displaced refugees, and another 25 million are forced to leave their homelands due to environmental causes.[6] Eighty percent of these people are women and children.[7] In the U.S., one of the most prosperous nations in the world, there are at least 300,000 homeless,[8] though the nature of homelessness makes it impossible to get an accurate count.

In the West, the convenience of running water and hot showers are so common that we take them for granted, yet most major U.S. cities have hidden pollutants in their water supplies,[9] while 14 billion plastic water bottles a year adds to the problem of waste. In the still darker shadow, 20 percent of the world's population (1.5 billion people) lack access to safe drinking water, with 12 million deaths *annually* due to contaminated water.[10] (That's double the 6 million Jews that died in the Nazi Holocaust.)[11]

Meanwhile, medical advances have extended life expectancy worldwide to nearly twenty years longer than just half a century ago (from 46.5 years in 1950 to 65.4 in 2005).[12] In the same time period global infant mortality decreased by nearly one third (from 157 to 56 deaths per thousand births).[13] Yet *20 million children* are orphans who lost their parents to AIDS.[14] Despite the fact that 44 million Americans have no health insurance,[15] there are free clinics in most major cities, making medicine more accessible. Drugs are available for a huge variety of ailments, many at fairly reasonable costs. Yet chronic pain plagues 43 percent of American households, with an annual cost of $90 billion[16] and incurable diseases like AIDS ravage whole continents, with 31 million deaths since 1983, and an additional 73 million people infected.[17]

While the standard of living and life expectancy has increased for a greater number of people, *quality* of life in terms of meaning and enjoyment is in jeopardy. The World Health Organization states that 450 million people worldwide suffer from mental health problems, with 120 million complaining of chronic depression.[18] Meanwhile, the "just-say-no-to-drugs" culture jams our e-mail inboxes with ads for Viagra and Cialis, while anti-depressants are marketed to our children.

In the realm of science, we've explored, studied, and catalogued more of the natural world than any time in history. Yet predictions say that 37 to 50 percent of existing species are likely to be extinct by 2050, in the greatest mass extinction since the dinosaurs.[19] Ninety percent of the large ocean fish are gone, due to overfishing and ocean pollution.[20] Perhaps science's most important contribution to the current situation is the enormous amount of data it has contributed on global warming, toxic waste, plankton disappearance, topsoil depletion, weather disturbance, ozone depletion, air quality, water quality, and the diminishing sperm count across species.[21] Thanks to the wonders of science and technology, our impact on the environment can be measured and quantified, interpreted and broadcast. But the picture isn't pretty, so most people turn the other way.

What about crime? Violent crime has been in steady decline since

1994, reaching the lowest level ever recorded in 2003. (Homicide down 70 percent in New York City, 74 percent in San Diego, with big margins in other major cities.)[22] Yet reporting of violence still dominates the news, and prison sentencing has increased nearly threefold, with the taxpayer footing the bill. The U.S. has the largest percentage of incarcerated population of all first-world countries, 80 percent of which are victimless crimes.

Our technology is creating a world-wide neural net that brings each individual into increasing connectivity with the rest of the world. Yet people feel disconnected from each other, no longer spending as much intimate time with family and loved ones. We have more freedom to go where we want, whenever we want, while remaining connected to the vast web of consciousness that is blanketing the globe. Nearly a fifth of the world's population is now hooked into the World Wide Web, [23] and the numbers are rising rapidly. This growing neural net continually dissolves the previous barriers of time and space, while creating a monumental reorganization of education, commerce, politics, and entertainment.

New York Times columnist Thomas Friedman, in his recent book, *The World is Flat,*[24] tells us that access to information technology is leveling the playing field between First World nations and India or China. The Internet is enabling open-sourcing, out-sourcing, in-sourcing, and in-forming, changing the nature of all our relations. The speed of computation has gone from an already mind-boggling 60,000 instructions per second (IPS) in 1971 to 10.8 billion IPS.[25] Now, with fiber optics, all the information in the world could be transported in a matter of minutes. Consciousness is traveling every-where at once, instantaneously. The old lines of power are being replaced by increasing relatedness. Friedman states:

> "This is why I introduced the idea that the world has gone from round to flat. Everywhere you turn, hierarchies are being challenged from below or transforming themselves from top-down structures into more horizontal and collab-orative ones. "[26]

"Clearly, it is now possible for more people than ever to col-
laborate and compete in real time with more other people on
more different kinds of work from more different corners of
the planet and on a more equal footing than at any previous
time in the history of the world – using computers, e-mail,
networks, teleconferencing, and dynamic new software."[27]

The number of choices available is so great as to be dizzying. I have
even heard the term "choice fatigue" to describe the wearying effect
of trying to navigate through all this complexity. Humans are changing and the planet is changing, along with the climate, the gene pool,
and most elements of daily life. In a world of accelerating change, we
cannot expect the values created in a former era to stay the same. We
are, as Jean Houston has said, entering the "jump time," where "every
given is quite literally up for grabs."[28] Life as we know it is transforming on every level, demanding new skills, behaviors and policies. Like
our ancestors in previous eras, we are facing challenges never before
imagined. How do we navigate our way through this confusing complexity? How do we find sustainability in a consumption-addicted
economy? How do we create unity, yet honor diversity? How do we
find meaning in an increasingly impersonal world, where even dating
occurs electronically? How do we find stability in ever-accelerating
change? How do we wage peace in this final clash of empires? And
how do we shift from local isolation and centralized control to local
organization and a globally conscious civilization?

Evolution is the gods' way of creating more gods. Like gods, we have the
powers of both creation and destruction, now on a global scale. We
can fly to the moon, influence the gene pool, render species extinct,
shift the climate, or irradiate the planet with nuclear warfare. Like a
cancer, we can continue to expand our population, creating wars and
epidemics as a balance, or we can use birth control to stabilize population and live sustainably. Indeed, if we are finally exiting our glorious
adolescence, stabilizing growth is a natural and necessary task. Can we
hold the powers of creation and destruction in reasonable balance? To
become like gods, our growth must now be spiritual, not material.

In all our previous mythologies—from the organic limits of the Great Mother to the worship of god-kings; from the Islamic obedience to the Koran and the stern Father God of the Christians—*humans have been in a childlike relationship to parental gods.* The original thesis of the Great Mother with her son-lover has now been balanced with its antithesis: the Great Father and his daughter-wife. We have experienced the Static Feminine, the Dynamic Masculine, the Static Masculine, and now the Dynamic Feminine. Archetypally, each aspect has made its contribution. To mature, each gender has had to free itself from the domination of the opposite-sex parent.

June Singer, in her book, *The Power of Love to Transform Our Lives and Our World,* points out:

> "In the process of coming to a transpersonal perspective, the ego must first release itself from all those internalized authorities, from the parents to those in the wider world. As these have an inhibitory function they need to be allowed to ebb away, leaving a space for something new to enter."[29]

We've been children for a long time. As infants in the primordial garden, Mother Nature was nurturer and teacher. As children in ancient times, we offered sacrifices and obedience in exchange for protection and favors. In the Christian era, values were dictated by parental priests passing on the word of an alternately loving or angry Father God. Our obedience was based on fear of repercussion, and the repercussions were severe. Disobedience was punishable by death for well over a thousand years, and millions died in wars and witch hunts for lapses in that obedience. This fear lodged its claws deep in our collective bones, passed down through the generations, as human parents taught their children to keep safe by submitting to authority. In the scientific revolution, we found certainty in rational study, weaning ourselves from parental influence, yet the social and political world was still ruled by the patriarchal figureheads of kings, popes, professors, and presidents.

We've been growing up, but have not yet matured into adult

responsibility. Instead, we enact the shadow side of this childlike obedience: adolescent rebellion and an egotistical inflation of our own power. Our culture exhibits a great love of this power, a compulsion to move toward it, even to the endangerment of all we hold dear. Isn't there a better way?

THE LOVE OF POWER

For the past five thousand years, the central organizing principle for human culture has been built on force, backed by the threat or presence of violence. The origin of the word violence comes from *violare*–to bear upon with force.[30] One could argue that any action that forces another's behavior through threat of violence is, on some level, a violent action, whether or not any harm is actually done. A street gang needs only to flash their weapons to get you to hand over your wallet. A police officer need not use his gun, but the fact that it hangs from his belt is enough to keep crowds in line.

In that age-old maxim that "might makes right," moral correctness has been equated with force. The more potential there is for violence, the greater the force. We express the strength of our military (our armed *forces*) in terms of the number of troops, tanks, or bombs. Force is measured by the amount of damage that can be done, not by the level of wisdom, moral fiber, or benevolent result. Even troops whose job is to keep the peace are called peacekeeping *forces* and are usually armed. We are so inured to the presence of force that we scarcely flinch at the violence in movies, video games, and television. It is said that an average teenager witnesses thousands of murders and 100,000 acts of violence on TV by the time they reach adulthood. In newspaper publishing, the motto is: "If it bleeds, it leads."

Violence or its threat is the foundation of a dominator paradigm.

And the human result? Most often, the threat of violence creates passive obedience. Do what you're told and you won't get hurt. Children learn this quickly from violent parents, until the voice of the parent is instilled in the child's own mind, to haunt them forever after. There have always been movements to overthrow this domination: revolts and uprisings from the downtrodden, rebellion from the counterculture, and deconstruction from the philosophers. Yet force still remains the central organizing principle of our society today.

This is an old model based on domination and control. Yet the fact is—and has always been: there are more people submitting than there are dominating. In reality the dominant paradigm is a *submissive paradigm,* in which the majority of humans are trained from an early age to submit—to parents, to teachers, to clergy, police, and government. Though this happens peaceably in most instances, it is the model under which most collective efforts organize themselves in the world today—from families to schools, from corporations to the military. If we wonder why there were so few voices in the U.S. Congress who were willing to speak out against the invasion of Iraq, perhaps it is because the deeply internalized nature of the submissive paradigm has silenced our voices.

The submissive paradigm is built on relationships that are inherently unequal. Like parent to child, they are often a thinly veiled variation of master to slave—one person or group calls the shots while another fulfills them. There's no doubt that this works—and works well—as long as the rulers at the top rule wisely and the system in question remains simple enough for control to be maintained. There is, however, a robbery that occurs. Control systems strip people of their autonomy, and use their disowned wills as collective entities, such as armies and corporations, which can then wield tremendous force. These forces are blunt instruments that lack sensitivity, to say the least. They can only function by maintaining a certain level of detachment and rigidity. They are also subject to the wisdom of those on the top. If the highest offices lack that wisdom, the whole system can crash. Hazel Henderson points out that the man at the top becomes like a dinosaur brain—much too small for the complexity of the beast he rules.[31] Are we to follow the dinosaurs and become extinct?

FREEDOM AND RESPONSIBILITY

For children in a family, it is necessary that parents maintain control and protection—until the child is mature enough to direct his or her own life with wisdom. The cry of adolescents in general, and indeed the cry of an adolescent society, is a cry for freedom. To hold that freedom responsibly is a sign that the adolescent is becoming an adult. The adolescent needs their own power in order to mature. But we hope that they will use that power wisely, in service of something greater than their own ego.

Struggle between power and love is not an either-or struggle. We do not give up our autonomy, our self-interest, or our technological power, to get to the heart. We merely use these gifts for increased awareness and relatedness, exchanging information and connection in as many ways, and between as many different kinds of people, as possible. The flat world is enabling this capacity at lightning speed.

Only with appropriate awe and humility for the magnificence and complexity of the creation can we enter the young adulthood that is our next step as a species. Only then can we retool our relationship to the divine as one of co-creative partnership, rather than procreative obedience. We are, for the first time since the Neolithic, able to enter into relationships of equality, just as adolescents do when they first begin to date. And like adolescents, we are naïve about how to form and sustain equal relationships.

Co-creative partnership depends on mutually respectful relationship. This kind of relationship is a new form on the planet. Like elementary school children, men and women have played in different realms—men on the battlefield, women at home, men in the workplace, women with the children, men creating, women sustaining. But now, for the first time, each gender is entering fields that were previously the other's domain. Men and women are working side by side in the workplace, in the home, in organizations, schools, banks, and markets. For the first time, they have at least the *possibility* of meeting on an equal level, in terms of power, education, and economics, even if great disparities do still exist. Like budding adolescents, we barely know how to form this kind of relationship—a relationship based on autonomy and authenticity rather than roles.

As any therapist can tell you, the vestiges of childhood remain strong in the psyche long after their purpose has been served. In both politics and religion today, we are still following a father figure, often blindly. We have not yet awakened from the trance of obedience to higher authority—even when that higher authority proves itself to be dishonest, unwise, or dangerously manipulative. Dishonesty in elections, false intelligence to start a war, corporate scandals, and appointments of corrupt officials all suggest that Big Daddy is flawed, and may not have our best interests at heart. We are much like children in a violent or alcoholic family – realizing that the father's behavior is dangerous to the family. Yet the system we live in is structured on a top-down, father-controlled, military model. Its power is still organized through a chain of command with the *lugal,* or "big man" at the top—a carryover from the first days of the ziggurats five thousand years ago. When imperial power is the goal, the ends justify the means. Damage to the environment and losses of human life are regarded as just "collateral damage." When and if those at the top become corrupt, the whole system is threatened. This kind of power seeks to preserve itself at all costs.

We are becoming aware of a glaring truth: *At the heart of the power paradigm, there simply is no heart.*

FROM POWER TO LOVE

This is a very old story uttering its time-worn plot with a desperate last gasp. Unfortunately the breath that it takes to support that last gasp may consume everything it has created, unless we listen deeper. Beneath the battle cry, a new story is emerging. Its characters are not children, but emerging young adults, still naïve, but rapidly growing in strength, ability, and understanding. The old story of one part fighting against another—whether as mind over body, male against female, humans against Nature, or nations battling each other—must give way to a new story that no longer denies but instead *integrates* previously divorced principles. We can no longer waste our precious energy on the fight between us and them, Republicans and Democrats, progressives and conservatives, right wing and left. Our dueling dualisms only squander our precious resources.

Deborah Tannen, in her book *The Argument Culture,* points out that the language of conflict permeates all our news and therefore our framework. We have a war on drugs, a war on poverty, a battle of the sexes. News about political parties reads more like the sports page than a cooperative dialog of the issues. "Republicans Win Six Seats from the Democrats," "Environmentalists Attack Industry." Talk shows try to feature opposing views on any subject, but with the eye of seeing which is better, not for a dialogue of integration. The global brain is electrified by dueling polarities. But does it have heart?

The products of rationality, social coordination, laws, and technology have united our world on the outer planes. They have given us the means to communicate, translate, bargain, negotiate, and coordinate. They have given us cell phones and computers, automobiles and jet planes, surround sound systems and living Technicolor. But, as Ken Wilber has pointed out, they have ignored the interior world. Because of this denial we have not yet risen to a level of consciousness that allows the heart to awaken on the inner planes—fostering compassion, empathy, altruism, synergy, and elevated consciousness. We have not yet learned how to elevate love beyond the sphere of our personal relationships. In the realm of mainstream memes, love is not even mentioned as a value. Many consider it a utopian fantasy, a naïve holdover from the days of the flower children. At best, values of the heart are seen as mushy and feminine, lacking the valor and heroism of the masculine, and therefore discounted.

The masculine values, at their best, brought us the heroic impulse. In earlier times, heroism was the ability to succeed in conquest and domination. Today heroism is defined in terms of dying for your country, denying your fear, holding to an ideal in spite of obstacles. We now need a new definition of heroism, and a new task for the Hero. We need a heroism brave enough to face its shadow, a heroism that can expose corruption, halt pollution, and fight oppression. We need a heroism with the courage to stand up, speak out, and tell the truth.

It is time for us all to be heroes. Each of us plays a part in outgrowing and overthrowing the power paradigm whose organizing principle is ultimately based on force. It is incumbent on each of us to play a role. We can no longer wait for an outside power to do it for us. The new order cannot emanate from a single source, but must reflect the multiplicity of the many variables that make up our world, and remain flexible while we weather the changes.

Values and morality need a massive overhaul. In the third chakra era, obedience to authority held a high value in both the military, and society in general. While it brought social order, its shadow side was that it required us to deny emotion, longing, and woundedness. In denying our feelings, we lost our moral compass of connection and compassion. In denying longing, we overruled the part of our psyche that works for something better. In denying our wounds, we have perpetrated those wounds on others.

The sexual morality of a religion that burned deviants at the stake must be replaced by a collective morality that holds the larger totality in perspective. This is not an arbitrary set of rules created by a parental authority, but a co-creative agreement that arises out of the needs of the present and a vision of the possible, one that puts right and wrong, good and bad, in terms of its literal cause and effect on our collective future. It takes essential aspects of the upper chakras to accomplish this: communication, vision, and a spiritual revolution. While these things have always been happening in some form or another throughout time, what is different now is that we have the technology—and the necessity—to use them in the service of a global awakening.

The need to repress the qualities of the lower charkas—earth, body, sexuality, and emotion—has run its course. If its evolutionary purpose was to push us upwards in the chakras and to develop a technology that offers a shared realm of consciousness, then it has fulfilled that goal. We now have instantaneous global communication (fifth chakra), the ability to transmit images through this network (sixth chakra) and a vast field of information accessible throughout much of the world (seventh chakra). The plethora of spiritual books and metaphysical centers shows us we are undergoing a spiritual revolution.

The heart chakra is the central integrator between the upper and lower chakras, requiring at least some awakening in each end of the spectrum in order to be integrated into a balanced whole. We are only now, for the first time, able to approach that integration on a global scale. As we enter a disembodied, high-tech world, we find increased need to reclaim the body and sensuality, (first and second chakras) with what James Nesbitt dubbed "hi-tech–hi-touch."[32] Rising up from millennia of oppression, we fight for our freedom, power, and sovereignty (third chakra), We can now reclaim the vital qualities of the lower chakras, termed by Jay Earley as "ground qualities",[33] and combine them with the "emergent qualities" of our modern achievements to bring the dawn of a culture that allows us to be both healthy and happy.

It is only recently that our species has had enough power to have global impact. Where the past has focused on issues of private morality, we now must concern ourselves with what one country can do to another country, what a business can do to the environment, and what technology can do to save or damn our future. We now need to carve out a morality based on shared responsibility for the global effects of our collective action. In the words of former State Senator Tom Hayden: "It's not that the common man has to overthrow the ruler, but the paradigm of needing an outside ruler."[34] But if we are to overthrow the present control paradigm, what is the basis upon which order and morality can be maintained?

The electronic network forms a global brain. The planet is our shared ground. What's missing between them is the global heart. Just as the mind can have many thoughts and the body has many distinct parts, a single heart beats at the core of each of us. If we are to survive as a global organism, we must find our collective heart. Relationship is the crucible through which the new paradigm will be forged.

But first we need to find a new organizing principle.

ESSENTIAL POINTS

• We live at a time of genius and lunacy, opportunity and crisis. Humans are both better and worse off than ever before, with wide disparities between achievements and pitfalls in most aspects of life.

• In the archetypal paradigms of the past, humans have been in a childlike relationship to parental gods. Both genders have had to dynamically overthrow the static aspects of the opposite sex parent. We are now ready to enter mature relationships based on authenticity and autonomy, rather than roles and obedience.

• The old organizing system was based on force. The dominant paradigm has really been a submissive paradigm, where there are more people submitting than there are dominating.

• We have denied the lower chakra values in order to develop the upper chakra values. This development has now been achieved, with a global network of communication that can relay images and information. It is now time to go back and reclaim the denied lower chakras related to our physical reality, our need for sensual pleasure, and sovereign personal power, and integrate them with the upper chakras of communication, imagination, and spiritual understanding, for a true integration of the heart.

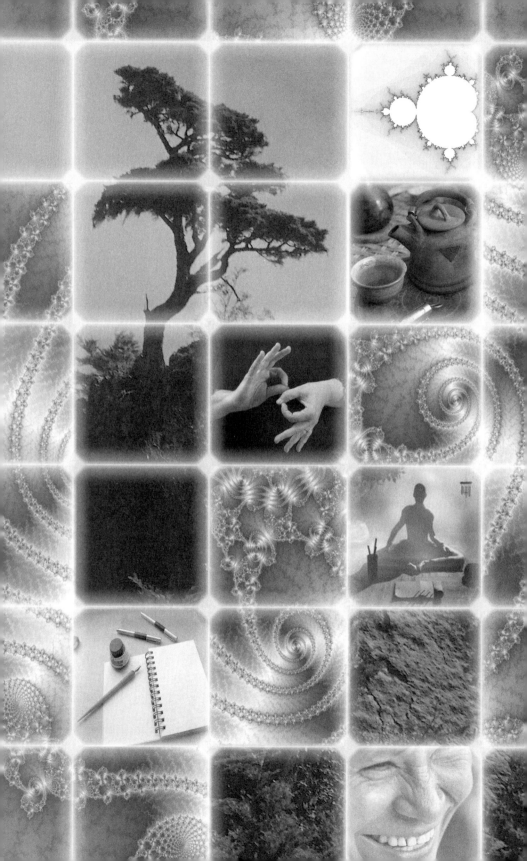

CHAPTER 14

DON'T AGONIZE,
SELF-ORGANIZE!
Better Living through Living Systems

Step by step, from the juvenile earth onwards, we have followed going upwards, the successive advances of consciousness in matter undergoing organization. Having reached the peak, we can now turn round and, looking downwards, take in the pattern of the whole.[1]

—Pierre Teilhard de Chardin

Whenever I step off an airplane, I am always amazed at the miracle of social coordination that greets me. Even before I've stepped into the airport, an array of trucks and personnel arrive to transport the luggage. Once inside the terminal – no matter where I land – people are brewing coffee, selling newspapers, cleaning bathrooms, and driving taxis and buses. How is it that in every major city, and most major towns, you can find schoolteachers and garbage collectors, restaurant workers and laundromat owners, truckers of supplies and merchants to sell them, nurses, doctors, dentists and hairdressers, so that somehow the basic necessities of human society get met? How does this happen? No central authority dictates where people should live or what profession they should follow, yet society somehow organizes itself miraculously.

In a similar example of how social systems self-organize, Paul Hawken, in a talk given at the Bioneers Conference in San Francisco in 2004, reported that as many as *two million* non-governmental organizations have sprouted worldwide to address issues of social justice and environmental sustainability.[2] In an earlier article, he speaks of the mindset behind this phenomenon: "No one started this worldview, no one is in charge of it, no orthodoxy is restraining it."[3] These organizations have risen and multiplied, despite the fact that they are marginal, have little funding, and their members are overworked and underpaid. How does a movement like this happen, seemingly all by itself, with no central authority telling people what to believe, what to do, or how to organize? What is the organizing principle that makes this possible?

In Chapter Nine we followed the history of science from the study of material objects and their movements to the discovery of forces and fields (matter, movement and energy: chakras one, two, and three). As science progressed, tools were created that enabled us to peer into the mysteries of Nature's ever-smaller building blocks; first cells, then molecules, then atoms, and finally subatomic particles. And while this produced fascinating and important discoveries about the nature of matter, examining the infinitely small didn't tell us much about how something behaved as a whole. It's as if we were trying to understand economics by analyzing the ink printed on the dollar. These things can only be understood as a collection of elements in a larger context. After a long period of splitting things apart, we finally began to look at how things go together.

Even as we examined smaller and smaller particles, we found that matter was mostly empty space, more like a *system of relationships* than a group of things. In the quantum world, this is called *relational holism,*[4] a term that describes how whole systems are created by the relationship among subatomic particles.

> "Subatomic particles come into form and are observed only as they are in a relationship to something else. They do not exist as independent "things." There are no basic "building blocks." . . These unseen *connections* between what were previously thought to be separate entities are the fundamental ingredient of all creation."[5]

Systems theory looks at the way groups of things—such as molecules, families, co-workers, or ecosystems, organize themselves into larger entities. Cells are made up of organelles, which are made of molecules. Cells form tissues and organs, which in turn form a physical body that becomes part of a family, a community, and a nation. What makes this occur? What are the guiding principles? What keeps an ecosystem in balance? What makes life grow into greater order and complexity, rather than running down into nothing, as predicted by the second law of thermodynamics?

A system is a set of relationships that forms an identity as a whole. These relationships occur within the system (such as a sibling relationship as a subset of a family) as well as between the system and its environment (such as between the family and its community.) The kids go to school, the parents go to work, and they all go to the store, to the movies, and watch television. They take in from the environment, and they give back to it, watching news, spending money, eating food, learning, teaching, and producing garbage.

Systems exist on all levels, from the micro to the macro. A human body is a *living system,* as is a family, a corporation, a school, or a planet. Each of them are made from smaller parts that work together in service of the larger identity. All of this occurs through *relationships.*

The internal organization of a system occurs through the agents within the system. Arthur Koestler termed these agents *holons*[6]— as they describe discrete, whole entities at any level of the system—a whole cell, a whole organ, a whole person, a whole family. Each holon is made up of smaller holons and is *simultaneously* part of a larger holon. From the smallest subatomic particles to the universe itself, it's holons all the way up and down. This series of nestings is called a *holarchy.*

Through contact and connectedness, holons affect each other. They change and evolve, just as we, ourselves, grow from our relationships with each other. Together, holons create something greater than what they are by themselves. Our glands excrete chemicals; the heart pumps oxygen, the stomach digests food, yet your body as a whole is something entirely different from the organs that comprise it. By some miracle, you experience yourself as a single being, a dynamic living system capable of growth and change, living in a larger, dynamic system that is capable of providing food, rain, beauty, and stimulation.

Fritjof Capra observes:

> "In order to solve any single problem, we need systemic thinking, because these are all systemic problems, interconnected and interdependent." Heart cells work together as part of a larger living system. If we are to awaken the global heart, we must learn to think systemically.

Living systems are inherently *self-organizing.* There's no outside force making sure these agents do what they are supposed to do— their behavior arises spontaneously from within the system—through interactions with the larger environment, and between the holons themselves. Erich Jantsch, in his landmark book, *The Self-Organizing Universe,* shows that self-organizing dynamics occur throughout the entirety of creation. And it's a good thing, too, for imagine if we had to tell each tree how to grow its branches, each bird how to fly, each ecosystem how to balance itself out, or even tell each heart how to beat. These systems are far too complex to be managed in this way, yet without human interference they run remarkably well, and did so for billions of years before humans arrived on the scene.

From the first microbial mats to a species capable of flying to the stars, the dynamics of self-organizing systems have kept the magnificently intricate system of the Earth in a balance optimum for life. Wow! It only took four billion years to create a species capable of noticing this, but now we can see that these principles are inherent to our very being. They apply not only to chemical and biological systems, but to social organization as well. They describe essential values that we would do well to adapt if we are to model ourselves along principles that are evolutionary rather than stagnant, self-regulating rather than externally imposed, and resilient rather than fragile. What are the essential principles of self-organization that make this possible?

A BRIEF OVERVIEW OF SELF-ORGANIZING DYNAMICS

The first condition that must be met in order for self-organizing dynamics to occur is that the system needs to be *open*. An open system is one in which energy enters and leaves the system, creating change as it passes through. Our planet, though finite, is an open system because it receives energy from the sun. Trees are open systems because they use solar energy to produce food and make compost from their leaves. Humans are open systems because we consume energy from our environment and turn it into activity and waste.

A closed system is one in which there is no exchange between the system and its environment. Without added energy or input, a closed system eventually runs down. If you don't feed a caged animal it eventually dies. If I don't read books or have conversations, I run out of ideas.

Secondly, a system needs to be in a state of *non-equilibrium.* Open systems tend to be in a constant state of non-equilibrium, because things are always changing. Equilibrium, by contrast, is the final state of a *closed system,* a condition where all the forces have cancelled each other out, a point where nothing else can happen – no change, no evolution, no life. Therefore, stability and equilibrium are *not* desirable states for a living system, especially one that is under stress.

The challenges of disequilibrium force a system to evolve. The challenge of survival stimulated organized efforts at hunting, gathering and farming. As population expanded, agrarian cultures were faced with a new challenge—how to feed and coordinate larger numbers of people—and this produced the advances of writing and mathematics. The Christian vision of a unified family of brothers and sisters was an answer to the Greco-Roman melting pot of diverse races and cultures. The challenge to understand anomalies in science produces new discoveries and paradigm shifts.

Rigid structures and control tactics destroy a system in transition. The systems by which we live are *all* under stress right now: economics, politics, environment, education, social communities, families, and individuals. Try as we might, we can't predict the way events will unfold. It may seem frightening, but from a systems perspective, this kind of stress can be seen as good news, because it hastens evolutionary change.

In the words of Margaret Wheatley, author of *Leadership and the New Science: Discovering Order in a Chaotic World:*

> "anything that disturbs the system plays a crucial role in helping it self-organize into a new form of order. . . . disorder can be a source of a new order. . . growth appears from disequilibrium, not balance."[7]

As population soars and technology creates greater choices and challenges, chaotic patterns result. The complexity of our world surpasses the capacity of the ruling paradigm. Like a single parent with too many children, the ruling father becomes overwhelmed, especially as the children grow older and wilder. Unfortunately, a common reaction to this disequilibrium is to heighten control: restrict freedom, make rules, and rigidly enforce them – all in the understandable effort to maintain order. As a therapist, I've seen this many times in large families. The attempts to curtail individual freedom may work for a while, but the result is a lack of energy due to submission, or chaos due to rebellion. Either way, the system eventually breaks down. All war, on some level, results from an attempt of one group to impose structure on another, or a rebellion against such control.

When we have moved too far away from the natural process by which things occur, the result is fear. Fear results from losing contact with what is fundamental: security, safety, the Earth, our bodies, and our inner experience. Losing touch with what is fundamental, we court its shadow side: *fundamentalism.* Fundamentalism stems from the desire to create stability through control. As life becomes ever more unpredictable, we see a rise in fundamentalist values. As the Progressive Left tries to break the stranglehold of the Static Masculine system, the Conservative Right clamps down with more rigidity. And the more we move toward diversity and freedom, the more we see people waving the banner for conformist values. Fundamentalism restricts the creative potential of a system to evolve.

Fundamentalism can also be seen as a resistance to initiation, a resistance to the unknown disequilibrium state so necessary for evolution to occur. Fundamentalism is a going backward, a regression to an earlier stage, an attempt to return "home" to the familiar, to safety, to first chakra ground values. In the chaos of escalating complexity, fundamentalism is a search for simplicity—values, meaning, and identity—all elements that make or break an unstable system's ability to transform to a new level.

The cry for values is a necessary one. Values organize complexity, steering its self-organizing processes. But values can become restrictive when they are projected onto "things," rather than dynamic processes. We give value to cars, houses, computers. But do we take into account the process by which they are created? What about the workers, the materials, the waste, the energy expended? When values are fixed on maintaining stasis, they make a system less flexible and therefore less resilient.

If we are becoming evolutionary agents in the creation of our future, we must remain open and flexible. We must learn to embrace uncertainty, to let go of outcome, and instead pay attention to the *process* by which things evolve. If we can accept stress as an evolutionary factor, we can weather the intense changes that appear to be coming on the road ahead. Like the initiate, we must relinquish control and attachment. Erich Jantsch states: "What evolution seems to maximize is not efficiency or productivity, but flexibility to persist." [8]

Given a state of openness and non-equilibrium, the next set of conditions apply to the holons themselves. In order to self-organize, holons must have a minimum of four properties: *the capacity for self-renewal, self-autonomy, relatedness,* and *self-transcendence.* Below, we will examine these elements more closely.

THE CAPACITY FOR SELF-RENEWAL

Holons in the system need to maintain their basic integrity long enough to make more of themselves. Called *autopoesis,* this refers to basic survival and reproduction – elements of chakras one and two. For human culture to evolve, we had to learn to survive and procreate in order to pass on our learning to subsequent generations. A single generation doesn't evolve very far. Cells in the body replace them-selves regularly–the stomach lining every three days, white blood cells every ten days, the entire body every seven years. Without this capacity for self-replication, there is no continuity.

AUTONOMY AND FREEDOM

This important principle tells us that holons in the system need to be free to act according to their own nature. The heart must be free to pump blood, the stomach to digest food, and the lungs to breathe. If any organ were forced to do another's job–the lungs to digest food, for example–we'd be in sorry shape. Each organ is uniquely designed for its particular job. Freedom maximizes the contribution that can be made by the holons. The stomach, for example, needs to be free to digest food when it is eaten, not on a schedule.

Ultimately the evolutionary trend through history has been toward increased freedom and autonomy for individuals: freedom from dic-tatorships, freedom from slavery, freedom to determine our own lives. As we saw in the last chapter, technology has greatly increased that freedom. Cars grant us the freedom to go where we please; personal computers the freedom to pursue research, shopping, or cyber-sex. Cell phones give us increased freedom to talk to anyone, anytime, anywhere. Within the limits of your personal economics, you now have the freedom to go where you want, when you want, how you want. Even the desire for money often masks the desire for freedom, for enough money increases sovereignty over our time. The fight for freedom from parental control is one of the main issues in adolescence. Beneath the "me-first" mentality of the baby-boomer generation is a cry for individual autonomy.

The United States was founded on principles of freedom. As the American Revolution was a rebellion against the authority of England, it could be said that America produced some of the first cultural adolescents. America's Constitution assures its citizens freedom of speech, freedom to assemble, freedom of religion, freedom to own property, even freedom to bear arms. Until recently, the U.S. has been a world leader in granting its citizens freedom to act, speak, spend, move about, and live largely as they choose. Despite the U.S. government's hidden agendas, the public rhetoric about the U.S. invasion of Iraq has been that America is bringing freedom to the Iraqis. Even if that motive is questionable, the concept of freedom strikes a deep chord in the psyche of the Western world.

Fundamentalism fears freedom, but the paradox in systems theory is that freedom actually brings about greater stability and greater resilience. As Erich Jantsch describes: "The natural dynamics of dissipative structures teach the optimistic principle of which we tend to despair in the human world: the more freedom in self-organization, the more order." [9] Freedom enhances resilience, because we are free to respond to the stresses and changes in our environment—in short, we are free to evolve.

You might be asking: If we support freedom for individuals, then how do we stop the consuming nature of greed? How do we keep people from killing each other, stealing, or harming the environment? These are certainly important questions, but it must be pointed out that our current system of controls isn't doing a very good job of stopping these things!

Freedom isn't limitless, nor does it exist in a vacuum. Instead freedom is best utilized within an external boundary that defines the system. The digestive enzymes of the stomach are contained by the sack of the stomach or there would be no digestion. The boundaries of the Tigris-Euphrates valley forced innovation in the early civilizations. The finite resources of our planet pose necessary limitations to our personal freedom. As population grows, we are hitting what

Duane Elgin calls the "evolutionary wall."[10] By hitting our limits, we are forced to evolve. Perhaps this will enable us to at last define ourselves as a collective entity.

Freedom is the maturing of the third chakra concept of power. To move from the love of power to the power of love requires moving from a society of masters and servants to one of sovereign, autonomous individuals. This is the difference between adults and children. Children are told what to do because they don't understand the world well enough to make their own choices, whereas adults, as much as they can, make more informed choices. If a young teenager shows himself to be oblivious to the rights of others – playing his music too loud, driving recklessly, or leaving messes in the kitchen– that teenager may lose privileges or have his freedoms restricted. Maturity is based on a balance between personal will and social responsibility, just as the evolution of a system is enhanced by a balance between autonomy and integration. This requires integrating the individual back into the whole. Having achieved the first two principles: *self-renewal* and *autonomy,* we now look to the principles of *relatedness* and *transcendence.*

RELATEDNESS

If there is one continuous theme throughout creation, it is the fact that everything comes into being through relationships. From the conception of a child, to building a house or starting a business, relationships are the portal from which everything new emerges. If we are to birth a new era, it will most certainly occur through networks of relationships.

In the book *A General Theory of Love,* the authors state: "Understand how a neural network functions, and you will know the innermost secrets of the intuitions that guide us to love."[11] Agents in a system need a high degree of interconnectedness. What survives is not necessarily the most aggressive and powerful but the most symbiotic and cooperative. In the past, we have tried to weave the connections between people into a single force, much like a rope, where individual threads are bound together, made to go in the same direction. An army is the best example of this: many lives, stripped of their individual wills, are forged into a powerful force with a single will. This also occurs in many corporations, families, schools, churches, and sub-cultures, where uniformity is encouraged, and diversity discouraged. Threads that are not part of the rope are seen as deviant, and cut off. Many threads certainly make the rope strong, but they also make it less flexible. When we liken the threads of the rope to a global population, trying to get them to go in the same direction is clearly unworkable.

If we instead think of our connections as a web, then each connection remains distinct and important. The overall web becomes stronger with each link, yet it still remains flexible and resilient. When we see relationships as a self-organizing web, we move from a linear chain of command to a multi-dimensional field of possibilities. Instead of power passed down through a chain of command we have information moving through a web of connection. A web can hold something together without binding it. It is non-linear, more like a womb or a field. It can encompass more area. A web forms a unity, yet preserves diversity, with each link in the web representing a distinct contribution to the whole.

Relationships are participatory. We participate in their engagement and they change the nature of the participants. You behave one way at a business meeting, another around children, still another in bed with your lover. Your role depends, not on who you are, but on who you interact with. Your power doesn't come from your role, but from the quality of your relationships. You have more power through positive connections than through negative ones—through people that care about you, like to do business with you, and believe in what you're doing. Ultimately, people serve what they love. Love inspires the will rather than coercing it. Relationships based on love and caring strengthen the web because they strengthen the points of connection, making the web strong.

Margaret Wheatley states: "The learning for all of us seems clear. If power is the capacity generated by our relationships, then we need to be attending to *the quality* of those relationships. We would do well to ponder the realization that love is the most potent source of power."[12]

Caring, loving relationships have strength. They endure. They share. They serve each participant by each enhancing the other. They cooperate and co-create, making less work for each. They are the basis of what we learned in kindergarten—to care for others and to share our toys. Individuality is not at odds with the whole, but a complementary principle that strengthens the whole.

Relationships enable the exchange of information. Cells exchange chemicals and genetic information. People in organizations visit each other's offices to deliver the latest piece of information. Telephones and e-mails transfer information. Meetings and conferences are mass exchanges of information, where more interactions occur in the hallways than the scheduled lectures. Life *forms* itself around information, whether it comes from the DNA in our cells, the blueprints for a house, or the evening news.

Margaret Wheatley advises us as to look at information, not so much as power, but as nourishment.[13] Through nourishment, a system gets stronger—and smarter. Through information, it gains resilience. Information is essential for the emergence of a new order for it tells us how to form (in-form-ation). As each holon reacts to information from its environment, it makes adjustments to the whole. Restricting, controlling, or distorting information chokes the system. Wheatley quotes Jan Carlson, former head of Scandinavian Airlines: "An individual without information cannot take responsibility, but an individual who's been given information can't help but take responsibility."[14]

If we want to couple freedom with responsibility, then we need to nourish ourselves with information. Our world is wired to distribute information like never before. Through the Internet and broadcast media, information travels round the globe at the speed of light. Where the Internet began as an information storage system, (retroactively called Web 1.0) it is now becoming an interactive information medium (Web 2.0). Web 2.0 is seen as a social phenomenon characterized by open communication, decentralized authority, freedom to share and re-use, and more highly organized content. It is a move away from static web sites, toward a more fluid system that can embrace the rapid influx and change of information. Because it is responsive, it is the feedback mechanism of an evolving global system.

Intelligence is often correlated with the speed at which one can process information and make it into meaning. Meaning comes from the ability to make connections and see the whole. If you look at a table of data, it only has meaning by connecting the bits of information into a larger context. As we gather more information, we gain the ability to see the whole.

Highly populated areas have always been on the leading edge of cultural sophistication. There are more opportunities for each person to exchange information, hence to learn and grow. The Internet and the communications industry have exponentially increased the opportunity for interconnectedness among humans, organizations, nations, economies, educational institutions, and governments, to name but a few. Information is free for the asking, available any time of the day at the touch of a fingertip. Though it seems doubtful at times, our collective system is actually getting smarter by the nanosecond. As we continually make connections between the enormous amount of information available, we are assembling an understanding of the whole. Can we turn this massive amount of information and knowledge into wisdom? Yes, if we hold this information in the light of a larger context.

SELF-TRANSCENDENCE

How does a child learn it is part of a family? How does an employee contribute to the mission of a company? How does a nation find an identity as part of a global civilization? If we are holons constellating a larger holon, what are we forming together and what is its purpose? These questions can only be asked by a *self-transcendent system*.

Pierre Teilhard de Chardin said, "Mind has been undergoing successive reorganization throughout the history of evolution until it has reached a crucial point—the discovery of its own evolution." Self-transcendence is the ability of a holon to recognize its purpose at a larger level, and to discover and influence its own evolution. Such realization gives us meaning, value, and connection. It is an organizing vision. Isolated people without goals or direction complain of a lack of meaning in their lives, whereas being part of a relationship, a family, or an organization creates meaning. If you understand the goal of your company, you can better contribute to it. You can bring your own will, enthusiasm, and creativity to that goal. This is especially true if your contribution is aligned with who you intrinsically are when you occupy your natural place in the web, operating through the connections that are nearest and dearest to you. What has meaning, we tend to love. Serving what we love gives us meaning.

It is important to realize who we are as individuals, to find our personal power and autonomy, and to learn to live authentically. But the complementary principle that *supports* that power comes from alignment between the individual and the larger system. Markets demonstrate this clearly – if you have a product that answers a larger need, both you and the culture will benefit. Gas-saving hybrid vehicles, for example, demonstrate the simultaneous benefit to manufacturer, consumer, and environment. The manufacturer benefits by skyrocketing sales. The consumer saves money on fuel. And the environment is served by reducing pollution and the use of resources. As an extra bonus, it contributes to the hope of peace by reducing dependence on foreign oil. It's a win-win-win-win situation.

When actions are *aligned* with a larger purpose, we say they have value. If an employee furthers the goal of your business, then you would say that employee has value. When someone is recognized as having value in their community, it's because they serve the larger cause of that community. In this view, *values* are defined by the relationship of the part to the purpose of the whole. *Values that serve ecological sustainability and social justice serve the whole as well as its parts.*

Self-transcendence is the capacity to not only recognize, but also transform oneself. At a personal level, self-transcendence is the ability to look at myself, decide that I'm not being very helpful or friendly, and then change my behavior to become more friendly. But where did I get the idea I wasn't very helpful or friendly? It can only come from the larger system. That might be somebody's feedback, or it might be my own projection. But even if it's a projection, there is something larger I am projecting onto in order for that to happen. Erich Jantsch says:

> "the self-reflexive mind not only relates the whole world to the individual, it also relates the individual to the whole world. From now on, every one of us assumes responsibility for the macrosystem. Not only for our societal systems, but also for the whole planet with its ecological order, and soon perhaps for space transcending our planet. "[15]

I know this may sound overwhelming. What, me, save the whole world? Isn't that the essence of hubris and grandiosity? Isn't that a fantasy? A job for others to do? Or maybe we should just leave it to some kind of self-organizing dynamic that will simply take care of itself? The answer lies in the difference between serving and saving. The proper relation of a holon to its larger matrix is not that the holon has to *encompass* the larger system, but merely to *serve* it. The stomach doesn't wrap itself around our outer skin, and it doesn't have to pump blood through the system, yet it does serve the whole body by being a healthy stomach. Through individual freedom we become more fully who we are. Through connectedness, we keep ourselves informed and learn about the whole. Through service to that whole, we open our lives to a larger purpose.

As we examine our own behavior and transcend our petty limitations, we enter the dance of the whole. As we find meaning and value in service to our relationships, we are simultaneously serving the whole. As we heal our wounds, expand our consciousness, soften our edges, and open our hearts, we are embracing—and are embraced in return—by the whole. Each person that wakes up to their purpose in the larger scheme of things vibrates with an intensity that is inspirational to others. These actions reverberate throughout the web, through all our relations, into the collective. We awaken ourselves by relating more deeply to what's around us.

In 1968 we launched a space vehicle that broadcast the first pictures of our planet hanging in space. For the first time in nearly five billion years of evolution, life on planet Earth had evolved to the point where it could see itself as a whole. We'd come a long way, from one-celled organisms to the planetary broadcast of our reflection. As pointed out in the Dynamic Feminine chapter, seeing our global reflection was accompanied by a rise in psychotherapy as a forum for self-reflection, increased popularity of transcendent spiritual practices such as meditation and yoga, and the general phenomenon of human consciousness finding it worthwhile to study human consciousness. All of these are evidence of a self-transcendent system.

Evolution becomes self-transcendent when it creates a species that can comprehend and deliberately influence its own evolution. When Darwin discovered the progressive patterns in the fossil record, we discovered that we were *products* of evolution. Now, with the ability to render species extinct or create new ones with genetic engineering, the capacity to change the climate through global warming, or release radioactive material, we are *agents* of evolution. But like Copernicus discovering that the Earth was not the center of the universe, but just one planet among many, it is an equally monumental shift to discover that humans are not the pinnacle of evolution, but only its latest model, perhaps the species capable of pointing the evolutionary arrow in a new direction.

Ultimately, self-transcendence points to a spiritual perspective. Individually, this perspective allows us to transcend our petty limitations, and move out of the center long enough to see the larger picture. Larry Dossey, in his book *Recovering the Soul: A Scientific and Spiritual Search,* describes consciousness as a vast, non-local phenomenon that is eternal and omnipresent. Our individual brains have the capacity to download awareness from this vast field, much as our personal computers can download information from the Internet.

Time honored spiritual traditions have long pointed to this transcendent unity as the ultimate underlying reality behind our phenomenal world of space and time. Known by many names, it is the Tao, Brahma, Divine Mind, Allah, God, Universal Spirit, endless void, or the Power of Now that can only be entered through expanded consciousness.

In the shift from power to love, we are moving from the death of hierarchy to the birth of holarchy.[16] From individuals to families, to communities, towns, states, nations, and our shared planet, we can see we are a nested holarchy of systems. On the physical level, we are nested in the biosphere itself, an intricate web, made strong by its diversity. The biosphere is the senior partner, the ground that holds us. To destroy it is to destroy our very selves. In the social and political world, we are holons in a vast interconnected system that involves the exchange of commerce, entertainment, ideas and information. To destroy this web by mistreating individuals and groups is to destroy the social network from which we evolve. At the level of consciousness, we are nested in a unified field of aware-ness that transcends our normal definitions of space and time. As we tap into this field by meditating, praying, asking for guidance, noticing synchronicities, or watching our dreams, we come to real-ize that it has a vast intelligence, compassion, and wisdom. And if that compassion seems to be sorely missing in our world today, it is only our own blindness that makes it so.

PUTTING IT ALL TOGETHER

What is essential about the principles described above is that they must all be present in order for evolution to occur. Once survival and continuity are established, there must be a balance between self-assertion and integration, autonomy and connection. Freedom and order, stasis and change, all become complementary principles rather than antagonistic.

"The seeming paradoxes of order and freedom, being and becoming, whirl into a new image that is very ancient – the unifying spiral dance of creation. Stasis, balance, equilibrium, these are temporary states. What endures is process – dynamic, adaptive, creative." [17]

So we are looking here at the elements of all the chakras. The ability of a holon to survive and procreate corresponds to chakras one and two. We see especially the need to balance the third chakra aspect of autonomy and power with fourth chakra relatedness. Evolving to the heart is *not* a matter of giving up our hard-won power, or of altruistically sacrificing ourselves through unconditional giving, but rather a matter of using that power *collaboratively,* in service of something larger and mutually beneficial. Humans will not give up self-interest, but when self-interest is served by a larger sense of meaning and purpose, behavior changes more easily. Chakras three and four, representing power and love, individuality and community, then become aligned. Relatedness and self-transcendence reflect the upper charkas: communication (chakra five); imagination (chakra six); and consciousness itself (chakra seven). Communication transcends distance, images transcend time, and consciousness transcends everything.

We have only just begun to have the evolutionary maturity for both freedom and relatedness. We have only just begun to have a network of information that can act as a global feedback mechanism to help us know who we are and what we are becoming as a collective entity. A common vision to save what we love can impel us to cooperate and innovate. Our rational, scientific systems can tell us *how* to do that. But it is our mythic framework that leads to the deeper meaning of the whole.

ESSENTIAL POINTS

• Nature and society operate as dynamic, self-regulating, living systems.

• In order for living systems to evolve, they must be open and flexible.

• Non-equilibrium hastens change. When a system is under stress it evolves more quickly, if it has the flexibility and resilience to do so.

• Rigid systems inhibit innovation and evolution.

• Agents of a system are called *holons*. For maximum evolution and health in a system, holons must have a high capacity for: self-renewal (autopoesis), autonomy, relatedness, and self-transcendence

• These properties are enhanced by an increased standard of living, the rise of personal freedom, global communication systems, and a spiritual revolution based on transcendence and service.

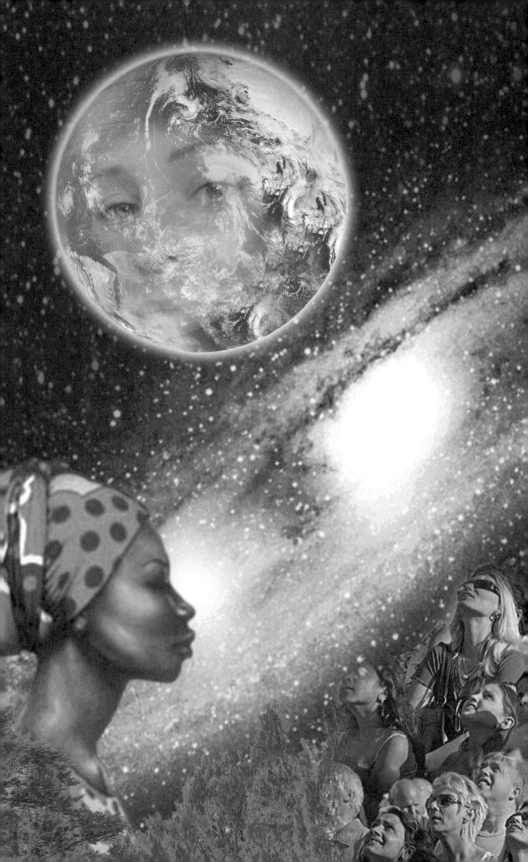

CHAPTER 15

I, THOU, AND WE

X, Y, and Z

> *The world is no more than the Beloved's face.*
> *In the desire of the One to know its own beauty, we exist.*

—Ghalib

Humans are a brutal bunch. Ancient kings blinded slaves by the thousands and impaled their prisoners alive. Romans watched gladiators mutilate each other for sport. Zealous Christians tortured and burned women at the stake. White Americans chained black Africans together on slave ships, then whipped them into submission on the plantations. Nazi gas chambers exterminated Jews and other minorities, while the U.S. dropped an atom bomb on Hiroshima and Nagasaki. And these are just the better-known atrocities.

On a more personal scale, we know that some parents violently abuse their children. Over 25 percent of Americans are victims of childhood sexual abuse,[1] and Third World children are marketed for prostitution by organized criminal cartels. Knowingly or unknowingly, most of us have bought products made by workers in sweat shops. Unwittingly, we are part of a culture that strips indigenous peoples of their cultural heritage, and renders species extinct by destroying their habitats. We have clear cut ancient forests, and deafened whales with sonic testing. We have killed birds and marine life with oil spills, and polluted the gene pool with genetically modified plants. The list goes on and on.

Often these atrocities are reported as a rational accounting of statistics, with no more inflection than we'd use reading a laundry list. The news speaks daily of the number of dead soldiers (ours, not the enemy's), then follows with a report on the stock market, in the same emotionless tone of voice. Issues are too often examined in terms of their financial costs, ignoring the cost to the soul, to the environment, to the quality of life, and to the future of us all.

Most of us have been on the receiving end of some kind of dehumanization as well. We have experienced the indignity of being treated as a number, slamming down the phone in frustration at voice routing systems. Few people have escaped being forced to do something they found distasteful in the name of religion, work, school, or military service. Most women know what it's like to be treated as a sexual object, and now it happens to men as well. People of color, gays, children, and the elderly all know what it is to be treated condescendingly.

We even treat ourselves as an objects. Too often, we push our bodies to exhaustion, ignore our inner signals and force ourselves to endure situations that deaden our souls and compromise our health. We make ourselves conform and perform, ignoring our individuality in order to fit in. We quiet our inner voices, and distract ourselves with the acquisition of more objects to fill the emptiness.

Are we hopeless as a species, or is there something wrong with our worldview?

All of the above are examples of an *I-it* relationship. The objectified "other" is treated as less than sacred, and certainly less important than the subjective "I." An *I-it* relationship denies the interiority of the other. It denies or diminishes their experience, their feelings, their point of view, and their consciousness. If the "other" is rendered lifeless and soulless, then it becomes morally permissible to do whatever we please to "it" for our own benefit. As long as we regard the Earth as an inanimate object, we can justify treating her like dirt – taking whatever we need with little regard for the consequences. As long as we regard an enemy population as a statistic, we can justify genocide as collateral damage. As long as we see plants, animals, people, and countries as *objects,* they have no other purpose than to serve our needs. Our relationships are primarily narcissistic – based on the primary subject alone.

RATIONAL, MYTHIC, AND EVOLUTIONARY SYSTEMS

In his book, *Design for Evolution,* systems theorist, Erich Jantsch describes three levels of systems: the *rational,* the *mythic,* and the *evolutionary.* [2] Each one is a mode of inquiry, and a framework through which we experience relationship. All of them are essential to maintaining a balanced view of the world. These three levels of systems are described below.

1. The Rational System

The *rational system* operates in the context of an *I-it* relationship. Its goal is to be "objective. " To maintain objectivity, it suppresses "subjective" values or experience, which are believed to either distort the facts, or simply be irrelevant. The rational system assumes separation between subject and object. We are most familiar with this kind of system in the way we study science, mathematics, economics, military tactics, and the statistics of social behavior. These systems focus on observable *exteriors* of objects and groups – their size, their shape, their numbers, or their properties. In social systems, they tell us how many teenagers commit suicide, or how many African Americans live below the poverty line, but they say nothing of the despair within these groups. (In Ken Wilber's four quadrant theory, this would be exterior individual and exterior collective– *it* and *its.*)[3]

The rational system began with the ancient Greeks and became the standard mode of inquiry during the Scientific Revolution. Its basic organizing principle is logic. It deals with precise measurements, laws, and empirical facts. If we were talking about a river, the rational system would measure the temperature of the water, the number of fish that swim in it, and the height and speed of the water at different times of year. If we were building a dam, this type of information would be essential for making sure that the dam was built safely. If the building of a dam were proposed on a ballot, its value would be measured in terms of financial cost and benefit to taxpayers. But in the rational system, the sacred value of the river for its local population would be ignored, as it cannot be measured objectively.

The rational system tells us *how* to go about something. It gives us information in the form of data: the nuts and bolts of technology and science. Rational systems argue about points that can be proven or disproven. They are exacting, deterministic, predictable, and dependable. If you want to build a house, you need to know that the engineering is sound. If you want to ingest a medicine, you need to know that it's been adequately tested and will produce the expected results. For questions of "how" it is good to approach things through the rational system.

2. The Mythic System

The mythic system implies a subjective experience. If, while measuring the temperature of a river, you slipped and fell in, you would suddenly jump from the rational level to the mythic level. Once you're immersed in the river, the water temperature is an *experience,* ("brrrr") not a number (50° F). If you're fighting for your life in whitewater, the speed of the water as a statistic doesn't tell you how to paddle, but the experience does.

The *mythic system* operates within a framework of an *I-Thou* relationship. Where the rational system tells us "how," the mythical system tells us "what" or "who." It looks at the larger identity formed by a collection of rational data. It recognizes the larger holon made of the holons inside. The mythic system is bi-directional. It establishes a feedback link between two subjects. It is determined by qualities, not quantities. Its power comes through feelings and resonance, not measurement. As we look at the way the observer influences the experiment in quantum physics, we are seeing how rational data, when examined closely enough, reveals a deeper, responsive system.

Far from being a flight of fancy, the mythic system is what gives us identity and meaning. It puts the rational data in an experiential context. It's holistic—it tells you *what* something is as a whole. If I gave you a table full of measurements, you would need to know what I was measuring to make sense of the data. To say it's a measurement of water isn't enough. Is it rainfall, ocean tides, the depth of a well, or the speed of a river? The identity of the whole puts the data into context. In the mythic system, the river is given a name. It gives or takes life. It has a spiritual value in the history of the people and animals that live along its banks. This meaning transcends its temperature or volume.

We think from a rational perspective, but our behavior is influenced from the mythic context – for better or worse. In religion and politics, figureheads such as the Pope or the president hold mythic identities as father figures. For many people, this archetypal identity holds more power than the rational statistics that show that figure's failures or shortcomings. The Ganges River in India, for example, is regarded as a sacred river of purification. Despite the fact that it is polluted with dead bodies and other toxic waste, people still bathe in the Ganges for spiritual reasons. To call our planet Gaia, after the Greek Earth goddess, is to give *it* a mythic reality and begin to think of the planet as a sentient *Thou*. We treat our planet differently if we see it as a divine entity, rather than an inanimate object.

The *I-Thou* relationship is not narcissistic, but interactive. It is not a subject acting on an object, but two subjects mutually influencing each other. I can place an object, such as a chair, anywhere on the floor, and have it stay put, but I can't do that very well to a cat. But if the cat sits on my lap I *can* stroke her fur and *encourage* her to stay. We can influence an *I-Thou* relationship, but we can't control it.

The mythic level comes from the stories we tell ourselves about the nature of reality. These myths guide our behavior, define our purpose, and shape our world. Yet they are often unconscious, or seen as less important than the rational system, when in fact their influence on the psyche is far stronger. Statistics about our world, while instilling fear and concern in those who read them, have not yet changed our behavior. Only a change in the mythic system—a change in how we view the world as a whole—can steer humanity in a new direction.

3. The Evolutionary System

The *evolutionary system* moves from *I and Thou* into *We*. Instead of just adapting to change as we do in the rational and mythic systems, an evolutionary system has the ability to both anticipate and shape that change. This takes place through a co-creative embrace, a dance of mutuality and reciprocity, where both *I* and *Thou* mutually influence each other in a process of escalating feedback. The river can erode the stream bank, which may in turn change the course of the river—that's feedback. But in the evolutionary system, people build levees or dams to shape the river, and maximize it for safety, irrigation, or ecological balance. That's evolution.

The evolutionary system tells us "where" something is headed. *Where* directs the future. It tells us what we are becoming. It is purposeful, teleological, visionary. If you fall in the river, it matters greatly where the river is headed. If it's going over a waterfall, you're not going to lay back and float downstream, especially if you have the data or the experience that communicates a powerful current. The evolutionary system looks, not only at the mythic level of *what* something is, but what it is *doing,* while the rational system tells us *how.*

In the evolutionary system, we function by design. We anticipate what might happen and design our systems accordingly. It is future-oriented—but the goal is collective utility, not personal gain. An evolutionary system would not cut down the last stands of redwood trees for profit, but realize that they have a larger function as recreational cathedrals and ecological storehouses. Economics is a rational system of checks and balances, but it is influenced by the feedback between markets and consumers. An *evolutionary* economics would design itself unto the "seventh generation" for maximum networking, sharing of resources, and social benefit.

The evolutionary system is co-created between *I* and *Thou.* The passage from third chakra to fourth chakra is pulled forward, not only by communication from the fifth chakra, but also by our creative potential. When we learn to create more of what we love in the world, the heart will sprout wings and fly to new realms. Barbara Marx Hubbard, in *Conscious Evolution: Awakening the Power of our Social Potential,* talks about how we are now coming to the "eighth day of creation," where we wake up (presumably after the seventh day of rest) and discover that *we* are the ones responsible for what gets created.[4] This is the beginning of our maturation as a species. It is the foundation of participatory democracy.

RATIONAL	MYTHIC	EVOLUTIONARY
I – it	I – Thou	We
Subject-object	Subject-subject	Inter-subjective
How	What	Where
Physical	Social	Spiritual
Science	Humanities	Future Design
Experimentation	Analogy	Modelling
Logic	Experience	Creation
Quantities	Qualities	Influence
Laws	Values	Purpose (teleos)
Behavior	Individual Ethics	Group Ethics
Objectivity	Subjectivity	Creativity

RELATIONSHIP: WHERE IT ALL HAPPENS

Relationship is the crucible through which evolution occurs. Authors Lewis, Armini, and Lannon, in their book, *A General Theory of Love,* tell us, "The evolution of the limbic brain 100 million years ago created animals with luminescent power of emotionality and relatedness, their nervous systems designed to intertwine and support each other like supple strands of a vine. . . what we do inside relationship matters more than any other aspect of human life."[5]

The rational, mythic, and evolutionary systems all work together. Each of these system levels reflects how we regard relationship. They tell us *what* we are, *where* we are going, and *how* to get there. If we are to create a new story for how we live together on this planet, it must be simultaneously rational, mythic, and evolutionary.

The symbiotic enmeshment with Nature in the early Static Feminine was an unawakened *we.* There was, theoretically, little or no separation between humans and environment, but one fused identity, akin to an infant child and its mother. There was quite obviously a mythic identification, yet it did not have a developed rational system.

The Dynamic Masculine era split off from the *we* into an individuated identity. As the Dynamic Masculine solidified into the Static Masculine, the rational system replaced the older mythic system. Through discovering the laws of Nature, we began to work the details of out *how* things occurred. Social laws gave us the *how* of social coordination. Science gave us the *how* of technology.

To see matter and Nature as an *it* was a great relief, as it lessened its power over the psyche and redefined that power by equating it with knowledge. An *it* could be controlled, manipulated, and used, restoring power to the individual. However, by getting stuck in the *I-it* mentality of the rational system, we lost both our mythic ground and the evolutionary purpose of our future. As Fritjof Capra and others have suggested, the rational data of our sciences are pointing to an underlying mythic reality that parallels many of the teachings of Eastern religions.[6] The progressive values of the Dynamic Feminine movement are using all three levels: by examining the rational data that tells us our world is in danger; by seeking to articulate a different mythic framework from which we might survive; and by weaving together multiple disciplines that are capable of designing systems that will serve us into the future.

Even though our rational system tells us that extreme change is on its way, we still operate under the mythic system of "parental imperialism." This system wasn't designed to serve a society at our current level of complexity. Imperialism is based on a social model of kingship that equates heroism with domination (e.g. war heroes). It arose out of millennia of separating from Nature, getting the rain off our heads and the dirt out from under our feet, finding medicines to combat disease, and developing machinery to do our work. For these developments it was helpful to regard the rest of our world as an *it*. But having been steeped in the rational *I-it* system of thinking, we cannot get to an evolutionary *We* without first coming to a deeper understanding of *I* and *Thou* .

I AND THOU AS AUTHENTIC RELATIONSHIP

Since both civilization and Nature are built on relationships, the real question is *what kind?* Is it an unconscious fused relationship, or is it differentiated? An *I-It* relationship or an *I-Thou?* Is it modeled after the parent-child relationship, or formed on the basis of cooperative co-creation? Do we regard ourselves as the dominators of the world, or as part of a complex web? And, the biggest question of all—with what are we *in* relationship? Who is this person we refer to as *I?* Who or what is the larger *Thou?*

To awaken the global heart is to fall in love with the world once again—or perhaps for the very first time. To fall *in love* with the world is to realize that everything around us is a living, sacred essence, a *Thou,* not an *it.* Trees, people, animals, mountains, oceans, and other cultures—all have a mythic reality, an intelligence, and a unique purpose. Each carries important information that feeds the whole. They have stories to tell, notes to sing in the grand symphony of life.

Each are essential pieces of the puzzle we must solve to see our world as whole again. Their integrity must be preserved for their role to be fulfilled. We can obviously love an *it*—just like some people love their cars or jewelry—but without a sentient response, we can't be *in love*.

If we are to pass through adolescence into a responsible realization of the evolutionary power that rests in our hands, we must shift our *primary* way of relating from the rational *I-it* to the mythic *I-Thou* relationship. Only then can we begin to entertain the notion of an evolutionary *We*. This certainly doesn't mean that we abolish the rational, for it forms an essential ground of our reality. It allows us to manipulate matter and exert our will, an aspect of maturity that allows us to combat the helpless dependency of children. But if we are merely counting (or felling) trees and failing to save or even perceive the forest, then we are destroying the larger mythic reality before we even understand what it is — and ultimately what *We* are.

How do we shift this framework in our relationships?

The basis of *I-Thou* relationships is *authenticity*. Authentic relationships can only occur between two or more subjects, not objects—each recognizing the subjectivity and sentience of the other. This requires deep introspection into our own nature and truthful communication of that nature to another. Authentic communication is a practice where one speaks truthfully from one's interior, listens empathetically and respectfully to the other, withholds nothing, and brings one's full awareness into the present. Authentic communication is essential for forging deeply authentic relationships between the interior reality of two different beings. We could say that authentic communication is a vital aspect of the fifth or throat chakra, located just above the heart. Communication, both personal and global, is a skill that we can consciously develop to help open, stabilize, and balance the heart.

Martin Buber, who wrote extensively about the *I-Thou* relationship in the 1930s, [7] describes *I-Thou* relationships as direct, open, mutual, and present. He makes the point that *Thou* is not just another object with an interior, but an actual relationship, and that every particular *Thou* (meaning anyone with whom you can enter such relationship) opens to an *eternal Thou*, which is divine source. This occurs through a process of dialog that Buber calls, "Turning." This process embodies the essential elements of authentic communication described above. He states: "The *I-it* is the eternal chrysalis, the *I-Thou* the eternal butterfly."

It is important to remember that we do not lose the *I* in this process. Just as an onion in the soup works best when it retains its unique flavor, the individuated *I* adds more to the whole by retaining its distinct qualities. Buber disdained the mystic idea of completely losing the self, for it precluded genuine relationship. We cannot connect to a deep awareness of the other until we have an authentic connection to the self within.

AXIS MUNDI AND ANIMA MUNDI–
THE PRIMARY RELATIONSHIP

"Who am I?" This question has occupied human consciousness since the beginning of time. Its answer cannot be satisfied by listing the rational data of height or hair color, a statement of our occupation, or even speaking our name. It cannot even be answered in words, for ultimately the question leads to the deeper mystery of consciousness itself. But the very act of asking indicates the ability to look inside and bring the focus of attention toward the core of the self – an awakening of self-reflexive consciousness.

Both initiation rites and mystical practices are designed to awaken the sacred, interior world at the core of the self. Called the *axis mundi,* or axis of the world, this core channel of energy runs through each one of us, connecting Heaven and Earth through the center of our very selves. Mircea Eliade describes the axis mundi as representing "one of the oldest religious means of . . . participating in the sacred order to transcend the human condition."[8] In initiation rites, it is awakened through a combination of descending to the underworld, and ascending to higher levels of understanding; stretching this axis out in both directions, above and below. For those who undergo this encounter with both ends of the spectrum, Heaven and Earth become united within the self. The initiate "has become holy, sacred, numinous through his encounter with the archetype in himself and his consequent ability to constellate it for others."[9]

The initiation stages of separation and loss force consciousness into the deep interior of the self, no longer able to focus on the usual distractions outside. Once this center is established, the initiate is given ordeals and practices designed to develop core strength, and raise energy up the spine. From this higher state of consciousness he or she can reconnect to the world as a divine being. All this serves to strengthen the essential *I*.

In the philosophy of *kundalini yoga,* the deep interior core of the body forms a vertical channel of energy that runs through the center of the body, called the *sushumna.* The seven major chakras are located along this column, regarded as the stepping stones along the axis mundi. The chakras themselves act as portals between the inner and outer worlds, acting as centers of organization for the operation of consciousness in its various levels of manifestation.

Ladders with seven steps appear on ancient temples in Egypt and Mesopotamia. They are found in the *coniunctio,* the creative union of the archetypal King and Queen.[10] The axis mundi causes consciousness to reach upward, toward the vast beyond, yet retains roots for the soul and body. The axis mundi aligns universal spirit and individual soul, valuing both equally, and seeing them as a continuum of consciousness that is indivisible. Then, and only then, can we integrate upper and lower realms within the balance of the heart. In English, the letter "I" reflects this central axis, with its feet on the ground, its crown in the heavens, and the central, vertical core that connects them.

To awaken the essential *I* requires that we find our way to our core experience. Here we find the heart of the matter, the center of the world, the holy mystery within. Even the word *core* relates to the heart as the center, as in the French word for heart, *le coeur,* or the Spanish word, *corazon.* It is from this core that we enter the *I-Thou* relationship.

If the axis mundi is the essential core of the self, the sacred *I*, then the intricate web of the outer world is the *anima mundi.* The anima mundi is the soul of the world, a matrix that is living, animated, and sentient.[11] The anima mundi is a very large *Thou,* which surrounds us at all times.

We could call it God, Goddess, Gaia, Brahman, Sunyata, non-local mind, universal soul, *purusha,* the Tao . . . all names which give it a mythic identity as a unified conscious entity. Whatever you call it, the main point in the shift from a rational to a mythic system is to realize that the anima mundi is *sentient.* The trees and the mountains, the rivers and the valleys, are subject, not object, animate not inanimate, intelligent not random. It is not an abstract field that we are immersed in, but a responsive one. It, too, is evolving, right along with us, as a result of our actions and consciousness. The evolution of the Internet into an interactive medium is an example of that evolution. As we interact with each other in cyberspace, both the Internet and the user evolve.

THE SECOND ENLIGHTENMENT

The shift from an I-it *to an* I-Thou *relationship is one that is so radical it could be considered a second enlightenment.* It is an essential realization if we are to co-evolve with our environment to become a sustainably designed *We.* It is part of the initiatory experience, an essential enlightenment in the process of becoming Gods. For in this realization, we are no longer passive recipients of reality as we find it. Nor are we ego-driven dominators, driving ourselves to extinction. Nor do we have to solve our problems in isolation, unaided. In understanding the eternal *Thou* of the anima mundi, we have an immense reservoir of help. We can see Nature as our guide, spirit as our teacher, and our inner experience as a feedback mechanism to help steer the way. We learn the lessons of Nature in part through the study of science. We gain the guidance of spirit through processes like meditation, hiking, writing, communing, loving, praying, or dreaming. And by the evolution of our own consciousness, we become more responsive and versatile as navigators along the journey.

In its deepest form, awakening to both the intelligence and soul of the anima mundi makes war impossible, and treats all life as sacred. Just as we would have difficulty cutting off our own arm, ecocide and genocide become equally inconceivable. While the scientific enlightenment brought us knowledge, the relationship between the axis mundi and the anima mundi is the source of wisdom. It is the realization, not of what we are *made of,* but of what we are *part of.* Ultimately, this should tell us what we are *made for.*

Teilhard de Chardin tells us it is easier to love if it is personalized, rather than abstract:

> "If the universe assumes a face and a heart, and so to speak personifies itself, then in the atmosphere created by the focus of the elemental attraction it will immediately blossom." [12]

The axis mundi and anima mundi form the most basic relationship there is—the relationship betweeen consciousness within and the world without. It is the primordial division through which the universe sees itself. Its dynamic flow of energy creates what is said to be the basic creative matrix, the torus, as shown in the opposite diagram.

AS EASY AS X, Y, Z

The poetic and the veridical, the proven and the unprovable, the heart and the brain——like charged particles of opposing polarity——exert their pulls in different directions. Where they are brought together the result is incandescence. [13]

—Pierre Teilhard de Chardin

What are the realms that need to be united with this perspective? What divorced entities need to be brought back into relationship once again to achieve the integration and wholeness of the heart?

We have correlated the Static Masculine era with the sign of the cross, which can either unite or divide, depending on how you look at it. If we look at the lines of the cross as drawing divisions, then it separates above and below, left and right. If you look at the lines of the cross as drawing connections, then it unites these aspects. Georg Feuerstein has suggested that the cross of crucifixion was a symbol of

Axis Mundi and Anima Mundi

Axis Mundi

Anima Mundi

Anima Mundi

Axis Mundi

an axis mundi intersecting with the horizontal world axis.[14]

This was the initiation symbol of the Static Masculine era—but it is time now to take that cross and give it another dimension. It is time to add a Z axis to the already existing X and Y axes. We can use these axes, not as separation, but as a means of joining. In that burst from flatland to three-dimensional space, we enter the spiral of the Dynamic Feminine, which moves beyond the linear separation of the arms of the cross and opens a three dimensional spiral of expansion. That which has been separated is rejoined and made whole again, the linear made circular, and flatland made mountainous.

Let's examine the possibilities that can be created by synthesizing dualities along these lines. (See diagram p. 284.)

THE VERTICAL Y AXIS

The Y axis integrates above and below, which represents mind and body, Heaven and Earth, spirit and matter, science and religion. It is to strengthen the axis mundi that comprises the core organization of the self. This vertical axis gives the other two axes a place to anchor.

Mind and Body

We have described the vertical core of the self as the axis mundi—the central *I* that runs through each one of us, extending from above the crown to the roots below. This is the Y axis, awakened by moving both downward and upward: through the Underworld journeys that break down and reconstitute the soul, and through the upward ascension to higher consciousness. When mind and body are separated, however, this axis is severed. The top can't get to the bottom; the bottom cannot rise to the top. Like social strata, they remain separated, unable to influence or join with each other.

As individuals, the healing of this breach occurs through the integration of mind and body, which I consider the cutting edge of personal healing. We are now learning that chronic emotional states can cause physical disease, and that illness is strongly influenced by beliefs. We are discovering that the mind works better in a healthy body, and that yoga postures affect consciousness. We know without a doubt that chemistry alters awareness, for better or worse, whether through antidepressants, food additives, coffee, or recreational drugs. As a twenty year practitioner of somatic therapy, I have been witness to the profound changes that occur when insight is connected to the body, and body sensations are awakened into conscious realization of their meaning.

To reclaim the severed connection between mind and body is the awakening of embodied truth. In a world that denies the body, we live disembodied lives—spending much of our working life typing on a computer, driving a vehicle, bombarded by noise, eating things that can barely be called food, harming ourselves and each other out of numbness and ignorance. By integrating mind and body, we heal the primary relationship *within* the self that precludes any other relationship. Together, mind and body become a *Thou*.

Heaven and Earth

To join the realms of above and below on an outer level is to reunite Heaven and Earth. The Chinese book of wisdom, the *I Ching*, says much about the importance of this relationship. In Hexagram 12, (called Stagnation), the symbol for Heaven is above, and the symbol for Earth below. Its interpretation is not optimal:

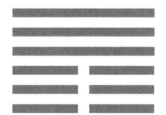

"Heaven is above, drawing farther and farther away, while the earth below sinks farther into the depths. The creative powers are not in relation. It is a time of standstill and decline." [15]

In hexagram 11 titled T'ai or Peace, Heaven is below and Earth is above.

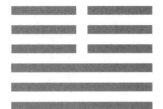 "The Receptive, which moves downward, stands above; the Creative, which moves upward, is below. Hence their influences meet and are in harmony, so that all living things bloom and prosper."

To bring the kingdom of Heaven down to Earth is to turn our spiritual reverence toward the exquisite harmony, beauty, and perfection of Nature. The Earth *is* divine. As believed in the era of the Great Mother, the Earth is infused with spirit, animate and living. As Jesus tried to teach us, the divine kingdom of Heaven *is* right here on Earth. It is intelligent, conscious, with a vitality beyond appearances. There is no contradiction. Healing this fundamental split leads to wholeness.

Science and Religion

To integrate Heaven and Earth is to validate the relationship between spirit and matter. As such memorable books as Fritjof Capra's *The Tao of Physics,* or Ken Wilber's *The Marriage of Sense and Soul* have suggested, science and religion are beginning to converge. The deeper we look into the cosmos—be it micro or macro—the more science looks like mysticism. Many sciences grew out of mystical traditions: chemistry grew out of alchemy, astronomy from astrology, physics from natural philosophy.[16] Essentially, science and religion are trying to do the same thing: explain the mysteries of creation and give us guidelines for how best to live.

About their separation, Ken Wilber says this: "So here is the utterly bizarre structure of today's world: a scientific framework that is global in its reach and omnipresent in its information and communication networks, forms a meaningless skeleton within which hundreds of sub-global, premodern religions create value and meaning for billions; and they each—science and religion each—tend to deny significance, even reality to the other.... This is exactly why many social analysts believe that if some sort of reconciliation between science and religion is not forthcoming, the future of humanity is, at best, precarious."[17]

In Wilber's analysis, science gives us truth without personal meaning, while religion gives us meaning, without empirical truth. The commonality, says Wilber, resides in the fact that they both describe a Great Nest of Being, a holarchy of self-organization, from subatomic particles to galaxies and from primitive to expanded states of consciousness. In Wilber's view, this takes place in the realm of four quadrants, two of which represent the interior *I* and the external *It,* and two of which represent the plural *We* and external *Its.*[18]

Science and religion are discovering the relationship between spirit and matter. Quantum physics has shown us that the observer influences the experiment. Emotional states have chemical correlates; chemistry affects consciousness. There is now statistical evidence that distant prayer can effect healing.[19] Physician and author Larry Dossey has done extensive investigation into this phenomenon. He describes three eras in medicine—the first being "mechanical medicine," the second "psychosomatic medicine," and the third based on non-local mind. In double-blind studies with AIDS patients and heart patients, significantly more healing resulted in the groups that had received prayer. This power of positive intention affects even mice and bacteria! [20]

Consciousness and Matter

Matter and consciousness are two ends of the spectrum that inform our reality. Without consciousness, matter would remain inert. We would be unaware of its beauty, its usefulness, or its guidance along the signposts of life. Without matter, consciousness would have nothing to focus upon, no edges to contemplate, no challenges to solve. Duane Elgin states this beautifully: "Without matter to push against, consciousness . . .would remain undisturbed and unknown. Matter makes life specific, tangible, and undeniable. The... mirroring qualities of consciousness are anchored by the concrete reality of the material dimensions."[21] He follows this to say: "Without an observing potential, matter would never know of its own existence and would not have the ability to pull itself together into an organic system and evolve to higher levels of self-referencing and self-organized functioning."[22]

Both matter and consciousness are partners in a dynamic dance of mutual influence and co-creative evolution. Each informs the other, each is enhanced by the other. Together, they form an integration that reflects the essence of who we are.

THE HORIZONTAL X AXIS

The horizontal X axis unites aspects of a single thing that has polarities. For example, the terms rational and intuitive both describe modes of thinking; masculine and feminine are two aspects of human expression; progressives and conservatives both represent political value systems; God and Goddess are both aspects of the divine. It is important to realize that these things are not separate entities, but exist along a continuum. There are progressive conservatives, for example, and rational intuitives, masculine women and feminine men. You can't have one without the other as they are inherently unified, or even defined by their opposite.

However, we often get caught up in trying to sort out which one is the right one, trying to land squarely on one side or the other. Is rational better than intuitive, is white better than black? Do we vote Republican or Democrat? Conservative or progressive? Are you male or female, strong or weak? Or as George Bush once stated, "You're either with us or you're a terrorist." Such polarized thinking takes us away from the core, away from the vertical axis, away from integration. It fools us into thinking such dualities can be solved. Because they are, in fact, unified, the more we favor one, the more the other tries to get our attention. We have seen how the bright light of Christianity cast an equally dark shadow. We are seeing how the tug of war between political factions creates gridlock in our political process. We narrow our range, and throw ourselves out of balance, whenever we feature only one side.

To come back to center, we need to see the essential qualities of both sides of a continuum. We need to value our enemy's perspective, look for the commonalities, and transcend differences, moving to a place where they are integrated at a higher level. This does not collapse them into an homogenized sameness, but honors both polarities as expressions of a higher unity.

Masculine and Feminine

The balance between masculine and feminine is one of the most basic and necessary social healings we can make at this time. Emerging from the last five thousand years of our collective middle childhood, where "boys" and "girls" played in separate realms, we are now like adolescents, just beginning to create equal, authentic relationships–in the home, in the workplace, in government, religion, and education.

Clearly, we have a long way to go to achieve this balance. Women still earn far less than men. They only won the right to vote as recently as 1920, and still comprise a small percentage of government in most countries, while in other countries, they cannot even show their faces in public. Most educational institutions are founded almost entirely on Static Masculine principles, developing intellectual intelligence more than emotional, and teaching by linear logic more than by experience. In the religious realm, this divide is most marked of all, at least in the mainstream. Roman Catholics still do not allow women to become priests, and the church hierarchy that sets moral standards argues against birth control, abortion and divorce. Jews are just beginning to accept women rabbis. Islam seems farthest behind of all, with some sects inflicting heinous attitudes of brutality toward women, such as the Taliban in Afghanistan. The elite class, politically and financially, is still an "old boy's network," much as it was in ancient times. To succeed in such a world, women often become masculinized – forfeiting their innate rhythms and social style for power in the male world.

Volumes have been written on this subject. What I have tried to show in these pages is that history has progressed as a developmental process from our own childishness and naïvete. We can waste precious energy blaming men for the war machine into which they were indoctrinated so long ago in order to protect their families. We can blame women for not stepping up to the plate, forgetting the millennia of oppression that kept them down. Both genders have been oppressed. Both have essential contributions to make to the whole. And both males and females can be damaging when they have absolute power, unbalanced by the other.

With the oppression of women over the last five thousand years, we have seriously robbed the world of the feminine contribution. Not only women, but men have also suffered as a result of this. Men have been robbed of the softness, the balance, the beauty, and the renewal that the feminine can bring. Their work lives are often hard and cold, inhumane and competitive. Urban environments so often lack beauty and harmony that we shut down our senses in order to live there.

The archetypal Sacred Marriage or *hierosgamos* is an integration of masculine and feminine, God and Goddess, and in many ways of all polarities within the self. This is not predicated on gender. Both men and women have internal opposites to integrate. It is not about male-female intimate relationships, but about the qualities brought to any relationship—gay, straight, brothers and sisters, co-workers, and co-creators. Just as this integration occurs within the self as a part of maturation, it needs also to occur within our organizations, families, communities, governments, educational, and financial institutions in order to stimulate our social maturation.

A global era of the heart is one in which men and women work and play together as equals, each enhancing the other. In order to retain the individuality that both masculine and feminine can bring, however, it is necessary for each gender to be strengthened by contact with their own kind. Women's groups, men's groups, and time alone for each person, can strengthen their remembrance of their inner nature, so that it does not get lost when brought into relationship with the opposite. This is especially true for women,

	STATIC FEMININE	DYNAMIC MASCULINE	STATIC MASCULINE	DYNAMIC FEMININE
CENTRAL ARCHETYPES	Mother-Son	Warrior-king	Father-daughter	Partnership
ORGANIZING PRINCIPLE	Nature	Kingship	Written Law	Self-organizing systems
VALUES	Birth, Magic, Nature, Body, Tribe, Cycles, Tradition	Conquest, Trade, Wealth, Sacrifice, Dominion	Obedience, Control, Rationality, Industry	Freedom, Creativity, Participation, Community, Ecology
ACCOMPLISHMENTS	Cave Art, Prehistoric Sculpture, Tools, Farming, Pottery, Weaving	Writing, Mathematics, Militarization, Trade, Architecture, Empires	Philosophy, Literacy, Industry, Education, Science, Middle Class	Global Communication, Visual Media, Information, Human Rights, Gender equality
CHALLENGES	Survival	War, Slavery	Poverty, Pollution, War	Maturity, Complexity
ERA	Paleolithic and Neolithic	Bronze and Iron Ages	Antiquity to Christian Era	Information era to scientific revolution

who get subsumed into the masculine culture, and can easily forget who they are. Both *I* and *Thou* need to retain their distinct character for a true relationship.

Static and Dynamic *(see chart pp. 279, 281.)*

Our collective history reveals four distinct social patterns among static and dynamic, masculine and feminine archetypal dynamics. We began with the Static Feminine, back in the times of the Great Mother. This was followed by the overthrow of the Mother by the aggression of the Dynamic Masculine in the creation of early civilizations. We saw how the Dynamic Masculine then evolved into the Static Masculine rigidity of law and order. We finally looked at the newly emerging Dynamic Feminine, with its free-flowing creativity, and its emphasis on relationship and community.

None of these archetypal patterns ever rule by themselves. There are always elements of each quality in any given time period and stage of life. Each pattern has its positive aspects, each has its shadow, as shown on the opposite page. What is important is to integrate all four aspects into our evolving social system. The Static Feminine provides nourishment and stability, with respect for Nature and her limits. The Dynamic Masculine provides power and innovation. The Static Masculine provides order and knowledge. And the Dynamic Feminine provides freedom and creativity. Thus the static and dynamic fluctuations in a system behave as complimentary principles for balancing stability and innovation, constancy and change.

East and West

The Chicago meeting of the World Parliament of Religions in 1893 marked the first formal gathering of Eastern and Western spiritual traditions. It is recognized as the birthplace of worldwide interfaith dialog. Master yogi Swami Vivikenanda, a student of Ramakrishna, attended the gathering, and later traveled throughout the U.S. to spread the yoga tradition. In the nineteenth and twentieth centuries,

Positive and Negative Characteristics of Masculine and Feminine Eras

Dynamic Masculine

Positive	Negative
Assertive	Dominating
Commanding	Violent
Adventurous	Reckless
Powerful	Tyrannical
Transformative	Destructive
Heroic	Egotistical
Innovative	Disrespectful
Differentiating	Negating

Static Masculine

Positive	Negative
Stable	Rigid
Ordering	Controlling
Systematic	Bureaucratic
Detached	Dissociated
Sets Standards	Disempowers
Benevolent	Punishing
Intellectual	Heady

Static Feminine

Positive	Negative
Sustaining	Devouring
Stable	Restrictive
Cyclic	Boring
Wholeness	Infancy
Unified	Unconscious
Grounded	Limited
Good Mother	Bad Mother

Dynamic Feminine

Positive	Negative
Transformative	Chaotic
Creative	Undisciplined
Erotic	Indulgent
Playful	Irresponsible
Egalitarian	Indiscriminate
Inclusive	Boundary-less
Holistic	Undifferentiated
Imaginative	Unrealistic
Free	Unfocused

many Eastern texts were translated, and even Jung explored the chakras in his book *The Psychology of Kundalini Yoga.* [23]

As we saw in the Dynamic Feminine chapter, the psychedelic revolution opened some minds to the miracle of consciousness and the need for a healthy body, reviving interest in yoga and meditation. The Dalai Lama's forced exile from Tibet has brought his wisdom more prominently to the West. Yoga centers are sprouting up everywhere and books on Buddhism, Hinduism, Zen, and other Eastern traditions are numerous enough to fill whole bookstores.

The East has a rich spiritual tradition, but is marked in many places by material poverty. The West has a strong material base, but it could be argued that it suffers from spiritual poverty. The Eastern traditions reflect the values of the upper chakras, while the Western lifestyle is more centered on the lower chakras. To combine the two is to echo all that we have been saying about the heart—both the integration of left and right, upper and lower realms, balanced and integrated in the heart.

The Z Axis

The Z axis runs forward and backward through the center at right angles to the other two axes. I think of this axis as integrating the inner self and the outer world, the individual and the collective, as well as past and future. Here we see the importance of balance between unity and diversity, collective welfare and individual rights, activist extroversion with mystic introversion, community needs and self-interest. The Z axis represents the basic *I-Thou* relationship between the inner world and the outer.

Neither can be held at the cost of the other. Each holon needs to be whole in itself, and each needs to be in service of a larger whole. It is not I *or Thou* , but I *and Thou* . Our individuality is a contribution to the whole, one that serves diversity and supports unity. We cannot change the world by merely sitting alone in meditation, nor can we change it without renewing our own center through contemplative practices. When spirituality includes appropriate activism, and activism is informed spiritually, we are integrated along the Z axis.

The Z axis also aligns past and future, whose center is, of course, the present. By understanding our past, we can become more conscious of the dangers and possibilities in our future. Those who have brought the past to light have a better chance of freeing themselves from its unconscious dictates. Facing forward, we define ourselves by how we orient to the future. Where we are going defines who we are, what we're about, and what we are becoming. The heart at the center is the moment of now, the moment of experience, the only moment in which we can create change.

A RETURN TO WHOLENESS

If these three axes are brought into balanced and integrated relationship, we have the basis for a self-organizing system of relationship that could transform our severed society into wholeness once again. In a complex world that seems to be falling apart, this rejoining is the coming together that can bring us to the peace of the heart, through aligning the elements of the world and our psyches in right relationship.

The key archetypal symbol in the heart chakra (see p. 285) is two intersecting triangles, one pointing up and one pointing down—also the symbol of the sacred marriage, or *hierosgamos*. Mythically, this occurs between a God and Goddess, equal archetypes of masculine and feminine divinity, who enter into a balanced and cooperative relationship based on love. But it also occurs along each of these axes: The Y axis uniting above and below, The X axis uniting polarized expressions of one kind of thing, and the Z axis aligning within and without. This integration restores an original wholeness that opens the realms of the global heart.

Unification of
X, Y and Z Axes

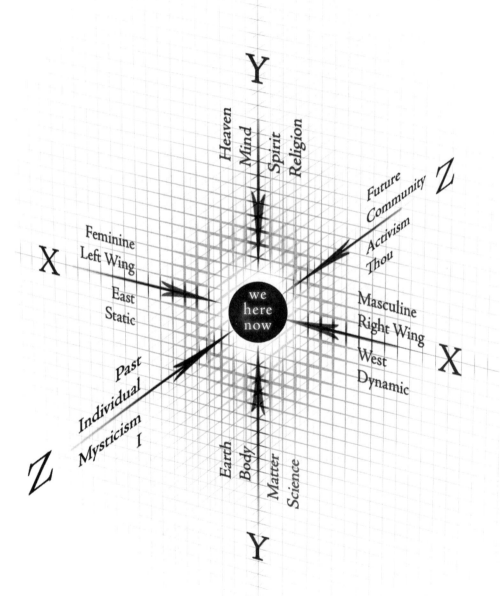

ESSENTIAL POINTS

• We can examine living systems through three basic modes of inquiry: the *rational, mythic,* and *evolutionary.* These levels are based respectively on the relationship of *I-it, I-thou,* and *We.*

• To get to the evolutionary *We* requires understanding the world as a sentient *Thou.*

• The *I and Thou* relationship can be described as occurring between the *axis mundi* and the *anima mundi,* or the vertical channel within each of us and the soul of the world.

• This kind of relationship can be used to reunite severed realms into an integrated wholeness. These realms include Heaven and Earth, mind and body, science and religion, spirit and matter, masculine and feminine, East and West, static and dynamic, inner and outer, individual and community, and past and future.

• The integration of these three levels of systems inquiry, and the synthesis of divorced polarities, can lead to a paradigm of wholeness, at the center of which lies the heart.

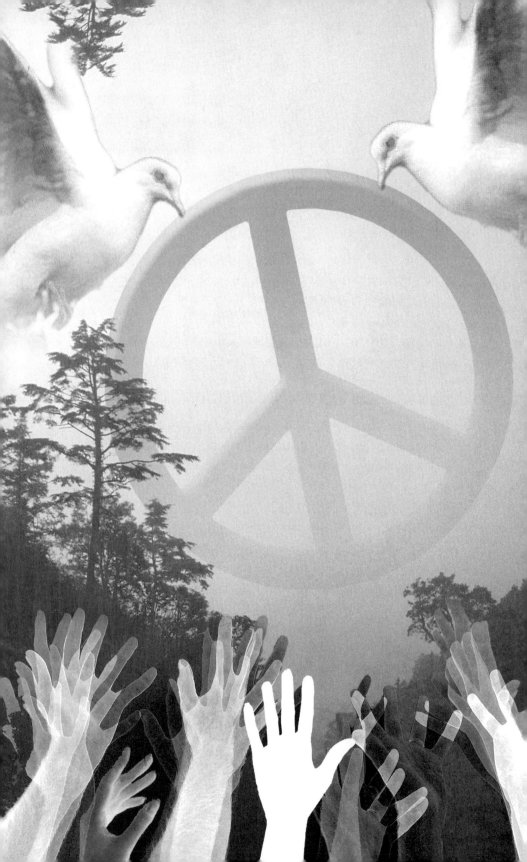

CHAPTER 16

REALMS OF THE HEART

Opening the Global Chambers

> *No matter how upside-down it all may temporarily appear, we will have no fear because we know this secret: Life is crazily in love with us — wildly and innocently in love with us. The universe always gives us exactly what we need, exactly when we need it.... Love is an act of heroic genius.*[1]

—Rob Brezny

We are the first beings with the intelligence to grasp how much we are loved. The eternal *Thou* has been courting our love with incredible gifts of abundance and beauty since time began: a planet with the perfect balance of temperature, gases, and gravity for our form of life; the immeasurable beauty of mountains and flowers, trees and birds, even in remote places we might never see, and a food supply of unending variety. The heavens provide fluffy clouds to shade the sun and make glorious sunsets by evening, followed by a canopy of stars to remind us of eternity, with a single white moon to light our way in the dark. Our bodies are exquisitely designed for the journey. Our brains surpass anything we've encountered in other species. Not only can we perceive the many colors and sounds, smells, textures, and tastes of the world around us—we can penetrate their mysteries.

We are the first animal with the capacity to contemplate the vastness and complexity of this creation. Without wings or fast legs, we've created means of transportation to traverse the whole garden, with a long life in which to travel. The Gods have been good to us. The World Parents have been kind. The greatest gift we can give in return is to mature into glorious beings, worthy of our inheritance. It is time to walk into an *I-thou* relationship and allow ourselves to experience profound love.

How do we embrace the eternal *Thou* in a relationship of sacred reciprocity? How do we open our own hearts? How do we serve the global heart? What are its realms and its requirements? What can we do to help birth the emerging Age of the Heart?

BEGIN THIS AT HOME

Waking the global heart begins with you. It radiates outward from your daily thoughts and actions. It begins with awakening your capacity to really love, with the joy of giving service, and the inclusion in a higher purpose. It begins with your daily offering, your way of making something–anything–a little better than you found it.

It is there, with arms open, at any moment you stop and witness the amazing miracle of creation swirling around you. Each time you remember, the trees will whisper to each other that it is beginning. The wind will carry the word. Somewhere, someone will breathe a little deeper.

No matter how elaborate the theory, the question always remains: What can I do differently, today and tomorrow? The following points outline some of the major areas in which the heart flourishes. It is a place to begin, a daily practice to develop. For each of our hearts is a cell in the global heart, giving and receiving love. Each time we create an act of love, we inspire others to do the same.

Gratitude
Imagine that you are giving a gift to each of two children. One claps delightedly, thanking you, and runs off to play, enjoying and appreciating her gift. The other plays with the gift briefly then tosses it aside, or complains, "This isn't what I wanted!" Which child opens

your heart? To which child do you want to give more? The *Thou* to which we relate, whether it is a person, a workplace, a garden, or a community, responds no differently.

The heart opens when you truly appreciate the many gifts of your life. The food you eat each day that someone else grew, harvested, trucked, and sold; entertainment at the flick of a switch; instant access to the world's information; clothing that's just your size, a climate-controlled shelter to sleep in—all these are here to support you in making your contribution. They take away the struggles of survival so that you can see farther, higher, longer, so that you can give more of your gifts. Can you receive these blessings and say, "Thank you!" with all of your heart?

Now for the harder part: Can you be just as grateful for your challenges? Think back on the difficulties you've faced in the past. How much did you grow? What did you learn? Where did they lead you? To curse the world is to separate from it. To thank your fate is to move through the lessons more quickly. When tragedies occur, simple things that we take for granted become as precious as life itself: water, food, shelter, clothing, legs that can walk, hands that can reach , eyes that can see, friends or strangers that help us out. To those who have lost these things, their return is a rich blessing, each one met with immense gratitude.

What we appreciate appreciates. Gratitude is a remembrance of all that we have received. It inspires us to give something back.

Generosity
A common question often asked at cocktail parties is, "What do you do for a living?" We might better ask, "What do you offer the world?" or perhaps, "What is your give-away?" For some people, their work and their offering are one and the same. For others, work is just an exchange in order to receive a paycheck that allows them to then *get* what they want.

If gratitude opens the heart, then generosity gives it wings. The real test of character—that which lasts beyond our brief life—is what did we leave behind? What did we improve? There is freedom and lightness when an act is done without the purpose of reward. We work hard to *get* the things we want. What if that effort went equally into giving?

Success occurs when you leave something better than you find it. If you have a relationship, and your partner is better off because of your influence, that relationship has been a success, whether or not it lasts forever. If you work at a business, and each day you leave it in better shape because of what you've offered, your work has been a success. If you visit someone's house and leave it cleaner than you found it, you have left behind a gift of grace.

You have an opportunity to give at every moment. Whatever you can create as an offering, whatever help you can give, whatever compassion and empathy you can extend beyond yourself, do it now. Contribute to the future. Make it a priority. Ask what you can give rather than what you can take. Even if it is just a daily prayer, or a small act like picking garbage off the street, do something *daily* to improve the world around you.

If you have money, contribute to struggling organizations that are working to save this world. Help someone go to school, get out of debt, start a business. If you have time, volunteer at a non-profit you believe in. If you have influence, use it to create change, inspiring others to work from the heart. If you have artistic talent, make an offering where it is most needed – singing in a retirement home, beautifying your street, or reading poetry to prisoners. If you have more than enough of something, give some away. Even if you think you could sell them, see what it feels like to just give some of your possessions away.

Think of something wild and crazy to do as a surprise for someone. Create a special present: clean their house, babysit for their children, mow their lawn, leave cookies on their front porch. If you really want to challenge yourself, do this for someone you scarcely know—or even someone you dislike!

Empathy and Compassion

Empathy is the connective tissue of an *I-thou* relationship. If generosity gives the heart wings, then empathy gives the heart its ground. It occurs whenever we can see and feel another's experience. It is the glue of relationships, the sacred connection with another person's interior, the key to *I* and *thou.*

Empathy is the building block of compassion. It begins by learning to listen with the heart. Here we drop all judgment and preoccupation with our own dramas. We simply extend our awareness to include and appreciate another's experience. Much of this happens on a feeling level, for feelings are the texture of experience. When we feel *with* another, we open to compassion, which literally means to feel someone's suffering. The opposite of compassion is judgment , which only comprehends the outer behavior, not the inner experience. Compassion is the warp and woof of the heart's tapestry. The Dalai Lama tells us:

> "As long as you have compassion, you will be free of the deepest anxiety. The capacity to devote yourself to the welfare of others yields otherwise unobtainable power and potentional for good. Generate great compassion, and you become a friend to all sentient beings, a companion to all other altruistic beings and a cherished child of the enlightened."[2]

The next stage of moral development rests on the cultivation of compassion. It begins by being in touch with your own wounds and longings. It expands by being in touch with the suffering of others. It is expressed in the dedication to relieve that suffering as much as you can. As natural disasters and tragedies are blasted through the media, and as the Internet connects more people from disparate parts of the world, we have ample opportunity to practice compassion.

Acceptance

Gratitude, compassion, and forgiveness all lead to acceptance. The heart says "yes" when you settle into acceptance of how you are right now, so that you can truly be here fully, in this moment. The heart purrs approvingly when you apply that acceptance to others, and appreciate their beauty in spite of their flaws. Each person you see struggles against gravity each morning; each one has faced troubles and loss, obstacles and lessons. Each one is doing the best they can with the tools they have. If you find yourself criticizing others, ask instead how you can help. For each of us truly wants to live the best way we can—we just need a little help in doing so.

The heart's sweetest blessing—and one that brings waves of gratitude—is the realization that what is here is enough, that we don't need more. It is amplified by reflecting the light we see in another back and forth until it is bright enough to light the world and herald a new dawn.

Forgiveness

In my former role as a therapist, I often told my clients, "Resentment is like drinking poison and hoping the other person will die." Resentment anchors us in negativity without changing our reality. Forgiveness, by contrast, frees the heart to love again.

Forgiveness is not the same as condoning. It doesn't mean that what someone did to you was OK. It just means you are releasing yourself from the past and letting go of blaming your more difficult teachers. It doesn't mean you have to go back into relationship with the person who harmed you, but it does create more freedom to love, by letting go of that relationship and moving on. Forgiveness allows us to practice compassion and acceptance.

Often, forgiveness can only happen when the emotional work of healing the wounds has been done. For those wounds need to be felt and grieved. Anger may need to be appropriately expressed, then released. Once the emotional clearing has taken place, forgiveness completes the healing process.

When we, ourselves, have been the wrongdoers, forgiveness is courted through genuine apology. This can only come from taking the time to see the harm we caused—not as a criticism we must defend against—but from a place of empathy and compassion, seeing the other's reality from an *I-thou* perspective. Too often we say a hollow, "I'm sorry," without taking the time to empathize deeply.

Celebration

The realm of the heart is filled with what you love and the things that make you happy. It is made from the willingness to not only protect what you love, but to enhance it—polish it until it shines, feed it your lavish attention, and bring it into the center of your life. Make yourself happy! If you love the wilderness, spend as much time there as possible. If you love music, play it often; listen to it even more. If you love children, find ways to spend more time with them.

Let what you love occupy the center of your life. Make the fulfillment of your longing your highest priority. When your longing is answered, you will have cause to celebrate.

The heart is nourished by celebration and play, pleasure and beauty, creativity and laughter. These are the seeds of love. They are the ground from which it grows, and they are present in every new relationship. It is not a loving act to wish suffering on anyone. Why would the *anima mundi,* the soul of the world, wish suffering upon humankind? Joy is a sign that the heart is open. Contentment is a result. Foster the age of the heart with glorious celebration, creative collaboration, and passionate production of continuous delight.

TAKE IT TO THE WORLD

By living the values of the heart—in all our choices, large and small—we steer the course of civilization toward the next age. These values are based on love more than power, on relationships more than things, on contribution more than acquistion, on cooperation more than competition, on networks rather than markets, and by becoming co-creative contributors, rather than individual consumers.

What is possible is beyond our wildest imaginings. Yet the seeds of it are already planted, within our deepest dreams and desires. Each of us has a longing that is urging us on; each of us carries a piece of the grand puzzle. We can name the trends that we wish to see, calling others to join us. We can choose the values we wish to live by, and continually reflect on who we are, where we are, and what we are becoming. The tendrils of these dreams are already sprouting. Even now their shoots are poking above the ground!

The following five categories describe essential realms that comprise a global era of the heart. They are existing trends that have been growing for some time. They are all moving in the direction of the values we have discussed: freedom, compassion, ecological sustainability, service, creativity, relatedness, and transcendence. May the various factions and organizations within these trends recognize each other as imaginal cells in the emerging butterfly, and join forces cooperatively. May you, the reader, find resonance with these trends and help them come into being. And may our shared values of a possible future replace the fundamentalist values of the imperial past.

PEACE

The holiest of all spots on Earth is where an ancient hatred has become a present love.

—Kokoman Clottey and Aeeshah Ababio-Clottey[3]

World peace is the most essential outer realization of our time. As great as the invention of writing or mathematics, airplanes or computers, greater than the discovery of subatomic particles or the creation of the great cathedrals, the accomplishment of world peace will produce blessings we can barely imagine. By harvesting the resources tragically wasted in aggression and defense, we can redirect our intelligence, capital, creativity, and collaborative efforts toward solving our many problems. It is doubtful we will solve them any other way.

The Sanskrit name of the heart chakra gives us a clue to its secret.

Anahata means "sound that is made without any two things striking," also translated as "unstruck or unhurt." This implies a direct correlation between opening the heart and refraining from causing harm. Only when people are not being harmed can they be free of defenses, free to be their true self, and therefore make their unique offering to the whole. This requires a level of sophistication that transcends third chakra aggression and domination as a way to solve problems, and moves toward communication and cooperation.

Peace is not merely the absence of warfare, any more than true health is simply the absence of disease. Nor is peace simply a quiet state of equilibrium–impossible to achieve in an evolving system. Though refraining from harm is an essential first step, lasting peace is created by actively redressing harm already done. Peace is a creative process of actively joining *I* and *thou* into a co-creative *we*. It requires authentic communication, empathetic listening, and wildly creative solutions.

Communication and creativity–related to the throat chakra directly above the heart–is a way of lifting us out of power and into cooperation, a way of fostering empathy, compassion, and forgiveness. For the first time since the military mentality of the first civlizations, we have the means of global communication. When conducted through an autonomous self-organizing system such as the Internet, we have the technological means of experiencing a global group mind. As communication technology gets ever more sophisticated, we need to simultaneously increase our skills at communicating. Colleges and universities now offer programs in conflict resolution, peace negotiation, and mediation.

Michael Nagler, author of *The Search for a Nonviolent Future,* advises us to overcome the habit of using violent language in our communication, much as we sensitized ourselves to sexist language in the past few decades. To speak of a war against poverty, a war against drugs, a battle of the sexes, combatting racisim, even the fight for freedom, is to continue a way of thinking that is based on conflict. While these issues are all important, we need to focus on solutions rather than battle. Instead we can speak of healing poverty, rehabilitating drug users, integrating the sexes, honoring minorities, and claiming our freedom.

When the news continually directs our attention to stories of violence and gore, when we incessantly focus on what's wrong in each other (or ourselves), when we pit one side against another in all our debates, we are only affirming the old story. In truth, our age is not nearly as violent as the five thousand years of sibling rivalry that has led us to this point. We are simply more *aware* of the violence, and find it ever more intolerable. It permeates not only our language, but our thoughts, our games and entertainment, and of course, our actions.

The movement toward peace has been in process for a long time. That there is such as thing as a war crimes tribunal is progress. That the invasion of Iraq was debated as long and widely as it was, is progress. That fewer died in the first *year* of the Iraq war than in a some *days* during the First World War is actually progress. It may not be fast enough to stave off the insane perpetuation of suffering that occurs daily, but it is clear that there is a worldwide trend away from war and towards peace. This is part of our maturation as a species.

On February 15, 2003, ten million people around the world marched for peace. Not just in Washington and San Francisco, New York and Boston, but in Paris, London, Madrid, Rome, Berlin, Copenhagen, Tokyo and Mexico City—and many others. Many of these nations represented were not going to war, but their people turned out in record numbers to plead with the U.S. to avoid the debacle that has driven young Iraqi boys to such desperation that they explode themselves in suicide missions. There is only one way to end terrorism, and that is to create a world in which it has no purpose.

When we make elements of peace into something triumphant and sexy; when good deeds are celebrated on front page headlines; when the wars within us find resolution, we create peace day by day. We direct attention to the fact that it *is* possible, that it *is* occurring, and by this act, we help it increase. We can make peace a central value in our emerging mythic system—something we are moving toward, that draws us inexorably through to the future.

War not only takes valuable resources from where we need it most but it perpetuates wounds for generations. For the other implication of the name *anahata* as "unstruck," or "unhurt," is that we must heal our own wounds for the heart to truly awaken.

No one escapes being hurt somewhere along their journey. Wounding and betrayal, abuse or trauma, disappointment and loss—these painful demons come to us all, and leave their marks upon the heart. In response, we tend to wall off our hearts. We create a separation inside, a kind of war within ourselves, which, like all wars, creates suffering, numbing, and wastes precious energy. War against Nature, war within our own nature, war against others, and war against nations—it's all been around for so long that many people believe that war is simply an inevitable fact of human nature. The maturation process that is now being asked of us is to change that belief and find another way to solve difficulties.

When forces that have been locked in struggle and aggression find their way into peace, there is a vibration of harmony that can be heard by all. So many times in my past therapy practice, when someone integrates warring parts of themselves, or resolves a deep conflict with another, there are cries of relief and tears of joy—the sound of a soul coming back home to its natural state of wholeness. This results in a deep peace that comes—not from self-control, laws, or regimentation—but from deep, inner healing. When old battles are resolved and wounds are healed, there is more room for the heart to truly open and love.

What would be the sound of "no two things striking" heard round the world when at last arms are laid to rest, nuclear weapons dismantled, and the newspapers no longer feature violence on the front page? What would be the sound on the radio that announced that humanity, had, at last, put an end to war as a means of solving differences? What kind of programs could be supported by our tax dollars? What kind of news might we talk about instead? Does this sound Utopian? Perhaps, but it is necessary nonetheless.

The achievement of global peace is a survival imperative. For the escalation of weapons will surely make war obsolete—either by eliminating the species that persists in it, or eliminating the weapons themselves. In the larger world, the sound of no two things striking is the chorus of harmony rising from the masses, the great unfurling of evolution, set once again on its course of synthesis, after thousands of years of divergence. For when society is ordered around violence and militarism, enormous energies and funds are squandered that could otherwise be used creatively.

In the words of Michael Nagler, professor of nonviolence at the University of California at Berkeley: "Nonviolence is a creative force that contains within itself the principle of creative order." The creative potential that is awaiting us when we no longer spend the bulk of our energy and tax dollars in battle with other parts of our collective selves is literally beyond our imagining. When we are no longer engaged in the duality of win-lose, we must instead invent creative solutions. When whole populations are no longer oppressed, then their creativity can be unleashed. The song that is waiting to arise is a harmonic, multi-symphonic masterpiece of creation singing the morningsong that signals the dawn of a new era.

At a party not too long ago, I met a man, Nick Turner, who claimed to channel a being from the future. Skepticism in hand, I asked him, just out of curiosity, what would happen after we achieved world peace (with the optimistic assumption that we would someday). His reply was immediate, and has always stayed with me: "Then this planet will be ready for membership in galactic civilization." Assuming that there is such a thing, it makes sense that a planet would have to achieve a level of maturity that transcends violence in order to interface with alien life forms. If, indeed, a galactic civilization exists that we have not yet had the technological or spiritual maturity to encounter, what gifts of knowledge await us with this discovery? This, I imagine, would be the start of the age that follows the age of the heart, perhaps a fifth chakra age of galactic communication. But this conjecture is far to the future, for there is much to solve on this planet before we are ready and able to survive contact with an alien *thou*.

In the words of Mahatma Gandhi: "There is no way to peace. Peace is the way."

To this I add: The way of the heart leads to peace. Peace, in turn, opens the heart.

A NEW SYNTHESIS

> *However far science pushes its discovery of the essential fire: and*
> *however capable it becomes some day of remodeling and perfecting*
> *the human element, it will always find itself in the end facing the*
> *same problem—how to give to each and every element its final value*
> *by grouping them in the unity of an organized whole.*
>
> —Pierre Teilhard de Chardin

Thesis, antithesis, synthesis. This is an old story, espoused by philosophers since the beginning of reflective thinking. From Socrates to
Jesus, Goethe, and Hegel, from Karl Marx to the integral world of
Ken Wilber, the song of synthesis has been sung again and again.
This dialectic is one of the basic rhythms of cultural evolution. The
pattern is clear: we begin with a basic thesis; then split off from it to
make something different; then reintegrate with the former thesis
again at a higher, more complex level. From the splitting of chromo-
somes in cell division to the bifurcation of social systems and political
movements, evolution proceeds by differentiation and reunification,
novelty and confirmation.

In our discussion of the X, Y, and Z axes, we see how each synthesis brings us back to the center, where we find the heart. In the
human story, we have examined the broad strokes of cultural history to see how the dynamics of masculine and feminine, static and
dynamic have influenced different areas of history. To recap this story
in terms of the synthesis occurring now, I offer this review:

We began with a basic thesis, as children in the primal garden of
the Great Mother, living in fused symbiosis. We grew and began to act
upon the natural world, planting seeds, irrigating, traveling, building
communities. We then walled ourselves off from Nature, ostensibly
in the name of security, but this began our differentiation and separation. We became ever more distant from our primal ground, instead
aspiring to invisible forces from above, lifting ourselves upward
toward the heavens. We moved from feminine values to masculine
values; from procreation to domination, from the Mother-son motif

to that of Father-daughter. We learned to write, calculate, build, mechanize, print, communicate, relay images, and compute information, until we built the means for a complex industrial society with a planetary communication network–a global brain.

Instead of finding our authority from below, we sought it from above. Instead of organic law, we followed written law. We developed democracy, personal rights, individualism and personal autonomy. Through science and industry, we transformed the world and ourselves. We gave birth to the ego. We even learned, as deconstructionists, to step back and critically evaluate our contemporary cultural milieu.

But in this process, we lost our ground, our health, and, many would say, our souls. We still lived as children under parental dictates. By differentiating, we were caught in an either-or paradigm, between the basic thesis and its antithesis, caught between Nature and civilization, instincts and socialization. The antithesis was necessary to develop our freedom and build a knowledge base necessary to understand the Earth as a whole–but we went so far into individualism that we began to sacrifice the whole, so far into reductionism that we became fragmented. We lost our purpose and our collective moral compass.

We adopted masculine values so completely that the feminine was forgotten. Fight and flight took precedence over tend and befriend. Conquest and achievement became more important than nurturing and care. Separation and detachment held higher value than compassion and connection.

Now, as masculine and feminine forces approach a mutual maturity, we are ready again for a grand synthesis. The archetypal Mother and Father have played their roles in our development. We who are alive today are their children, which means that, quite simply: *We are the synthesis.* We are now ready to enter relationships as adult to adult rather than parent to child, maturing to the point where we take back the reins, and steer the course of evolution in a new direction. As Barbara Marx Hubbard has said, we are moving from "procreation to co-creation," from the primary emphasis on the parent-child relationship, to one of mutual cooperation in the service of co-creating our future.

If the dance of thesis, antithesis, and synthesis has happened repeatedly, what's different now? At our current level of complexity, it is not only a *synthesis of dualities* that is occurring, but *a convergence of plurality.* Today's synthesis is not the creation of a third *thing,* but the process of throwing ourselves headlong into integration itself. Yes, there are many dualities to unite: the politics of left and right, the values of masculine and feminine, the balance between progress and sustainability, civilization and Nature. We must turn *us and them* into *I and thou,* and ultimately *we.* We must integrate mind and body, Heaven and Earth, inner and outer.

But the grandest synthesis in our world today is to to *find a common purpose for a plurality of beings,* a common identity in the holon of a higher order. This requires that we each retain our diverse natures, yet realize a collective identity as members of a global civilization. This grand synthesis does not lose the unique individuality of the parts but establishes *unity in diversity.*

Our growth and success as a species has pushed us up against what writer Duane Elgin, calls the evolutionary wall. He states: *"Our time is unique in one crucial respect: the circle has closed—there is nowhere to escape."*[4] For the first time in our history, the entire human population is confronted with a common predicament whose solution will require us to work together. Just as single-celled organininisms once banded together to make complex creatures; just as our ancestors banded together to create the irrigation projects in the Tigris Euphrates valley; just as there were cooperative efforts to rebuild Europe after WW II; the current crises will call forth global cooperation like nothing ever has before. It is *only* through cooperation that we will solve our collective crises, create a culture of peace, and begin the Age of the Heart. While this cooperation may be mothered by necessity, we may find it has hidden jewels. Learning to work with others different from ourselves can be deeply enriching, enlivening, and heartening.

We are hitting the boundaries of a planet of finite resources and infinite possibilities. Boundaries are the means by which we define something, and it is perhaps this very limitation that can give humanity a new definition as an evolving, global system. Our anxiety may be no less than the pressure of planetary convergence breaking down our isolated selves in the global cauldron that's cooking our collective soup for the next banquet of the gods.

INTERRELATEDNESS

> *Remain true to yourselves, but move ever upward toward greater consciousness and great love! At the summit you will find yourselves united with all those who, from every direction have made the same ascent. For everything that rises must converge."*
>
> —Pierre Teilhard de Chardin

As civilization grows more complex, it is simultaneously becoming increasingly interrelated. We are converging upon ourselves, and this is forcing us to *relate*. Throughout cultural evolution, the trend has been toward uniting larger areas of land, populations, and cultures. In the age of empires, war was a means of conquering differences and congealing them into a larger whole. But now this is happening without war, as humans are brought into increasing contact with each other.

In Europe, twenty-five countries, speaking different languages and living under varying social customs, governments, and economies, have joined together to form the European Union. What seems to be emerging from Europe is the values of a new kind of dream, one that is based on relatedness and the values of the heart. This dream, as Jeremy Rifkin states in his book, *The European Dream,* is quietly eclipsing the more ego-driven individualism of the American Dream. He states that the American dream is:

> "far too centered on personal material advancement and too little concerned with the broader human welfare to be rel-

evant in a world of increasing risk, diversity, and interdependence. It is an old dream, immersed in a frontier mentality, that has long since become passé." By contrast, the European dream: "emphasizes community relationships over individual autonomy, cultural diversity over assimilation, quality of life over the accumulation of wealth, sustainable development over unlimited material growth, deep play over unrelenting toil, universal human rights and the rights of nature over property rights, and global cooperation over the unilateral exercise of power.[5]

He describes one of the emerging differences as occurring between markets and networks. Markets work on thte basis of competition, and are designed to maximize self-interest, with little regard for their effects on other parties. Networks serve self-interest as well, but only by optimizing benefits to others and the group as a whole. Networks maximize creativity, as they come from a larger pool. They work through collaboration more than competition. On the Internet, for example, one's popularity on search engines is based on how much you give, reflected by the number of sites that link to yours. Networks focus on the principles of *sharing and belonging,* whereas markets focus on *ownership and manipulation.* In the shift from valuing things to valuing relationships, Rifkin describes Europeans as placing more value on "belonging than belongings."[6] They see the world less as a storehouse of objects to obtain, and more as a labyrinth of relationships, with value placed on access rather than acquisition.

> "In the new European Dream, freedom is to be enmeshed in interdependent relationships with others. The more inclusive and deeper the relationships, the more likely one will be able to fulfill his or her ambitions. To be included, one requires access. The more access one enjoys, the more relationships one can enter into and the more freedom one experiences."[7]

Modern technology has made possible a global network of consciousness. Information travels through this network at the speed of light. News of any major event reaches broadcasters in a matter of minutes, makes its way to a majority of listeners and readers within hours, and seeps into even outlying areas within days. If intelligence is measured by the speed at which information is absorbed, the global brain is getting pretty damn smart. If intelligence is defined by memory capacity, the Internet is the most colossal storehouse of information next to the biosphere itself, and both have their library doors open round the clock. If intelligence is defined by the ability to learn and evolve, the global brain—at least in geologic time—is organizing itself at lightning speed.

Higher states of consciousness have been defined as ones in which consciousness is omnipresent—everywhere at once. When I can download the weather in Australia from my living room in California, when I can talk to most locations on the globe from an airplane seat eight miles high, and when I can check my e-mail by cell phone while riding a chairlift up a ski slope, I have entered a neural net whose consciousness is simultaneously everywhere.

Pierre Teilhard de Chardin, writing in the 1950s with astounding foresight, named this growing layer of conscious connection the *noosphere*. The noosphere, as an organ of consciousness, is akin to Gaia growing a cerebral cortex. Communication has increased in speed, density, frequency, and connectivity. We are nearing one-fifth of the global population connected to the World Wide Web, and ultimately to each other. We have already learned that increased relatedness hastens evolution. What could happen when this group mind learns to gather its thoughts, focus, and concentrate on the issues at hand?

There are basically three levels in the human brain, which are responsible for different levels of consciousness. The reptilian brain is oriented to eating, sleep, and sex. It is the kill-or-be-killed mentality, and rules the sexual drive and survival instincts. The mammalian brain, or the limbic system, is largely oriented to emotion and bonding. It is the feeling sense, the emotions of rage and joy, envy and loneliness. The cerebral cortex, however, is what makes us distinctly human. It is this latest development of the triune brain that has evolved the intellect of the rational mind, the reasoner and the thinker. The cerebral cortex gave us the mother of invention and the father of abstraction. The frontal lobes of the cerebral cortex in particular are said to be responsible for the ability to plan for the future, and the capacity for compassion and moral behavior. As the authors of *A General Theory of Love* point out: "Emotions reach back 100 million years, while cognition is a few hundred thousand at best."[8]

If the Internet is analogous to a growing cerebral cortex for the planet as a whole, then perhaps the global brain is at last evolving to a state in which the *collective intelligence* becomes capable of future planning, moral behavior and acts of compassion.

Through the Internet, we are faced with a harmonized collectivity of consciousness equivalent to a sort of super-consciousness. Teilhard de Chardin described the noosphere as moving steadily toward a coalescence of consciouness, which he named the Omega Point, a supreme center of a higher order. He describes Omega as a "distinct center radiating at the core of a system of centers."[9] Within this system, each element of consciousness is at least partially centered upon itself. Even when looking outside, our waking consciousness is fundamentally self-referent. He believes that by centering within our own core, we automatically come into association with a greater center that encompasses us all. This is exactly the goal of the axis mundi in relationship to the anima mundi.

In the true sense of holons, each being centered within themselves, yet acting as members of a higher holon, centering brings us into alignment, not only with ourselves, but with our proper place in relationship to the whole. It is this aspect of self-transcendence that brings us to our next major aspect of awakening the heart: spirituality.

SPIRTUALITY

We are as gods, so we might as well get good at it. Stuart Brand

If evolution is God's way of making more gods, then we certainly have a long way to go. We don't look like gods, we certainly don't act like gods, and we don't treat each other *or* ourselves as gods. We are instead wounded, out of shape, unhealthy, insecure, and largely unconscious far too much of the time. *It thus becomes each person's responsibility to work on themselves.* Far from being a purely narcissistic impulse of the boomer generation, self-improvement is an imperative to realize our untapped potential as potential gods. The qualifying difference is whether we engage in this self-improvement from a place of ego—endlessly preening ourselves for a socially sanctioned beauty rating—or as an offering to the whole, creating ourselves as works of art, honing mind, body, and spirit into an expression of our glorious humanity.

It is no surprise that in the age of the couch potato, we have body builders. In the overwhelming glut of information, we empty our minds in meditation. In the massive wounding that seems to leave some piece of emotional shrapnel in every man, woman, and child, we have psychotherapy and self-help books. In a drug-addicted culture, there are twelve-step groups and treatment facilities in every major city. In an educational system that focuses almost exclusively on intellectual knowledge, we have exponential growth in yoga centers, experiential workshops, and dance movements like Gabrielle Roth's Five Rhythms.

We improve ourselves because there is *so much more we can be.* We can do this as an offering, not a taking, a way of bringing beauty into the world, a contribution of intelligence, artistry, or strength; not just for ourselves, but as a contribution to the marvelous reality we are creating together.

There is a profound spiritual revolution all around us. People are waking up to the underlying spiritual reality hidden in the miracle of life. They are leaving their churches to create spontaneous ceremonies in their back yards. They are leaving corporate boardrooms to take yoga retreats. They are voluntarily meditating, fasting, and reading books on spirituality—not to please God or avoid damnation, but to regain a sense of the sacred. Sales of books on spirituality are growing faster than any other category of the book industry, with billions in sales annually. Spirituality has even become an industry, as more stores and catalogs feature spiritual accoutrements, such as candles, incense, meditation cushions, yoga props, Tibetan bells, prayer flags, or statues of deities. Today's spirituality is not so much an act of worship, sacrifice, or petition, as it is a means of elevating one's consciousness to a place where an overarching spiritual reality becomes apparent. Through these practices we enter the ultimate *I-Thou* relationship. As Martin Buber said, this is how we become fully human.

The pre-dawn spiritual revolution cannot be contained by a church. It is not made from dogmatic beliefs. It does not have a dictatorial ethical code. It is not even a social movement, as was Christianity, but a movement that is more often intensely personal. It takes place deep in the interior of one's being. Its focus is not on gaining access to a far-away Heaven, but on transformation and awakening right here, right now. As a do-it-yourself road to higher consciousness, it's a direct interface with the divine, through meditation, prayer, chanting, hiking, gardening, circling, dancing, drumming, lovemaking, singing, study, contemplation, or psychoactive substances. When practiced in groups, it is co-creative, egalitarian, and spontaneous.

Pre-dawn spirituality is not born of the mind alone, for it recognizes that we are glorious beings in phenomenal bodies, living on an exquisite, material planet. This is not an either-or value system that pits one part against another, but an integrative spirituality, integrating Heaven and Earth, mind and body, and bringing them into the sacred center of the heart.

As we expand our own consciousness and enter the reflexive self-awareness of internal questioning, we become more and more aligned with the truth of our own nature. Indeed, one of the necessary requirements in today's busy world is to learn how to remain centered.

In the chakra system, the heart is the very center of a system of seven centers, with three chakras above and three below. The heart is seen, not as the source of consciousness, but as the prime integrator of consciousness. The more we come into our deep core center, the more we align with the axis mundi that runs through us all, spanning base to crown. The more deeply we honor the *I-Thou* relationship with the anima mundi, the closer we get to the realization of a single unity, a very large and wonderful *We*.

The spirituality of the emerging era is both immanent and transcendent. The transcendent aspect allows us to step away from our petty concerns, to detach and see things from a distance. If you were holding this book against your eyes, you couldn't read (and the older we get, the farther away we have to hold it!). We all know that distance gives perspective. Archimedes said that if he had a lever long enough and a place to stand, he could move the world. Ken Wilber points out that we need to be able to separate from something before we can operate on it. By separating from the instincts of our bodies, it became possible to override those instincts. By separating from matter, we have been able to inspect and dissect the material world, solving many mysteries. While this separation has the danger of leading to fragmentation and dissociation, it is a necessary part of the evolutionary pattern—to separate, differentiate, and re-integrate at a higher level.

The separation that is needed now is to take a step back from the culture itself. As long as we are unable to detach from the incessant cries of advertising and sensationalist media, we are hypnotized into the cultural trance that is consuming the biosphere. From that hypnotic state, we can do little to change the world. We need to be able to disengage from its more insidious qualities in order to imagine something new. That means turning off the TV and breaking the hypnotic programming that tells us to consume. We need to listen to the birds and the wind at least as often as the evening news. We need to read poetry as often as the newspaper. We need to go online and get news stories from other sources, conducting our own investigations into truth. We must transcend our culture in order to transform it.

As a vehicle for transcendence, meditation is by far the most ancient, tried-and-true, simple, effective, inexpensive, go-anywhere, do-anytime kind of practice there is. It is the vehicle for transcending the mental matrices that keep us behaving in unproductive patterns, beliefs, and habits. Meditation allows us to disengage the clutch of life long enough to shift to another gear, a shifting that is desperately needed at this time. Meditation allows us, in the words of Willis Harman, to shift from seeing external authority as the *source,* to discovering internal authority as a *resource.*[10]

Meditation is not, however, something that affects the individual alone. In studies conducted by the Transcendental Meditation society in twenty-four cities where one percent of the population meditated regularly, meditation was shown to be statiscally linked to drastically reduced crime, when compared to control cities of similar geographic region, population, and college membership.[11] Can the global brain meditate itself into a new world?

DEEP ECOLOGY

> *Environmentalism has been seen as a separate strand. In fact it is the fiber that all strands are made from.*
>
> —Hazel Henderson

Nature, we are learning, is not a force over which we must triumph but the medium of our transformation. Nature is the inclusive *Thou,* the larger holon in which we are but cogs. But unlike other species, we are cogs that have the ability to control Nature. This control has led to a dangerous dissociation, one that threatens the host body in which we live.

Ecology is literally the study of our home and the maintenance of its balance. How do we maintain our homes in daily life? Kids need to be told to clean up their rooms, whereas adults do it as part of their daily routine. If we are to mature as a species, we need to treat our world in the same way that we try to teach our teenagers at home: clean up after yourself; don't use up the last of something without replacing it; conserve energy by turning out the lights when you're not using them; recycle your garbage; think of others beside yourself, and treasure what's been given to you. Simple enough. Can we learn this as a species?

In living ecosystems, an immature species is by nature competitive, agressive, territorial, and free-riding. In a mature forest, the dynamic interplay of species has found cooperative balance with other life forms, using maximum employment, and recycling everything. In a mature ecosystem, no one species is in control, nor does the health of the ecosystem depend on any single species. It is a dynamic balance in which each part serves the whole.

The biologist Elizabet Sahtouris states: "Young species are found to have highly competitive characteristics: They take all the resources they can, they hog territory, they multiply wildly. Sound familiar? But a lot of species have managed to grow up, to share things and territory, to cooperate. It's what keeps them alive."[12] Can we learn this simple principle of cooperation? If so, we can save energy, heighten creativity, and assure the continuance of our place in evolution.

In the process of maturing as a species, we need to learn to cooperate not only with each other, but with the the limits and laws of Nature. When we mature as a species, we will pride ourselves on having a beautiful and healthy collective home. Pristine forests, undammed rivers, clean air and water, systems of clean energy and maximum recycling, would be values considered *before* the dollar, not after. Creating appreciation for the natural world would be a fundamental part of every child's education.

We are too far removed and far too numerous to return to Nature in the way we once lived so long ago. We cannot go back to our infancy and breastfeed, and we can't support the present world population by hunting and gathering in the wilds. But we can employ a *relationship* with Nature in all that we do. Schools can have beautiful gardens in addition to paved playgrounds. Children can take field trips to wilderness areas as often as to museums and factories. Urban homes can be built with rooftop gardens, and more suburban areas with community gardens. We can imagine every newspaper carrying a section on the environment equally as detailed as the sports or finance section—for which is more important to our survival—the winner of the latest football game or how to live sustainably with our environment?

History has come a long way since the environment was so extensive and abundant that our ancestors could not imagine its diminishment. The train of evolution has been accelerating its speed in a single direction—toward replicating ourselves and taking what we need to survive. That train has gained incredible momentum, and it is difficult for many people to believe that it can't go in the same direction forever.

The diverging paths of Nature and civilization must converge, or there will be increasing catastrophe for both. This is the greatest synthesis we can make at this time. It is time for us to become members of a mature ecosystem—one that lives with natural checks and balances, sharing resources equitably, recycling and fully employing all its members. Synthesis with Nature denies neither side of the equation. But it requires seeing Nature as a *Thou* rather than an *it,* an intricate feedback loop that weaves the living web of *we.* It is a co-creative partnership where we model ourselves along Nature's inherent principles, and integrate the needs of human evolution with the resources of the planet. In the final analysis, Nature is our teacher, our senior partner, and our model for the future.

ESSENTIAL POINTS

• Waking the global heart occurs on both a personal and collective level. Each of us are cells in the global heart.

• Personal practices include gratitude, generosity, empathy, compassion, acceptance, forgiveness, and celebration.

• Collective realms of the heart include the quest for peace, increased interrelatedness, synthesis of plurality, spirituality, and deep ecology.

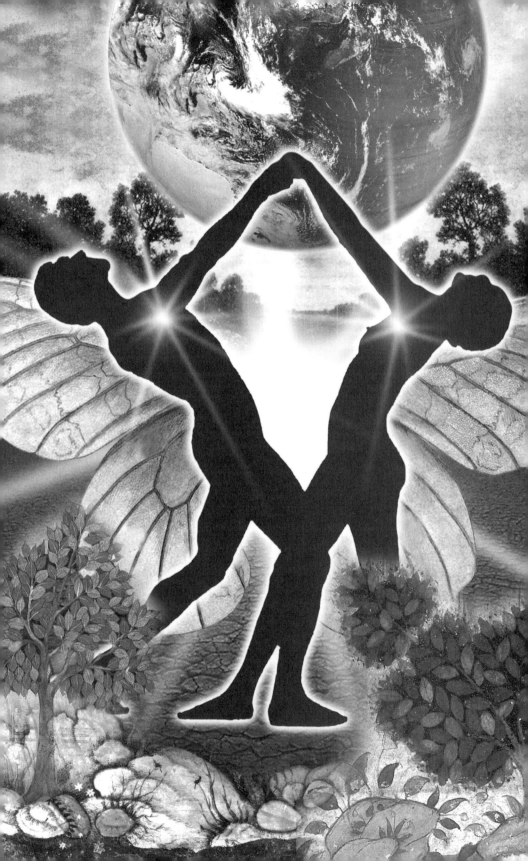

CHAPTER 17

WEAVING A NEW STORY
Coming of Age in the Heart

*Furthermore, we have not even to risk the adventure alone; for the heroes
of all time have gone before us; the labyrinth is thoroughly known;
we have only to follow the thread of the hero-path. And where we had
thought to find an abomination, we shall find a god; where we had
thought to slay another, we shall slay ourselves; where we had thought to
travel outward, we shall come to the center of our own existence; where
we had thought to be alone, we shall be with all the world.*

—Joseph Campbell

It is the month of May, that glorious window between hot and cold,
where the outdoors sings with color and shouts with birdsong. I
sit with my laptop on my back deck, surrounded by a hillside garden
nestled in the redwoods. I marvel at the tall trees, unmoving through
the winter, with their roots in the Earth, their branches high in the
sky. Unlike me, they are a testament to patient stillness, each one an
axis mundi, connecting Heaven and Earth. Some have been standing
for hundreds of years—since before Columbus discovered America.
Others in nearby protected areas have been standing even longer,
some since the birth of Christ or even Buddha. Still others are being
logged for lawn furniture and decks, resurrected, ironically enough,
so people can enjoy the beauty of the outdoors.

While these trees have silently stood their ground, human stories have changed many times. Whether these living pillars between Heaven and Earth will continue to stand, and whether the millions of people living in a cement world will get to see them, depends largely on the stories we tell ourselves. What will those stories be? And what are the changes in the present story?

In the times before written history, we can only guess at the stories our ancestors told around the firelight. We can project our ideas upon pregnant-bellied statues and make an educated guess that their makers worshipped a Goddess, a Great Mother, who was synonymous with Nature. Life and death and birth were one eternal cycle, over which they had no control. Nor do we know how our ancestors defined themselves, but from our present vantage point, we could say they were infants in the primal garden, mere babes in the woods, living in a state of magical wonder.

Later, in the early civilization of Babylonia, the story enacted each year was of the god-king, Marduk, slaying the Great Mother, Tiamat, then establishing a new order of men upon her dead body. At the end of the story, we are told that the gods created the race of humans to take on the drudgery of work. Our identity was named: slaves to the gods, or at best servants—a safe, humble role. We worshipped and paid tribute to human god-kings, who acted as intermediaries between the worlds, and kept the mundane world in order. Knowing little about how the world worked, we believed that our sacrifices appeased the gods and increased the chances that rain would fall, the crops would grow, and we would birth many children. Time passed, and we did birth many children, who prospered and multiplied.

In the Christian myth, humans had fallen from celestial realms to a lowly existence on Earth as punishment for sin, whether Adam and Eve's transgressions, or our own. We were no longer slaves, but sinners. God no longer needed our labors, but our obedience. We no longer sacrificed bulls, goats, or elderly kings, for the sacrifice of the Savior served to redeem us all. Christ died for our sins and rose from the dead to demonstrate His divine nature. In this story, the son of the Holy Father enters into the death and resurrection of initiation for the good of "mankind" as a whole. For this great act, the rest of us were spared the painful process of our own rite of passage. But without a personal initiation, an essential part of the mystery was lost.

It was believed that our sins were forgiven by the Savior's sacrifice—but they were not corrected. Penance was not the same as amends. We were not asked to address those we had harmed, but to address God instead. For Catholics, forgiveness occurred by merely confessing one's sins, along with saying a few Hail Marys and *mea culpas*. By the time of the Reformation, there wasn't much we could do but keep the faith and follow scripture. For Protestants, redemption was passive, occurring through God's grace—at least for the few chosen ones, who were privileged enough to live well. Our forebears were good, God-fearing folks who made the best of their times by keeping their heads bowed, working, learning, and reading the Bible. We continued to grow and our numbers doubled.

In the scientific revolution, humans gained power over their surroundings from knowledge gained through *observation* of Nature. We had a new identity, as discoverers, creators, manipulators. The world was our workshop and we were its artists. Nature's power was diminished and our power was heightened. Nature was an "it" from which we could take what we wanted. With power restored, we could do as we pleased, and from this we built a brilliantly successful—but non-sustainable—civilization. Our powers enabled us to grow exponentially, spreading across the globe, while retreating deeper into the indoors of buildings, cars, and cities.

As we follow the course of history from our embeddedness in Nature to its possible destruction, we see that it is not the *fall* where we went wrong, but perhaps the *rise*. By this I mean our separation from the Earth as the ground of our being. In this separation, Nature was first denigrated and is now degraded. This is the sin for which we must now make amends.

In the new story, it is the *collective* that is undergoing death and resurrection, along with many individuals, each in their own way. This death will also be for our sins, but on a larger scale. Not for the transgression of an illicit sexual fantasy, but for the rape of the environment; not for the killing of a brother, but for the bombing of a nation under false pretenses; not for the corruption of the money-changers, but for the rapacious greed of corporations; not for the worship of the old gods, but for allowing the false idols of the dollar and the Hollywood image to be worshipped as gods. Our sins have become global and there is no one else to clean them up.

When we were children, caring for the world, the environment, our health and prosperity, were taken care of by others. In our infancy it was the Great Mother who provided all our needs. In our toddler-hood it was the World Parents, pantheons of gods and goddesses who assured the stability of the seasons, the crops, and animals. In our middle youth, it was the Father, alternately wrathful or loving, who forged budding civilizations into empires, and empires into military-industrial complexes. As we grew in knowledge, we relied on science to provide the answers, and many still do, thinking that given enough time, science and industry will find solutions to all our problems. But the brilliance of science has given rise to many of the problems that need solving—and the scientific data tells us that time is running out.

We no longer have the luxury of remaining as children. The archetypal parents won't save us this time. Mother Nature is going bankrupt and can no longer be depended upon. The fish are disappearing from the oceans; the topsoil is being stripped from the land; urban air is filled with smog; the ice caps are melting. The cupboards are no longer well-stocked; they have not been replenished, and the masses are hungry and still multiplying. Children around the world are crying, with no mother to console them; millions of them grow up with no parents at all. Developing countries long for what the West has squandered.

And what has become of the Father? Ever more distant, his realm is rotting with corruption, getting ready to fall. Christian churches struggle with priests who molest children and right-to-lifers who commit murder. Muslims blow up themselves up in crowds and buses in a desperate attempt to glorify the name of Allah. Israeli Jews treat Palestinians as vermin, forgetting the atrocities of Nazi Germany. Heads of countries, heads of state, heads of corporations, and the news media that tells us all about them, spin webs of illusion to cover their actions. Truth is a rare commodity, seldom seen or heard. Like children, we are kept distracted from our pain with a constant supply of new toys and gadgets. And, like the many affluent children who suffered a similar fate while Dad worked a sixty hour week, we find that toys are no substitute for love. The single father just can't do it alone, and the children are left to fend for themselves. This makes for a pretty dysfunctional adolescence.

There are exceptions, of course. There are many churches who serve benevolent causes and genuinely inspire their congregations. There are Muslims who are peaceful, and agonize over terrorism in the name of Allah. There are Jews who reach out to Palestinians and work for peace. There are corporations that are working to save the environment, and handfuls of politicians who dare to speak the truth. There are listener sponsored-radio stations, like KPFA, that broadcast real news, and countries with duly elected officials.

Nor, when I speak about the corrupt Father, am I referring to the ultimate divine, which is far beyond masculine or feminine, and can never be corrupt. This realm is not the one that has abandoned us, but the realm that is beckoning for deeper discovery. This realm is right here within and around us if we can get out of our egos and the *maya* they create long enough to see straight. For the stories we tell ourselves are merely projections upon the archetypal realm; they model our understanding of the world as we grow and learn. Yet they form the reality by which we live.

A NEW IDENTITY

In each of these stories, humans had an identity. Now, once again, our identity as slaves, servants, sinners, or cogs in a wheel is changing, and change is the only thing we can count on right now. As a people going through an initiation process, we are caught between one form and another, with nothing to rely on but awakening to the process. In the new story, humans are the redeemers. *This is the resurrection side of the initiation.*

We are the redeemers, and what needs to be redeemed is nearly every facet of our civilization: the environment, economy, government, education, medicine, and our spiritual worldview. It's a big job, overwhelming to contemplate. Many find it easier to turn on the tube and zone out than to feel so small in the face of such challenges. The bad news is that these challenges won't go away. But the good news is that we don't have to do it alone. That was part of the old myth where we had to face our challenges in solitude, one person against the world. To go it alone would be pure hubris and dangerous arrogance today, a formula for certain failure.

In the new story we need to rename ourselves as global citizens. Benjamin Franklin once claimed that his greatest invention was of the term "American," back at a time when the early settlers were French, Italian, English, Dutch, or German. The name *American* embraced all the settlers in a higher order, allowed them to transcend differences, and identify with the new land they were calling home.

Elizabet Sahtouris has named the current younger generation the *Millennials*, which certainly seems more inspiring than Gen X or Y. *But it is not just the youth, but the entire collective that is coming of age.* I like the term *Gaians,* as it identifies us with a living, evolving system of the Earth. But many find that term to be too Pagan, too gender-specific, or they confuse it with a label for sexual preference. The term *Earthlings* is sweet, but does not embrace the non-physical world of consciousness and technology that are so much a part of our emerging identity. I toyed with the term *Globals,* but it seemed too impersonal, and vaguely reminiscent of a basketball team. None of these terms implies what we are to do together.

For me, the best way to think of who we are becoming in the world today is that we are all *co-hearts.* The term co-hearts emphasizes both a shared identity and a means of connection, a co-conspiracy of the heart, a camaraderie of many, partners in a creative enterprise. It can apply to any level of the system: an intimate relationship with a partner, or co-workers in a corporation. We can be democratic co-hearts, economic co-hearts, educational co-hearts, romantic, or spiritual co-hearts. It allows us to connect with those around us with tenderness and intimacy, while also recognizing a larger kinship and common work. It implies that love is the means to include and transcend each social holon in a larger holarchy.

Jesus described his vision of synthesis as the manifestation of a divine kingdom of Heaven on Earth. His vision of a human family transcended boundaries of race, gender, and status. It is no surprise that "kingdom" was the term he used, for it was the main social structure at the time. People lived in kingdoms. They served kings, were ruled by kings, and went to war for their kings. But to speak of a kingdom is to use a masculine term that places man at the top of a hierarchy, ruling over other men, women, children, slaves, animals, and plants. It is an imperial model that falsifies the true nature of our world, which is more like a living web than a pyramidal hierarchy, more like a network of intelligence than a chain of command. I prefer to call it a *kin-dom*—a world in which we are all kin to each other. Within our kin-dom we are all co-hearts, working together to mend the web of life wherever it has been torn.

We are not then, merely the brain cells of the planet, yet the Internet clearly gives us the means of operating a global brain. We are not merely Gaia's sperm, capable of seeding another world when we someday master space travel. We can no longer be consumers, destroyers, or *idiots* who live individual lives at the cost of others.

We are first and foremost the very heartbeat of a planetary civilization, the coordinators of an amazing evolutionary experiment, the dancers in a cosmic dance between the Earth and the Heavens. We are the parents of the future. Someday we will be the ancestors that I pray will be remembered with gratitude rather than resentment. As co-hearts, our identity is one of membership; our task is stewardship. The sense of belonging and purpose that is missing for so many people can now take on a new definition.

In the new story, we are part of an intelligent web, where everything known is accessible to an ever-growing number of parts. We are not dependent children, nor are we independent adolescents, but inter-dependent adults. In the new story, we are in a co-creative relationship to the divine—not with the arrogance of thinking we are equal, but the discipleship of being gods-in-training, starting our new employment with spirit in an entry-level position. We are not passive recipients nor dominant controllers, but active participants. We are not abandoning God, but rediscovering broader concepts of the divine: the simultaneity of immanence and transcendence , the passionate love between God and Goddess, the infinite realm of non-local mind, the awesome power and exquisite beauty of Nature.

We need not face these challenges alone because we are never really alone. Through meditation, we can find guidance. Through science we can discover ever deeper mysteries. Through the World Wide Web, we can join with others and exchange information. We don't have to invent a new way, weaving it out of whole cloth, superimposing it on everything around us. Nature models our living systems and has done so for billions of years. Nature *is* the way, but we need not give up our brilliant technology and go back to mud huts. We need only turn the focus of our technology toward redemption rather than consumption. We can use our colossal media to inform rather than distract. The global brain can organize its thoughts, and wake up from the nightmare, to dream a new dream.

If the Babylonian gods created humans to free them from labors, then we are in turn creating a world of machines to free ourselves from labor. This theme is echoed in many science fiction stories and presents its own set of challenges, based on how we use or program these machines. From machines that extend the body, such as power tools and automobiles, to computers that extend the mind, humans are entering a godlike stature by virtue of freeing our energy from time consuming and physically exhausting work. With machines we have the benefits of a slave society without being inhumane. We are freeing ourselves for something grand, but what is it?

In the emerging story, we are the caterpillar becoming the butterfly. We know that the caterpillar is dying, and yet, until the new form is birthed, it is all we know; it is what we are. The caterpillar represents the old body politic. Its identity is as a consumer, not a co-heart. Its spineless, wormlike body has voraciously consumed its environment since it was born – it's the only thing it knows. It has expanded its size and burst its skin a number of times, each time reorganizing in response to population growth. But now it has reached maximum size. It cannot grow farther in the same dimension. Soon the chrysalis will form.

By most realistic predictions, the disparity between decreasing oil production and increasing demand will create a crisis. Peak oil production is said by some to have occurred as early as 2005, after which production goes down while demands for consumption continue to rise. This can only raise the price of gasoline and all products transported by gas or made by petroleum products, including food. With transportation costs rising, the freedoms we now take for granted will be curtailed. Unable to push outward and move about with the same exuberance of our youth, communities will be forced into profound and possibly benevolent changes. They will be forced to fall back on themselves, to live, trade, and learn more locally, even as the Internet connects them globally. Staying home, they may actually get to know their neighbors, working together to improve the beauty and functionality of their shared neighborhoods. They may have time to read those books, watch all those DVDs, and practice their yoga. As gas prices rise, people will be forced to walk and bike more, improving their health. Front lawns may turn to vegetable gardens. Neighbors may rip up their back fences to make community gardens.

Smaller towns may choose to become self-sufficient. The town of Willits, in Northern California, for example, is already planning its shift toward total self-sufficiency, with an ad hoc committee called WELL (Willits Economic LocaLization) made up of elected officials, businesses, citizens, and experts in six major focus areas: food, energy, shelter, water, health and wellness, and social organization. They meet regularly to plan the shift to a community economy. They aim to be completely energy-independent by 2010, and to satisfy their food needs with local farming. In the realm of health, they are seeking to have the first green hospital. Examining the work habits of the current Willits community, they realized that 30 million dollars per year goes out of the area in transportation costs, with people driving to work or to purchase goods. Virtually none of the food currently sold is from local growers, adding to the cost of transportation, and supplying only a few days' worth of food at any given time. Their intention is to convert Willits' usable land to grow food locally for its own population, lessening the dependence on what currently gets trucked in. Oil shortage or not, this inquiry is leading the town into increased connectedness, local organization, and energy efficiency. One of the group's coordinators, Brian Weller, explains, "I'm helping WELL to understand the process as an emerging social organization. This process will be achieved through people, and people have have different perceptual filters and different agendas, both open and hidden."[1]

As the economy shifts, wealth will shift from the value of one's stock portfolio, real estate, or vehicle, to the environment. As air and water qualities worsen, those who live in more land-based areas will be seen as having a wealth that can't be measured in dollar signs. Spaciousness, clean air, running water, and beautiful scenery will comprise the wealth of an area, with our national parks valued as treasures beyond compare. Communities that foster these ideals by designing their spaces to enhance their environmental integrity will be models for others. Co-housing communities will become more common, as people find ways to balance resource sharing with maintaining the privacy of a personal living space.

This doesn't mean the picture is completely rosy, but it is important to realize the advantages that may be birthed by the coming transformation. Darker predictions of the coming changes foresee the possibility of 85 percent unemployment, massive population reduction, and increased crime, looting, and all the other behaviors humans resort to when survival is at stake.[2] No one knows just how this transformation will play itself out. But however it occurs, we each have the choice to be a villian or hero.

THE HERO'S RETURN

For the past several millennia, the Hero's quest has been a dominant myth in our culture. As stated in chapter six, the Hero's quest is an outward push into realms of excitement and danger. It is a conquest of the unknown, a triumph of conflict, where we build our personal power through slaying demons within and around us. It is the quest of individuation, achievement, and transcendence.

It is now time for the Hero to return home. Our success as a species has become our liability. We're so good at prospering that we are compromising the biosphere. We have the data that tells us our world is in danger. We have the technology, communication, networks and intelligence, to address this danger. We need only turn our attention toward home to make the journey complete.

To return home is to return to the Earth, to the self, to the community, and to love. As the caterpillar dies, the excesses will be peeled away—the endless toys and gadgets, the mindless television broadcasts, the constant search for new stimulation or distraction. In any initiation, the outward attention is directed inward, the former fragmentation rewoven into a web of wholeness, deep within the self.

A global oil crisis will force people to come back home. As the caterpillar body is held by the chrysallis, unable to move, the shift begins. Forcibly restricted from the old ways, new possibilities awaken and take hold of the imagination. The imaginal cells spontaneously appear. At first they are isolated and vulnerable, part of a different story. They vibrate to a different frequency. As they appear in greater numbers, they start to recognize each other. They begin vibrating together, forming clumps, organizing themselves along new lines.

Do we dare to become the imaginal cells of our changing societies and imagine a new world? Do we dare to stand up for new beliefs, new ways, new values, and the need to coordinate with others in a similar dance? Can we recognize each other in this new vibration, and join together, creating events, organizations, and communities? As we gather to exchange information, to dream, to dance, to plan, we are the living imaginal cells joining together to form a new body politic.

The butterfly is a wholly different creature from the caterpillar: two wings held together by a strong and vibrant core in the middle, the axis mundi. The left wing and right wing are both needed in order to fly. They are part of one organism. But they must be bound to a strong center in order to do so, neither dominating the other, but working together in concert. They must be held by the core, the center, the heart.

In the politics of left and right, both are holding essential values. The left is holding the values of the global community—working for equality, opportunity, service and diversity, often ignoring the individual in service of the greater whole. The right is reaching toward simplicity, seeing community as family, glorifying the individual at the cost of the larger whole. The right reveres authority that is drawn from above, handed down from our forefathers. The left serves the masses, and draws its authority from below, the family of children growing to adulthood.

It is the heart that connects them, just as it is the heart that connects us all. And just as the physical heart beats vital energy into every cell, so can the global heart coordinate the many facets of civilization and vitalize each one. The heart opens to the greater love and finds common ground in a larger matrix. The heart is the integrator that brings us together at a time when we seem to be falling apart. The heart is the center of the tapestry; the core value; the new organizing principle.

The power of love is the sustainable value, the power that makes things last. We take care of what we love, we protect it and serve it. What we love enlivens us, renews us, gives us strength and inspiration.

In a paradigm of the heart, the values of the divine feminine and the divine masculine are held in relationship. It is not an either-or but a logical embrace of both, a balanced integration of *I* and *thou*. As men and women we have much work to do. We need each other, we are enhanced by each other. Nature and civilization, Earth and sky, matter and spirit, each are cosmic partners in the *hierosgamos,* the sacred marriage of opposites.

The great divide that was made when we first walled our cities has now pinned us up against those walls. Until we master space travel, there is nowhere else to expand. But we *can* take down the walls between us and make better use of what we have. We can take fences down between properties and create local commons. We can get out of our cars, out of our offices, and find that simplicity and sustainability bring us closer to Nature as the greatest creative force of all. As Teilhard de Chardin describes it, our awakening is "not that we have mastered Nature but that we have become conscious of the movement carrying us along–and have realized the meaning of the reflective exercise."[3]

In a paradigm of the heart, we stop spending the bulk of our money on defense, and bring it back home instead. Even if we "bomb them with bread," as was suggested when we bombed Afghanistan after the September 11th attacks, we save billions of dollars otherwise spent on destruction. This money can be spent on education, job training, health care, urban renewal, scientific research, ecological restoration, and think tanks for the future.

If we stop pitting one side against the other and give up the fight, working instead toward integration, we save enormous amounts of energy. Precious life-force is wasted as we battle one part of our psyches against another, fighting our sexuality, our bodies, our instincts, and each other. Much-needed information about issues in the news is obscured by focusing on the most divergent viewpoints between opposing parties. In American politics, precious time, and taxpayer dollars, is wasted by the gridlock between Republicans and Democrats. We must say bye-partisan rather than buy-partisan. If we have to fight, we can fight *for* something, rather than against. If we must defend, we can defend our forests and oceans, our rivers and farmlands, from the ravage of a dominator paradigm.

The emerging myth is none other than a love story. It is the passionate meeting and falling in love between *I* and *Thou,* between the axis mundi and the anima mundi, *atman* and *Brahman*, Goddess and God, culture and Nature. This is the sacred marriage. This is the central symbol of the heart chakra, the two intersecting triangles of spirit and matter, the symbol that guides us to the manifestation of Heaven on Earth. This is our possibility,and our promise for a new world. Just as the Renaissance developed out of the depressed economy and bleak aftermath of the plague in Europe, so too can we have the vision of a new Renaissance, born out of the darkness of our times. We can invest in ideas that create things that last: the environment, sustainable community, health, and spiritual awakening.

In chaos theory, there is something called "sensitivity to initial conditions" which refers to the possibility that small actions create large and unexpected effects further on down the line. This is especially true when a system is in transition. Interestingly, it is sometimes called "the butterfly effect," because it has been demonstrated that the tiny flap of a butterfly wing in North America could potentially set off a storm in China, as the subtle changes magnify through the atmosphere.

This means that our actions at this sensitive time can have far-reaching and profound effects, ones that we may not be able to foresee–for better or worse. Thus it remains even more imperative to set our values upon solid soil, to wake up to both our positive and negative potential as quickly as possible, and to act consciously and carefully.

BACK TO THE GARDEN

The sun is now sinking behind the trees, casting long shadows. It is getting chilly, so I gather my things to go inside. My gaze lifts to the garden once again, in appreciation for its loveliness. As if in answer to my writing today, a butterfly floats by and lights upon a flower, then moves from one blossom to another. I watch, amazed and fascinated by the synchronicity. Then I pause with a terrible thought.

What if humanity goes through this difficult metamorphosis from caterpillar to butterfly, only to find the garden is gone? What if there are no flowers to light upon, no birds to dance with, no garden to play in? For what purpose will it have been to free our labors, to join together, to develop ourselves? What greater tragedy could there be? How then would we live?

For the final piece in our story is the garden itself. When the metamorphosis is complete and the initiation is over, when the Hero has fulfilled the quest, and the resurrection heralds a new dawn, we return once again to the garden from which we came. We return, not as children without knowledge or power, living in fused symbiosis. Not as servants or slaves, bound to our duties. Not as cogs in a wheel, empty and mechanical, nor as scientists, observing and measuring. We certainly don't want to return as consumers who see only money to be made.

No, we come back to the garden as *co-hearts* in a *kin-dom,* fertilizers and catalysts, exchanging information and ideas in a field of beauty and promise. We come back to be part of the beauty, as artists and co-creators, understanding the mysteries of the elements of earth and water, fire and the air, and the evolutionary flow of time that grinds these elements into the magic of life. We come back as awakened souls, awake to our possibilities and awake to a world we can create together. We come back to tend the garden, not because it needs us, but because *we* need the garden.

For the garden is the storehouse of possibility that is both teacher and provider. The garden is the workshop from which we create our dreams. Here we find freedom and responsibility, a place where roots belong in the soil and branches belong in the sky. Yet the roots are all intertwined with each other, and the branches make love in the wind.

We who tend the garden are creatures of beauty that fertilize ideas as they blossom into understanding. Our labors of love bring us treasures to share, sweet fruits to eat, the harvest of fresh vegetables, shade-giving trees, and colorful flowers, birds who fly and squirrels who hoard, even the worms who aerate the soil—all are part of a divine and perfect plan, unfolding each moment to teach us—someday—to become the gods and goddesses that we truly are.

Will me make it? I leave you, I think fittingly, with yet another quote from Teilhard de Chardin:

> "The world is too big a concern for that. To bring us into existence it has from the beginning juggled miraculously with too many improbabilities for there to be any risk whatever in committing ourselves further and following it right to the end. If it undertook the task, it is because it can finish it, following the same methods and with the same infallibility with which it began. . . . In the last analysis, the best guarantee that a thing should happen is that it is vitally necessary." [4]

ESSENTIAL POINTS

• Completion of initiation requires a new identity of who we are and where we live.

• As imaginal cells in the body politic, we are co-hearts in a kin-dom, co-creators in a living system, weavers of a living web.

• We are the redeemers of what has been lost. We are all called to be Heroes, but the next task of the Hero is to return home.

• To return home is to take all our wisdom, technology, and accomplishments, and apply them to the garden in which we live. For the garden is the true home of the emerging butterfly and the blessed ground of the future.

POWER PARADIGM CHARACTERISTICS	HEART PARADIGM CHARACTERISTICS
Hierarchy	Holarchy
Reductionism	Holism
Chain of command	Web of connection
Imperialism	Participatory democracy
Militarism	Peace and social justice
Competition	Co-creation
Growth and expansion	Sustainability
Markets	Networks
Fundamentalism	Pluralism, syncretism
Either-or	Both-and
Mind over body	Mind-body-spirit integration
Exploitation of Nature	Deep ecology
I – it	I – thou-we
Rational	Mythic-evolutionary
Ego-driven	Relationship driven
Male dominated	Partnership
Expedience	Aesthetics
Family	Community

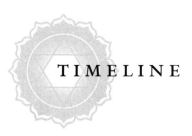

TIMELINE

BEFORE COMMON ERA

800,000	Control of fire
30,000	Goddess figurines
27,000	Last Neanderthals
25,000	Complex dwellings and storage structures
31,000–10,500	Cave paintings and bear cult shrines
9,000	Domestication of cereals in Levant, goats and sheep in Persia
8,000	End of Wurm glaciation
8350	Founding of Jericho
6850	Çatal Hüyük
6000	Farming reaches Europe
4500	Smelting of copper
4400	First Kurgan invasions of Goddess cultures
4000	Smelting of silver and gold
3500	Arches in architecture
3300	First writing
3100	Unification of Upper and Lower Egypt
3,000	Early Minoan and Egyptian dynasties Sumerian city-states Lagash, Uruk Invention of Abacus
2700	Epic of Gilgamesh
2500	Megaliths appear
2400	Unification of Sumer
2350	Urukagina's laws restricting women's sexuality
2296	Sargon I founds first empire

2000	Bablyonian mathematics (sexagesimal)
	Mohenjadaro, Harappa in Indus valley
2100	Earliest preserved law book (Ur-Nammu of Ur)
1800	Oldest known chariots
1700	Minoans develop Linear A
1686	Law Code of Hamurabi
1595	Hittites sack Babylon
1580	*Enuma Elish:* Babylonian myth of Tiamat and Marduk
1450	Eruption of Thera
1400	Hittite king rules much of Asia Minor
1379-1358	Rule of Akhenaten in Egypt (first male monotheism)
1250	Beginning of Iron Age
1200	Trojan War (Greece)
	Temple at Abu Simbel in Egypt
	Exodus of Jews from Egypt
	Collapse of Hittite Empire
	Start of Zoroastrianism in Persia
716	First Olympic games in Greece
753	Legendary Founding of Rome
725	Homer's Odyssey
700	Hesiod's Theogony
	First republics in India
612	Assyrian Empire collapses
600	Greek lyric poetry celebrating love
585	5/28/585 solar eclipse that stopped war between
	Lydians and Medes, Babylonians drew up treaty
	Pre-socratic philosophers
551-479	Life of Confucius

550	First aqueducts in Greece
539	Cyrus the Great, cylinder seal of human rights
537	Cyrus decrees Jews could return to Palestine (from Babylonian captivity)
533	Buddha's enlightenment (lifespan 563-483)
515	Pythagorean brotherhood
509	Roman Republic
508	Athenian democracy
500	Steel made in India
499	Persian wars begin
459–399	Life of Socrates
450	Peloponnesian war
427–347	Life of Plato
410	Hippocrates lays foundation of medicine
399	Trial and execution of Socrates
387	Plato founds Academy in Athens
384–322	Life of Aristotle
356–322	Alexander the Great
338	Phillip of Macedon conquers Greece
295	Euclidean geometry
270	First known heliocentric theory (Aristarchus)
146	Rome conquers Greece
44	Assassination of Caesar
31	End of Roman Republic
30	Death of Cleopatra
4	Birth of Jesus of Nazareth

COMMON ERA

29	Crucifixion of Jesus
35	Paul's conversion on road to Damascus
64–68	First Christian persecutions, Peter and Paul martyred under Nero
64–70	Gospel according to Mark
70	Jerusalem temple destroyed
80	Gospels of Mathew and Luke
95	Gospel of John
110–130	Gospel of Peter and Thomas
161–180	Reign of Marcus Aurelius
200	Patanjali's Yoga Sutras (India)
312	Constantine's conversion to Christianity
313	Legal protection of Christians by Edict of Milan
325	Council of Nicea
330	Christianity declared official religion of Roman Empire
386	Conversion of Augustine
391	Theodosius has Pagan temples destroyed, including Altar of Victory in Roman Senate and Alexandrian library
410	Visigoths sack Rome
476	End of Roman Empire (in the West), last Roman emperor deposed
570–632	Life of Muhammad
622	Beginning of Islam
674	First Muslim siege of Constantinople
800	Charlemagne crowned Holy Roman Emperor, first since 476

1095	First Crusade (Urban II)
1170	Founding of University of Paris
1209–1230	Albigensian Crusade in Southern France
1215	Dominican order established
1225–1274	Life of Thomas Aquinas
1250	Postal Service in Europe
1231	Establishment of Inquisition by Pope Gregory IX
1293–1530	Florentine Republic
1335	First public striking clock (Milan)
1337	Start of Hundred Years War between England and France
1341	Francesco Petrarch made Poet Laureate of Europe (lived 1304-1374)
1347–51	Black Plague sweeps Europe
1400	Coffee hits Western world
1412–31	Joan of Arc
1452–1519	Leonardo da Vinci
1453	Fall of Constantinople, end of Byzantine Empire
1454	Gutenberg patents printing press
1479	Start of Spanish Inquisition
1473–1543	Life of Copernicus
1492	Columbus reaches New World
1517	Luther begins Reformation by posting refutations on church door
1540	Jesuit order established
1543	Copernicus

1550	Glass mirrors
1564–1642	Galileo Galilei
1564–1616	Shakespeare
1580	Flush toilets
1596–1650	Rene Descartes
1561–1626	Francis Bacon (1597 Bacon's Essays)
1609	Dutch Republic, a haven of intellectual freedom
1600	Shakespeare's *Hamlet* Giordano Bruno executed
1602	Kepler's *On the Move*
1633	Galileo condemned by Inquisition
1648	End of religious wars in Europe
1665	Newton develops calculus
1677	Leeuwenhoek's discovery of microorganisms
1769	James Watt patents steam engine
1771	Dentistry
1775	American Revolution
1776	U.S. Declaration of Independence
1781	Kant's *Critique of Pure Reason*
1789	French Revolution United States Bill of Rights
1792	Denmark becomes first country to abolish slavery
1798	Malthus warns about population
1801	First railroad (England)
1802	Mass production (pulleys for the British Navy)
1804	Steam Railroad

1808	Goethe's *Faust I*
1823	Internal combustion engine
1824	Beethoven's Ninth Symphony
1831	Faraday discovers electromagnetism
1835	Telegraph
1840	World anti-slavery convention
1844	Birth of Nietzsche
1848	Seneca Falls Conference—beginning of women's suffrage
1854	Henry David Thoreau, *Walden Pond*
1855	Walt Whitman, *Leaves of Grass*
1859	Darwin's *Origin of Species* First commercial oil well
1860	Abraham Lincoln elected
1861–65	U.S. Civil War
1865	Slavery abolished in U.S.
1862	Machine guns
1863	First subway in London
1867	Dynamite
1871	Darwin's *Descent of Man*
1873	Maxwell's *Treatise on Electricity and Magnetism*
1876	Telephone (Alexander Graham Bell files patent) Refrigeration
1879	Edison light bulb First skyscraper (Leitner building, Chicago)
1880	First automobiles
1886	Wax cylinder recording

1891	Motion pictures
1892	Typewriters
1896	First Brownie camera by Kodak
1900	Death of Nietzsche Freud's *Interpretation of Dreams* Planck initiates quantum physics
1901	Transatlantic radio broadcast
1905	Einstein's theory of special relativity
1908	Orville Wright: one hour plane ride
1911	Television Color photography
1912	Jung's *Psychology of the Unconscious,* break from Freud
1913	Ford begins mass production of automobiles
1914	First airline passenger
1915	Theory of general relativity
1916	Einstein's General Theory of Relativity
1914–1918	World War One
1920	First public radio broadcast Women win the right to vote in the U.S.
1923	League of Nations
1926	Schrodinger's wave equation–quantum mechanics
1928	Penicillin
1929	Stock market crash in U.S.
1933	Hitler comes to power
1939	Hitler invades Poland, start of World War Two Antibiotics in use
1941	Bombing of Pearl Harbor

1942	Transistors
1943	Sartre's existentialism: publishes *Being and Nothingness* Albert Hoffman discovers LSD
1945	Hiroshima, Nagasaki bombed, end of WW II Founding of United Nations
1946	First digital computers
1948	Robert Graves, *The White Goddess*
1949	George Orwell's *1984*
1951	Witchcraft laws repealed in England
1953	Structure of DNA revealed by Watson and Crick
1954	Solar power: photovoltaic cells
1955	Fiber optics Teilhard de Chardin, *The Phenonmenon of Man* (lifespan: 1881-1955)
1957	Sputnik satellite launched by the USSR
1960's	Civil rights movement, rise of feminism, psychedelic revolution, peace movement, women's liberation
1961	First space flights Acid rain discovered
1962	Rachel Carson's *Silent Spring*—start of environmental alarm Founding of Esalen, human potential movement Kuhn's *Structure of Scientific Revolutions*
1964	Free speech movement in Berkeley
1965	Escalation of Vietnam war
1966	Endangered species act
1967	Summer of Love in U.S.
1968	Bertalanffy's General Systems Theory

1969	Moon landing James Lovelock's Gaia Hypothesis Ehrlich's *The Population Bomb*
1970	First Earth Day
1973	Abortion legalized in U.S. (Roe v. Wade)
1974	Gimbutas's *Goddesses and Gods of Old Europe*
1975	Fritjof Capra's *Tao of Physics*
1980	Personal computers common
1983	Computer viruses
1986	Carpal tunnel syndrome
1987	E-mail
1988	Prozac RU 486 (morning after pill) Nanotechnology
1989	Berlin Wall comes down, end of Cold War
1990–2000	Human Genome Project
1991	Persian Gulf War
1995	Clinton impeachment over Monica Lewinsky
2001	September 11th attacks
2003	Invasion of Iraq
2004	Tsunami in East Asia
2005	New Orleans flooded

SOURCES FOR TIMELINE

Bryan Bunch and Alexander Hellemans, eds., *The Timetables of Technology: A Chronology of the Most Important People and Events in the History of Technology.* New York: Simon & Schuster, 1993.

Chris Scarre, *Smithsonian Timelines of the Ancient World,* New York: DK Publishing, 1993, 1999.

Richard Tarnas, *The Passion of the Western Mind.* New York: Ballantine, 1991.

Bruce Wetterau, *MacMillan Concise Dictionary of World History.* New York: MacMillan, 1983.

Hammond Atlas of World History: The Ultimate Work of Historical Reference, London: HarperCollins, 1999.

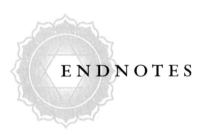

ENDNOTES

CHAPTER 1

[1] Joseph Campbell in conversation with Bill Moyers, *The Power of Myth,* New York: Doubleday, 1988, p. 32.

[2] Duane Elgin, *Promise Ahead: A Vision of Hope and Action for Humanity's Future,* New York: HarperCollins, 2000, p. 1.

[3] Lester Brown, Gary Gardner, Brian Halwell, *Beyond Malthus: Sixteen Dimensions of the Population Problem,* Worldwatch Paper 143, September 1998.

[4] Thomas Malthus, *An Essay on the Principle of Population, as it Affects the Future Improvement of Society with Remarks on the Speculations of Mr. Godwin, M. Condorcet, and Other Writers.* London, Johnston, 1798.

[5] Jean Houston, *Jump Time: Shaping Your Future in a World of Radical Change,* New York: Tarcher/Putnam, 2000, p. 1.

CHAPTER 2

[1] Rainer Maria Rilke, *Letters to a Young Poet,* New York: Norton, 2004.

[2] Joseph Campbell, *The Hero with a Thousand Faces,* Princeton, New Jersey: Princeton University Press, 1949, p. 51.

CHAPTER 3

[1] As quoted by John R. Van Eenwyk, *Archetypes and Strange Attractors: The Chaotic World of Symbols,* Toronto: Inner City Books, 1997, p. 139.

[2] Samuel Noah Kramer, *Inanna, Queen of Heaven and Earth: Her Stories from Sumer,* New York: Harper & Row, 1983, p. 127.

[3] *Ibid.,* p. 56 ff..

[4] One could argue that these roughly correspond to the chakras, from top to bottom.

[5] R. J. Stewart, *The Underworld Initiation: A Journey through Psychic Transformation.* Great Britain: Aquarian Press, 1985, p. 67.

[6] *Ibid.,* p. 23.

[7] Lion Goodman, "A Shot in the Light," *I Thought My Father was God,* Paul Auster, ed. New York: Henry Holt, 2001, p. 195 ff.

[8] Gregg Easterbrooke, *The Progress Paradox,* New York: Random House, 2003. p. 38.

[9] Thanks to Hari Meyers for pointing out this distinction.

CHAPTER 4

[1] Joseph Campbell, *The Hero with a Thousand Faces,* Princeton: Princeton University Press, 1968, p. 61.

[2] Marija Gimbutas, *The Civilization of the Goddess,* Harper Collins, 1991, p. 364.

[3] Richard Leakey, *Origins* New York: Dutton, 1977, p. 61.

[4] Gareth Hill, *Masculine and Feminine: The Flow of Oppposites in the Psyche* Boston: Shambhala, 1992.

[5] Sam Keen, audio tape, *Collective Myths We Live and Die By,* Mystic Fire Audio, 1994. He also said this was one of the rules of the Republicans and political conservatives.

[6] Michael Meade, *Men and the Water of Life: Initiation and the Tempering of Men,* Harper San Francisco, 1993, p. 12.

CHAPTER 5

[1] Michael Meade, *Men and the Water of Life: Initiation and the Tempering of Men,* HarperSanFrancisco, 1993, p. 12.

[2] Gareth Hill, *Masculine and Feminine: The Flow of Opposites in the Psyche,* Boston: Shambhala, 1992.

[3] Hesiod's *Theogony* translated by Norman O. Brown, Indianapolis, Indiana: Bobbs-Merrill, 1953, p. 15.

[4] Alain Danielou, *The Gods of India,* New York: Inner Traditions, 1985, p. 312.

[5] Erich Jantsch, *The Self-Organizing Universe* Great Britain: Pergamon, 1980, p. 137.

[6] Marija Gimbutas, *Civilization of the Goddess,* San Francisco: Harper Collins, 1991, p. 257.

[7] Mircea Eliade, *A History of Religious Ideas, Vol. 1,* Chicago: University of Chicago Press, 1978, p. 40.

[8] *Ibid.,* p. 40.

[9] Erich Neumann, *The Origins and History of Consciousness,* New York: Bollingen Foundation, 1954, p. 117.

[10] Anne Baring and Jules Cashford, *The Myth of the Goddess: Evolution of an Image.* London: Penguin Arkana, 1993, p. 75.

[11] *Ibid.,* p. 92.

[12] Estimates on the time frame for building Stonehenge vary greatly, spanning anywhere from 600 years to 2,000 years, depending on the source.

CHAPTER 6

[1] Catherine Keller, *From a Broken Web: Separation, Sexism, and Self,* Boston: Beacon Press, 1986, p. 65.

[2] A. N. Whitehead, *Process and Reality: An Essay in Cosmology,* ed. D. R. Griffin, and D. W. Sherburne, New York: Free Press, 1978, p. 340.

[3] Joseph Campbell, *Creative Mythology,* New York: Penguin Books, 1962, p. 420.

[4] *Science,* Vol. 304, April, 2004, p. 663.

[5] It is also possible, as Leonard Shlain has suggested, that the birth of alphabetic writing shifted the locus of activity from the holistic, image-oriented right brain to the more linear left brain. See *Alphabet vs. the Goddess: The Conflict Between Word and Image,* New York: Penguin Press, 1998. (That many have associated these brain states with feminine and masculine respectively may be more a comment on the periods in which they were favored than on actual gender qualifications.)

[6] Gerda Lerner, *The Creation of Patriarchy,* New York: Oxford University Press, 1986, p. 56.

[7] Ibid., p. 63.

[8] As quoted by Anne Baring and Jules Cashford, *The Myth of the Goddess: Evolution of an Image,* London: Penguin Arkana, 1993, p. 152.

[9] Circa 1580 B.C.E. This is the oldest proof of the contents of this myth, though its rewritten tablets date to about 1,000 B.C.E.

[10] As quoted by Joseph Campbell, *The Masks of God: Occidental Mythology,* New York: Viking Press, 1964, p. 77.

[11] Ibid., p. 79.

[12] "Epic of Creation," translated by E. A. Speiser. Ninian Smart and Richard D. Hecht, *Sacred Texts of the World: A Universal Anthology,* New York: Crossroad, 1982. P. 6.

[13] Ibid., p. 7.

[14] Ibid., p. 8.

CHAPTER 7

[1] *Epic of Gilgamesh,* Penguin edition, trans. N. K. Sandars, 1960, 1964.

[2] Ibid., pp. 114 - 115.

[3] Andrew Bard Shmookler, *Out of Weakness: Healing the Wounds that Drive Us to War,* New York: Bantam, 1988, p. 6.

[4] Hari Meyers, from a lecture given in Sebastopol, California, 2004.

[5] Andrew Bard Schmookler, *Parable of the Tribes: The Problem of Power in Social Evolution* Boston: Houghton Mifflin, 1984.

[6] Andrew Bard Schmookler, *Out of Weakness: Healing the Wounds that Drive Us to War,* New York: Bantam, 1988, p. 5.

[7] See Ken Wilber's works, especially, *A Brief History of Everything,* Boston: Shambhala, 2000.

[8] John Keegan, *A History of Warfare,* London: Random House, 1993, p. 304.

[9] *The Age of God-Kings,* Alexandria, Virginia: Time-Life Books, 1987, p. 63.

[10] *Barbarian Tides: TimeFrame 1500 – 600 B.C.* Richmond, Virginia: Time-Life Books, 1987, p. 17.

[11] Joseph Campbell, *The Hero with a Thousand Faces,* p. 40 ff.

[12] Ibid., p. 15.

[13] Ibid., p. 44.

CHAPTER 8

[1] http://www.brainyquote.com/quotes/authors/s/socrates.html.

[2] "The Grandeur of Imperial Rome," *Empires Ascendant: TimeFrame 400 BC-AD 200,* Alexandria, Virginia: Time-Life Books, 1987. p. 45.

[3] Ibid., p. 47.

CHAPTER 9

[1] Joseph Campbell with Bill Moyers: *The Power of Myth,* New York: Doubleday, 1988, p. 207.

[2] Christians worldwide: http://www.adherents.com/Religions_By_Adherents.html in the US: http://www.d.umn.edu/~mcco0322/history.htm

[3] According to Timothy Freke and Peter Gandy, in *Jesus and the Lost Goddess,* there is no record of a place called Nazareth. Instead, they suggest that he was called "Jesus the Nazarene," a word that means "initiate." Timothy Freke and Peter Gandy, in *Jesus and the Lost Goddess,* New York: Three Rivers Press, 2001, p. 102.

[4] John 10: 31-36 "Is it not written in your law, I said, 'You are Gods.'"

[5] The story of Jesus restoring eyesight to the blind can be interpreted as opening the eyes of the initiate, as non-initiates were called by the Greeks *mystae,* meaning "eyes closed," and initiates were called *epopteia,* meaning "those who could see."

[6] Elaine Pagels, *Adam, Eve, and the Serpent* New York: Vintage Books, 1989, p. 4.

[7] See Burton Mack, *Who Wrote the New Testament?* San Francisco: HarperSanFrancisco, 1995, p. 124 ff.

[8] Gareth Hill, *Masculine and Feminine: The Natural Flow of Opposites in the Psyche,* Boston: Shambhala, 1992, p. 16.

[9] Joseph Campbell, in conversation with Bill Moyers, *The Power of Myth,* New York: Doubleday, 1988, p. 199.

[10] Elaine Pagels, *Adam, Eve, and the Serpent* New York: Vintage Books, 1989, p. 82-83.

[11] An interesting footnote to Theodosius' reign was that he was originally protective of Pagan cults and shrines. His own crime, however, was to massacre seven thousand civilians in response to a tumult, for which he served eight months' penance. It was apparently after this that he changed his attitude about non-Christian religions and set out the decrees that led to their destruction. For more information, see: http://www.newadvent.org/cathen/14577d.htm.

[12] It wasn't until December, 1945 that an Arab peasant accidently discovered a jar containing ancient Gnostic texts near the town of Nag Hammadi. These texts, known as the Gnostic Gospels, had been buried to keep from being destroyed. They reveal a very different view of the Christian story from the orthodox view that has prevailed. See Elaine Pagels, *The Gnostic Gospels* New York: Vintage Books, 1989.

[13] See Burton Mack, *Who Wrote the New Testament? The Making of the Christian Myth,* San Francisco: HarperSanFranciscio, 1989, p. 82.

[14] a more common interpretation of sin is to "miss the mark," a term that comes from archery.

[15] Elaine Pagels, *Adam, Eve, and the Serpent,* p. 112.

[16] Ibid., p. 129.

[17] Ibid., p. 125-126.

CHAPTER 10

[1] Elaine Pagels, *The Gnostic Gospels* New York: Vintage Books, 1989, p. 34.

[2] J. N. Hillgarth, *The Conversion of Western Europe,* Englewood Cliffs, New Jersey: Prentice Hall, 1969, p. 44-48.

[3] For a discussion of chakras and the demons that arise from repressing them, see Anodea Judith, *Eastern Body, Western Mind: Psychology and the Chakra System as a Path to the Self,* p. 34-36.

[4] Charles Homer Haskin, *The Renaissance of the 12th Century,* New York: Meridian, 1927, p. 45.

[5] Jeffrey Burton Russell, *A History of Medieval Christianity,* New York: Thomas Y. Cromwell, 1968, p. 92.

[6] Ibid., p.165.

[7] James A. Haught, *Holy Horrors,* Buffalo, New York: Prometheus, 1990, p. 25-26.

[8] Henry C. Lea, *The Inquisition of the Middle Ages,* New York: MacMillan, 1961, p. 46.

[9] Helen Ellerbe, *The Dark Side of Christianity,* San Rafael: Morningstar, 1995, p. 42.

[10] Serenity Young, ed. *An Anthology of Sacred Texts By and About Women,* New York: Crossroad, 1993, p. 46.

[11] Karen Armstrong, *The Gospel According to Women: Christianity's Creation of the Sex War in the West,* New York: Doubleday, 1986, p. 71.

[12] St. Thomas Aquinas, *Summa Theologia,* (London: Blackfriars, Questions 92, 35.

[13] Karen Armstrong, *op.cit.,* p. 69.

[14] R. de Maulde-La-Claviere, *Women of the Renaissance*, and Jaccques Maritain, *Three Reformers,* as quoted by Leonard Shlain, *The Alphabet vs. the Goddess,* p. 329.

[15] Helen Ellerbe, *The Dark Side of Christianity,* San Rafael: Morningstar, 1995, p. 95.

[16] Jean Delumeau, *Catholicism Between Luther and Voltaire.* London: Burns & Oats, 1977, 438-39.

[17] William Edward Hartpole Lecky, *History of Rationalism in Europe,* London: Longmans, 1904, 1:387.

[18] Charles Beard, *The Reformation of the Sixteenth Century,* London: Williams and Norgate, 1907, p. 250.

[19] Helen Ellerbe, *op. cit.,* p. 88.

[20] Jean Plaidy, *The Spanish Inquisition,* New York: Citadel Press, 1967, p. 143.

CHAPTER 11

[1] Richard Tarnas, *The Passion of the Western Mind,* New York: Ballantine, 1991, p. 251.

[2] Jacques Maritain, *Three Reformers: Luther, Descartes, Rousseau,*New York: Scribner, 1950, p. 33.

[3] James Burke, *The Day the Universe Changed,* Boston: Little, Brown, 1985, p. 149.

[4] Fritjof Capra, *The Turning Point: Science, Society, and the Rising Culture*, New York: Simon & Schuster, 1982, p. 56.

[5] Rupert Sheldrake, *The Rebirth of Nature: The Greening of Science and God,* New York:

Bantam, 1991, p. 43-44.

[6] Ibid. p. 43-44.

[7] In *New Atlantis,* published 1624.

[8] It could be argued that the Gnostic Christians were aware of the powers of consciousness, but they were heavily repressed by the rise of orthodoxy.

[9] See the myth of Zurvan, p. xx) typsetter, set page #

[10] "Dualism in Descartes: The Logical Ground." Hooker, Michael, ed. *Descartes.* Baltimore: Johns Hopkins University Press, as quoted by Fritjof Capra.

[11] James Burke, *The Day the Universe Changed,* Boston: Little, Brown, 1985, p. 266.

[12] David Loye, *Darwin's Lost Theory of Love: A Healing Vison for the New Century,*Lincoln, Nebraska: toExcel, 2000, p. 5.

[13] James Burke, *The Day the Universe Changed,* Boston: Little, Brown, 1985, p. 261.

[14] As quoted by James Burke, p. 266.

[15] As quoted by James Burke, p. 272.

[16] As pointed out by Rupert Sheldrake, p. 10.

[17] Thanks to Leonard Shlain for this insight, *The Alphabet vs. the Goddess,* p. 390.

[18] From John Stuart Mill, *The Subjection of Women,* as quoted by Leonard Shlain, p. 389.

[19] Bryan Bunch and Alexander Hellemans, eds., *The Timetables of Technology: A Chronology of the Most Important People and Events in the History of Technology,* New York: Simon and Schuster, 1993, p. 283.

20 Ken Wilber, *The Marriage of Sense and Soul.* New York:Random House, 1998.

[21] Ibid.

CHAPTER 12

[1] Mark Morford "What's on your iGod?" http://sfgate.com/columnists/morford/archive

[2] Fees to attend this festival are paid in advance and range from $160 to $250 for the week, depending on when you buy your ticket. One you are in the gate, there is no vending or even bartering among participants. For more information about Burning Man, go to www.burningman.com.

[3] For pictures of this sculpture, see http://www.templeofgravity.com.

[4] Gareth Hill, Masculine and Feminine: The Natural Flow of Opposites in the Psyche, Boston: Shambhala, 1992, p. 17.

[5] Paul Ray, Cultural Creatives: How 50 Million People are Changing the World, New York: Harmony Books, 2000.

CHAPTER 13

[1] Thanks to James O'Dea, president of IONS, for this phrase. Christmas lecture on IONS campus, 2005.

[2] Joanna Macy, *Coming Back to Life: Practices to Reconnect Our Lives, Our World,* Canada: New Society Publishers, 1998, p. 17.

[3] Gregg Easterbrooke, *The Progress Paradox: How Life Gets Better While People Feel Worse,* New York: Random House, 2003, p. 80-81.

[4] Duane Elgin, *Promise Ahead,* New York: William Morrow, 2000, p. 99.

[5] Ibid., p. 12-13.

[6] Trends datasets/Population and Health/Refugees/International Refugees.html.

[7] Carolina Rodriguez Bello, "Refugees and Internally Displaced," 2003, Women's Human Rights Net, a division of Association for Women's Rights in Development (AWID) http://www.whrnet.org/docs/issue-refugees.html.

[8] Paul Hawken, "Possibilties." *Imagine: What America Could Be in the 21ˢᵗ Century,* Marianne Williamson, ed., Rodale, 2000, p. 4.

[9] http://www.nrdc.org/water/drinking/uscities/contents.asp.

[10] As quoted from World Watch Institute's CD Rom, *Signposts 2004.* From the article: *Behind the Scenes: Bottled Water,* by Paul McRandle.

[11] Another five million non-Jews died as well. http:www.jewishgen.org/ ForgottenCamps/General/FaqEng.html.

[12] Ibid., Worldwatch, Trends datasets/Population and Health/Life Expectancy.

[13] Ibid., Trends datasets/Population and Health/Infant Mortality.

[14] Ibid., Trends datasets/Population and Health/HIV and AIDS.

[15] "43.6 Million Don't Have Health Insurance" *USA Today*, 9/30/2003.

[16] http://www.chronicpain.org.

[17] Ibid. ,Wordwatch, Trends datasets/Population and Health/HIV and AIDS.

[18] Ibid., Worldwatch, Trends datasets/Population and Health.

[19] Jeremy Rifkin, *The European Dream: How Europe's Vision of the Future is Quietly Eclipsing the American Dream,* New York: Tarcher, 2004. p. 340.

[20] UN Global Report Millennial Equisystem Assessment: Living Beyond our Means, 2005.

[21] http://www.ourstolenfuture.org/NewScience/reproduction/sperm/humansperm.htm. A 1992 study in the *British Medical Journal* found that men in Western countries today have less than half the sperm production their grandfathers had at the same age. The report examined 61 separate studies of sperm count in men in many countries, including the U.S., and concluded that there has been a 42 percent decrease in average sperm count, from 113 million per milliliter (ml) to 66 million per ml, since 1940. (There are 4.5 milliliters in a teaspoon). http://www.alkalizeforhealth.net/Lspermdamage2.htm.

[22] Gregg Easterbrooke, *The Progress Paradox,* New York: Random House, 2003, p. 38.

[23] http://www.internetworldstats.com/stats.htm.

[24] Thomas Friedman, *The World is Flat: A Brief History of the 21ˢᵗ Century,* New York: Farrar, Straus, and Giroux, 2005.

[25] Ibid., p. 163.

[26] Ibid., p. 45.

[27] Ibid., p. 8.

[28] Jean Houston, *Jump Time*, New York: Tarcher/Putnam, 2000, p. 11.

[29] June Singer, *The Power of Love to Transform Our Lives and Our World,* York Beach: Nicolas-Hays, 2000, p. 62.

[30] Michael Nagler, *The Search for a Nonviolent Future:* Makao,: Inner Ocean, 2004, p. 31.

[31] Hazel Henderson, *Paradigms in Progress: Life Beyond Economics,* Indianoplis: Knowledge Systems, 1991, p. 6

[32] James Nesbitt, *Megatrends2000: New Directions for Tomorrow,* New York: Avon, 1990.

[33] Jay Earley, *Transforming Human Culture: Social Evolution and the Planetary Crisis,* New York: SUNY Press, 1997.

[34] Former State Senator Tom Hayden, speaking at the Praxis Peace Conference, June 2004.

CHAPTER 14

[1] Pierre Teilhard de Chardin, *The Phenomenon of Man,* New York: Harper Collins, 1955, p. 244.

[2] From a talk given at the Bioneers Conference, San Francisco, 2004.

[3] Paul Hawken, "Possibilities," *Imagine: What America Could be in the 21ˢᵗ Century,* Marianne Williamson, ed. 2000, p. 7.

[4] Margaret Wheatley, *Leadership and the New Science Discovering Order in a Chaotic World,* San Francisco: BerrettKoehler, 1999, p. 111.

[5] Ibid., p. 11.

[6] Arthur Koestler, *The Ghost in the Machine,* Hutchinson, 1967.

[7] Margaret J. Wheatley, *Leadership and the New Science,* San Francisco: Berrett-Koehler Publishers, 1999, 21.

[8] Erich Jantsch, *Evolution and Consciousness: Human Systems in Transition,* Erich Jantsch and Conrad Waddington, ed., Reading, Massachusetts: Addison-Wesley, 1976, p. 4

[9] Erich Janstch, *The Self-Organizing Universe,* Great Britain: Pergamon, 1980, p. 40.

[10] Duane Elgin, *Promise Ahead: A Vision of Hope and Action for Humanity's Future,* New York: William Morrow, 2000, p. 9-12.

[11] Thomas Lewis, et al. *A General Theory of Love,* New York: Vintage Books, 2000, p. 123.

[12] Margaret Wheatley, *Leadership and the New Science,* p. 40.

[13] Ibid., p. 101.

[14] Ibid, p. 107.

[15] Erich Jantsch, *The Self-Organizing Universe,* p. 177.

[16] Thanks to Brooks Cole for this phrase, www.holocosmos.com.

[17] Margaret Wheatley, *Leadership and the New Science,* p. 89-90.

CHAPTER 15:

[1] Google Scholar: http://www.ncbi.nlm.nih.gov/entrez/query.fcgi?cmd=Retrieve&db=PubMed&list_uids=7804768&dopt=Citation (This is based on reported cases. The actual number is likely to be higher.)

[2] Erich Jantsch, *Design for Evolution: Self-Organization and Planning in the Life of Human*

Systems, New York: George Braziller, 1975, p. 77 ff.

[3] Ken Wilber, *A Brief History of Everything,* Boston: Shambhala, 1996. (This theory is echoed in many of his works.)

[4] Barbara Marx Hubbard, *Conscious Evolution: Awakening the Power of our Social Potential,* Novato: New World Library, 1998, p. 99.

[5] Lewis, et al, *A General Theory of Love,* New York: Vintage Books, 2000, p. 191.

[6] Fritjof Capra, *The Turning Point* and other works.

[7] Martin Buber, *I and Thou,* Walter Kaufmann, trans. New York: Simon & Schuster, 1970.

[8] As quoted by Anthony Stevens, *Archetypes: A Natural History of the Self.* New York: Quill, 1983, p. 163.

[9] Ibid, p. 163.

[10] Ibid. p. 164.

[11] A term popularized by C. G. Jung, but originating with St. Augustine.

[12] Pierre Teilhard de Chardin, *The Phenomenon of Man,* New York: Harper Collin, 1955, p. 293.

[13] Ibid., Lewis.

[14] Georg Feuerstein, "Some Thoughts on Axis Mundi. http://www.yrec.info/contentid-132.html.

[15] *I Ching,* Wilhelm/Baynes version, New Jersey: Princeton University Press.

[16] Thanks to Richard Ely for these insights, published in the article, "Science and Mysticism: Siblings Under the Skin," *Pan Gaia,* Issue #16, Summer 1998.

[17] Ken Wilber, *The Marriage of Sense and Soul: Integrating Science and Religion,* New York: Random House, 1998, p. 4.

[18] The four quadrants of Wilber's Integral theory are expressed in a number of his books, perhaps the most basic being, *A Brief History of Everything,* Boston: Shambhala, 2000.

[19] For more on this, see Larry Dossey, M.D., *Healing Words: The Power of Prayer and the Practice of Medicine,* San Francisco: HarperSanFrancisco, 1993. The Instituate of Noetic Sciences is also doing research on this subject. See http://www.noetic.org/research/projects.cfm.

[20] Larry Dossey, *Recovering the Soul: A Scientific and Spiritual Search.* New York: Bantam, 1989.

[21] Duane Elgin, *Awakening Earth: Exploring the Evolution of Human Culture and Consciousness,* New York: Morrow, 1993, p. 295.

[22] Ibid., p. 295.

[23] Carl Jung, *The Psychology of Kundalini Yoga,* New Jersey: Princeton University Press, edited by Sonu Shamdasani, 1996.

CHAPTER 16

[1] Rob Brezny, *Pronoia is the Antidote for Paranoia,* Berkeley: Frog, 2005, p. 3.

[2] Dalai Lama, *How To Expand Love,* translated and edited by Jeffrey Hopkins, New York: Atria, 2005, p. 134.

[3] Kokoman Clottey and Aeeshah Ababio-Clottey, "Race Relations," from *Imagine: What America Could Be in the 21ˢᵗ Century,* Marianne Williamson, Rodale Books, 2000, p. 157.

[4] Duane Elgin, *Promise Ahead:A Vision of Hope and Action for Humanity's Future,* New York: Morrow, 2000, p. 9-12 (Italics his).

[5] Jeremy Rifkin, *The European Dream:How Europe'sVision of the Future is Quietly Eclipsing the American Dream* New York: Tarcher Penguin, 2004, p. 3.

[6] Ibid., p 377.

[7] Ibid., p. 279-80.

[8] Thomas Lewis, et al., *A General Theory of Love,* New York: Vintage, 2000, p. 228.

[9] Pierre Teilhard de Chardin, *The Phenomenon of Man,* New York: Harper Collins, 1955, p. 288.

[10] Willis Harman, "The Shifting Worldview: Toward a More Holistic Science," *Holistic Education Review,* September 1992.

[11] Transendental Meditation website: http://www.t-m.org.uk/research/46.shtml.

[12] Elisabet Sahtouris, adapted from *Understanding Globalization as an Evolutionary Leap* presented to the Institute of Noetic Sciences, July 2001.

CHAPTER 17

[1] Brian Weller, personal conversation.

To find out more, their website is: http://www.greentransitions.org/WEL/WillitsEconLoc.htm.

[2] Richard Heinberg, *Power Down: Options and Actions for a Post-Carbon World.* British Columbia: New Society, 2004.

[3] Pierre Teilhard de Chardin, *The Phenomenon of Man,* New York: Harper Collins, 1995 p. 237.

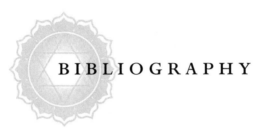

BIBLIOGRAPHY

American Museum of Natural History. *The First Humans: Human Origins and History to 10,000 B.C.* San Francisco: HarperCollins, 1993.

American Museum of Natural History. *People of the Stone Age: Hunter-gatherers and Early Farmers.* New York: HarperCollins, 1993.

Armstrong, Karen. *The Gospel According to Woman: Christianity's Creation of the Sex War in the West.* New York: Anchor, 1987.

Baring, Anne and Cashford, Jules, *The Myth of the Goddess: Evolution of an Image.* London: Penguin Arkana, 1993.

Buber, Martin, *I and Thou,* translation by Walter Kaufmann, New York: Simon and Schuster, 1970.

Barraclough, Geoffrey, ed. *Hammond Atlas of World History.* New Jersey: Hammond, 1999.

Bateson, Gregory, *Mind and Nature: A Necessary Unity,* New York: Dutton, 1979.

Burke, James, *The Day the Universe Changed.* Boston: Little, Brown, 1985.

Brown, Norman O. trans. *Hesiod: Theogony.* Indianapolis: Bobbs-Merril, 1953.

Campbell, Joseph. *The Way of the Animal Powers, Vol. I.* San Francisco: Harper & Row, 1983.

Campbell, Joseph. *Hero with a Thousand Faces.* Princeton: Princeton University Press, 1949, 1968.

Campbell, Joseph. *The Masks of God: Primitive Mythology.* New York: Viking Press, 1959

Campbell, Joseph. *The Mythic Image.* New Jersey: Princeton, 1974.

Campbell, Joseph. with Bill Moyers, *The Power of Myth,* New York: Doubleday, 1988.

Capra, Fritjof. *The Tao of Physics,* Berkeley: Shambhala, 1975.

Capra, Fritjof. *The Turning Point: Science, Society and the Rising Culture.* New York: Simon and Schuster, 1982.

Chopra, Deepak. *Peace is the Way.* New York: Harmony, 2005.

Dalai Lama, *How to Expand Love: Widening the Circle of Loving Relationships.* New York: Atria, 2005.

Dossey, Larry, *Recovering the Soul: A Scientific and Spiritual Search.* New York: Bantam, 1989.

Earley, Jay. *Transforming Human Culture.* New York: State University of New York Press, 1997.

Easterbrooke, Gregg. *The Progress Paradox,* New York: Random House, 2003.

Eisler, Riane. *Chalice and the Blade.* San Francisco: Harper & Row, 1987.

Eisler, Riane. *Power of Partnership,* Novato: New World Library, 2002.

Eisler, Riane. *Sacred Pleasure,* San Francisco: HarperSanFrancisco, 1985.

Eisler, Riane. (with David Loye) *The Partnership Way: New Tools for Living and Learning, Healing Our Families, Our Communities and Our Worl.* New York: Holistic, 1998.

Eliade, Mircea. *Rites and Symbols of Initiation: The Mysteries of Brith and Rebirth.* Putnam: Spring, 1958, 2005.

Eliade, Mircea. *A History of Religious Ideas.Vols.I, II, and III.* Chicago: University of Chicago Press, 1978.

Eliade, Mircea. *The Myth of the Eternal Return.* New York: Pantheon Books, 1954.

Elgin, Duane. *Awakening Earth: Exploring the Evolution of Human Culture and Consciousness,* New York: Morrow, 1993.

Elgin, Duane. *Promise Ahead: A Vision of Hope and Action for Humanity's Future.* New York: Morrow, 2000.

Ellerbe, Helen. *The Dark Side of Christian History.* San Rafael: Morningstar Books, 1995.

Freeman, Charles. *The Closing of the Western Mind: The Rise of Faith and the Fall of Reason.* New York: Knopf, 2003.

Freke, Timothy and Gandy, Peter. *Jesus and the Lost Goddess: The Secret Teaching of the Original Christians.* New York: Three Rivers, 2001.

Friedman, Thomas L. *The World is Flat: A Brief History of the Twenty-first Century.* New York: Farrar, Straus, and Giroux, 2005.

Gadon, Elinor. *The Once and Future Goddess,* San Francisco: Harper & Row, 1989.

Gimbutas, Marija. *The Language of the Goddess,,* San Francisco: Harper & Row, 1989.

Gimbutas, Marija. *The Civilization of the Goddess,* San Francisco: HarperCollins, 1991.

Gimbutas, Marija. *The Goddesses and Gods of Old Europe: Myths and Cult Images,* Berkeley: University of California, 1982.

Goodman, Lion, "A Shot in the Light," *I Thought My Father was God,* Paul Auster, ed. New York: Holt, 2001.

Hammond, Debora, *The Science of Synthesis: Exploring hte Social Implications of General System Theory,* Colorado: University Press of Colorado, 2003.

Heinberg, Richard. *Power Down: Options and Actions for a Post Carbon World,* British Columbia: New Society Publishers, 2004.

Henderson, Hazel, *Paradigms in Progress: Life Beyond Economics.* Indianapolis: Knowledge Systems, 1991.

Hill, Gareth S. *Masculine and Femine,* Boston: Shambala, 1992.

Hillman, James. *The Terrible Love of War.* New York: Penguin, 2004.

Houston, Jean, *The Hero and the Goddess: The Odyssey as Mystery and Initiation,* New York:

Ballantine, 1992.

Houston, Jean, *Jump Time: Shaping Your Future in a World of Radical Change,* New York: Tarcher/Putnam, 2000.

Hubbard, Barbara Marx. *Emergence: The Shift from Ego to Essence.* Charlottesville: Hampton Roads, 2001

Jantsch, Erich, *The Self-Organizing Universe,* Great Britain: Pergamon, 1980.

Jantsch, Erich. *Design for Evolution: Self-Organization and Planning in the Life of Human Systems.* New York: George Braziller, 1975.

Jantsch, Erich and Waddington, Conrad. *Evolution and Consciousness: Human Systems in Transition.* Reading: Addison, Wesley, 1976.

Jung, Carl. *Man and his Symbols.* New York: Doublday, 1964.

Keegan, John. *A History of Warfare.* London: Random House, 1988.

Kegan, Robert. *The Evolving Self: Problem and Process in Human Development.* Cambridge: Harvard University Press, 1982.

Keller, Catherine. *From a Broken Web: Separation, Sexism and Self,* Boston: Beacon Press, 1986.

Koestler, Arthur. *The Ghost in the Machine,* New York: Hutchinson, 1967.

Kramer, Kenneth Paul, *Martin Buber's I and Thou: Practicing Living Dialog.* New Jersey: Paulist, 2004.

Leakey, Richard, *Origins.* New York: Dutton, 1977.

Lerner, Gerda, *The Creation of Patriarchy,* Oxford University Press, 1986.

Lewis, Thomas, Amini, Fari, Lannon, Richard. *A General Theory of Love.* New York: Vintage, 2000.

Loye, Davd. *Darwin's Lost Theory of Love: A Healing Vison for the New Century,* Lincoln: toExcel, an imprint of iuniverse.com, 2000.

Mack, Burton. *Who Wrote the New Testament?: The Making of the Christian Myth.* San Francisco: HarperSanFrancisco: 1989.

Macy, Joanna and Molly Young Brown. *Coming Back to Life: Practices to Reconnect Our Lives, Our World.* British Columbia: New Society Publishers, 1998.

Mahdi, Louise Carus, Foster, Steven, and Little, Meredith. *Betwixt and Between: Patterns of Masculine and Feminine in Initiation.* La Salle: Open Court, 1987.

Meade, Michael. *Men and the Water of Life: Initiation and the Tempering of Men.* San Francisco: HarperSanFrancisco, 1993.

Merchant, Carolyn. *The Death of Nature: Women, Ecology and the Scientific Revolution.* San Francisco: HarperSanFrancisco, 1983.

Merchant, Carolyn. *Reinventing Eden: The Fate of Nature in Western Culture.* New York: Routledge, 2003.

Nagler, Michael N. *The Search for a Nonviolent Future: A Promise of Peace for Ourselves, Our Families, and Our World.* Maui: Inner Ocean, 2004.

Neumann, Erich. *The Origins and History of Consciousness.*, Bollingen Foundation, 1954.

Pagels, Elaine. *Adam, Eve, and the Serpent.* New York: Vintage, 1989.

Pagels, Elaine. *The Gnostic Gospels,* New York: Vintage, 1989.

Pfeiffer, John E. *The Creative Explosion,* New York: Harper & Row, 1982.

Prideaux, Tom. *Cro-Magnon Man,* New York: : Time Life Books, 1973.

Ray, Paul and Anderson, Sherry Ruth. *The Cultural Creatives: How 50 Million People Are Change the World.* New York: Three Rivers, 2000.

Rifkin, Jeremy. *Biosphere Politics: A New Consciousness for a New Century.* New York: Crown, 1991.

Rifkin, Jeremy. *The European Dream: How Europe's Vision of the Future is Quietly Eclipsing the American Dream.* NEW YORK: Tarcher/Penguin, 2004.

Sandars, N.K. trans. *Epic of Gilgamesh.* Penguin Edition, 1960, 1964.

Schmookler, Andrew Bard. *Out of Weakness: Healing the Wounds That Drive Us to War.* New York: Bantam, 1988.

Schmookler, Andrew Bard. *The Parable of the Tribes: The Problem of Power in Social Evolution,* Boston: Houghton-Mifflin, 1984.

Sheldrake, Rupert. *The Rebirth of Nature: The Greening of God and Science,* New York: Bantam, 1991.

Singer, June, *The Power of Love to Transform our Lives and Our World.* York Beach: Nicolas-Hays, 2000.

Singer, Thomas. *The Vision Thing: Myth, Politics and Psyche in the World.* New York: Routledge, 200.

Shlain, Leonard, *The Alphabet versus the Goddess: The Conflict Between Word and Image,* New York: Penguin, 1998.

Stewart, R. J. *Underworld Initiation: A Journey Towards Psychic Transformation.* Great Britain: Aquarian, 1985.

Stone, Merlin. *When God was a Woman,* San Diego: Harcourt Brace Jovanich, 1976.

Tannen, Deborah. *The Argument Culture: Moving From Debate to Dialog,* New York: Random House, 1988.

Taylor, A. E. *Aristotle.* New York: Dover, 1955.

Tarnas, Richard. *The Passion of the Western Mind.* New York: Ballantine, 1991.

Teilhard De Chardin, Pierre. *The Phenomenon of Man.* New York: Harper Collins, 1955.

Tolle, Eckhart. *The Power of Now: A Guide ot Spiritual Enlightenment.* Novato: New World Library, 1999.

Van Gennep, Arnold. *Rites of Passage: A Classic Study of Cultural Celebrations.* Chicago: University of Chicago Press, 1960.

Walker, Williston, and Norris, Richard A., Lotz, David W., Handy, Robert T. *A History of the Christian Church, 4th Edition.* New York: Simon and Schuster, 1985.

Wheatley, Margaret. *Leadership and the New Science: Discovering Order in a Chaotic World* San Francisco: Berrett-Koehler, 1999.

White, Michael L. *From Jesus to Christianity: How Four Generations of Visionaries & Storytellers Creation the New Testament and Christian Faith,* San Francisco: HarperSanFrancisco, 2005.

Wilber, Ken. *The Atman Project: A Transpersonal View of Human Development.* Wheaton: Quest, 1980.

Wilber, Ken. *A Brief History of Everything.* Boston: Shambhala, 2000.

Wilber, Ken. *Integral Psychology: Consciousness, Spirit, Psychology, Therapy.* Boston, Shambhala, 2000.

Wilber, Ken. *The Marriage of Sense and Soul: Integrating Science and Religion.* New York: Random House, 1998.

Wilber, Ken. *Up From Eden: A Transpersonal View of Human Evolution.* Wheaton, ILL: Quest Books, 1981.

Wilhelm/Baynes tr. *The I Ching or Book of Changes.* Princeton: Princeton University Press, 1950.

Williamson, Marianne. *Imagine: What America Could Be in the 21st Century.* Rodale, 2001.

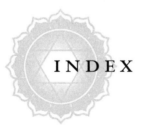

INDEX

A

Ababio-Clottey, Aeeshah, 294
abortion, legalization of (U.S.), *340*
Abu Simbel (Egypt), 114, *332*
acceptance, practice of, 292
Adam and Eve, 154–155
Adam, Eve, and the Serpent (Pagels), 154
adolescence
    awakening, 20–22
    chakra of, *31*
    cultural, 245
    exodus from, 226
    freedom from parental control and, 244–245
    humanity's, 20–25
    identity crisis, collective, 25
    initiation, 20–25
    nature of, *23*
    passing from, 266
    war games of, 24
adulthood
    chakra of, *31*
    interdependency of, 319
    nature of, *23*
    passage into, 20–25
    responsibility of, 22, 248
affection, displays of, 204
Afghanistan, 42, 53
Age of Power, 33
Age of the Heart, 301
Age of the Hero, 119–121
ageism, 207
aggression, militarism and, 94–95, 110, 114–117, 122
AIDS, 224
Akhenaton, *332*
Albigensian Crusades, 165
Alexander the Great, 114, 117–118, 133, *333*
Allah, 253
Alphabet vs. the Goddess (Shlain), 94, 206
Altar of Victory, Roman, 150, *333*
altered states, 209
alternative healing practices, 204
Amaterasu, Sun Goddess (Japanese mythology), 96
Ambrose, St., 153
Amenhotep, Pharoah, 119
American Dream, 302–303

American Revolution, 245, *336*
Amini, Fari, 246, 264, 305
An, Sky God (Sumerian mythology), 96
anahata (heart) chakra, 294–295, 297
anarchic societies, hierarchical vs, 114
anarchy, 113
Anaximenes, 130
ancestral beginnings, chakras of, 28
anima mundi, 267–270, *271*, 305, 308
animal rights movement, 191, 207
Anman, Otto, 185
Anthony, Susan B., 188
anti-Semitism, 166
anti-slavery convention, World, *337*
anti-war movement, 206
Anu (Babylonian), 102
Aphrodite (Greek mythology), 135
Apsu, Great Father, 100–101
aqueducts, *333*
Aquinas, Thomas, 170–171, *335*
Archelaus, 141
archetypal identity, power of, 261
archetypal realms, polarization of, 104
archetypes, central, *279*, 280
Archimedes, 308
The Argument Culture (Tannen), 232
Aristarchus, *333*
Aristotle, 127, 131–132, 133, *333*
arrows, symbology of, 88, 99
art
    Burning Man and, 201
    cave paintings, 60, *331*
    Dark Ages, 163
    goddess figurines, 80, 82, *331*
    mother-son images, banning of, 170
    prehistoric, 60
    Renaissance, 168
    Roman Empire, 135
Artemis (Greek mythology), 135
Artharva Veda, 73
Aryans, 99
Asia Minor, 127, *332*
Assyrians, 99, *332*
atheists, early Christians as, 149
Athens, Greece, 127–128
attraction, Eros and, 73
Atum (Egyptian mythology), 97

Augustine, St., 153–156, 170, *333*
Aurelius, Marcus, *334*
authenticity, 32, 266–267
authority, obedience to, 233
auto-immune diseases, 53
autonomy, freedom and, 192, 244–246
autopoesis, 244
awakening
    adolescent, 20–22
    collective/global, 28, 32, 233
    individual, 28, 32
    spiritual, 43
axis mundi
    alignment with the, 308
    and anima mundi, 267–269, 270
    defined, *271*, 272
    goal of the, 305
axis of evil, 133

B

baby-boomers, 245
Babylonia, mythology of, 97, 99–104, 314, *332*
back-to-the-land movement, 206
Bacon, Francis, 182, 183, *336*
Bad Mother/Good Mother, 75
balance, need for, 19
base instincts vs rational mind, 131–132
beauty as spiritual value, 73
Beck, Don, 209
Beethoven, Ludwig von, *337*
behavior, mythic system and, 261
Being and Nothingness (Sartre), *339*
beliefs and assumptions, exposing our, 27
Berry, Wendell, 39
Bertalanffy, Ludwig von, *339*
Best, David, 201
Bible, 169, 170
Biblical authority, 185
Bill of Rights, U.S., *336*
Bioenergetics, 205
biology as destiny, 64
Bioneers Conference, 237
biosphere
    capacity of the, 22
    compromise of the, 323
    consumption of the, cultural trance and, 308

    intricate web of, 253
    threat to the, 105
Biosphere Politics (Rifkin), 187
birth
    balance between death and, 66
    initiation and, 57
    sacredness of, 74
Black Death plague, 167, 168, *335*
Blake, William, 189
Blue level of Spiral Dynamics, 209
Bocaccio, Giovanni, 168
bonding, mammalian brain and, 304–305
boys, need for differentiation in, 89
Brahma, 253
brain, levels of human, 304–305
Brand, Stuart, 226
Brezney, Rob, 287
Bronze Age
    cities, 99
    human consciousness leap in, 95–96
    mythology of, 96–98, 99–104
    social and environmental chaos of, 95–96, 99
    temples, 99
    third chakra of, *30*, 93
    transition from Mother to Son, 96
brotherhood, Christianity and, 145
Bruni, Leonardo, 168
Bruno, Giordano, 181, *336*
Buber, Martin, 266–267, 307
Buddha, 142–143, *333*
Buddhism, 47
Burning Man, 199–202
Burning Times, 170, 180, 183
Bush (George W), administration of, 53
butterflies, 35–36, 40–41, 51, 53, 323–324
"butterfly effect", 326
Byron, Lord, 189
Byzantine Empire, *159*, *334*

C

the call, 39–43, 45
Calvin, John, 172–173
Campbell, Joseph
    blunders as suppressed longings, 40

future myth, nature of the, 17
"Great Reversal", history's, 89
hero-path, following the thread of the, 313
The Hero with a Thousand Faces, 120–121
innate
    myth, images of, 141
    passages, threshold, 57
    The Power of Myth, 149
    innate releasing mechanisms, 58
Capra, Fritjof, 240, 264, 274, *340*
carcinogenic environments, creation of, 192
Carlson, Jan, 248
Cartesian rationalism, 183
Çatal Hüyük, 78, 79, 82, *331*
caterpillars, metamorphosis of, 35–36, 41, 50, 51, 323
Cathars, 165
cathedrals, Dark Ages, 163–164
Catholic Church
    alliance with the state, 150, 156
    authority of, 155, 164
    ban on Darwin's theories, 185
    civil wars with Protestants, 171
    corruption of, 169
    culturally instilled terror of, 167
    curia council, 164
    domination of society, 167
    indulgences, selling of, 164, 169
    Papal Inquisition of, 166–167
    Pope, power of, 164
    prohibited books, list of, 181
    Protestant Reformation and, 169
    punitive authoritarianism of, 166
    questioning absolute authority of, 166
    Renaissance and, 169
    scientific discoveries, opposition to, 181
    stories of, 315
    taxes of, 169
    Virgin Mary and, 143, 163, 188
    wealth of, 164, 166–167, 168, 169
    women and the Roman, 277
cave paintings, 60, *331*
celebration, practice of, 293
centered, remaining, 307–308
cerebral cortex, 305
chakra theory, 28
chakras. *See also individual chakras*

ascendant spirituality and, 47
balance of third and fourth, need for, 254
communication, 28, 31
elements of, 130, 254
evolution and, 27
evolutionary system and, 262–263
as formula for society's wholeness, 27–28
global awakening and upper chakras, 233
heart as center of system of, 308
integration of upper and lower, 234
levels, *30–31*
lower. *See* lower chakras
need to reclaim first and second, 234
as organizational centers, 268
origin of concept of, 130
as portals between inner and outer worlds, 268
repression of lower, 233
survival instincts and, 58
sushumna location of seven, 268
upper. *See* upper chakras
Chalcolithic era, *85*
Chaos (Greek mythology), 73
chaos theory, 204, 326
chariots, *332*
Charlemagne, *334*
child abuse awareness, 207
childhood. *See also* chakras; *individual chakras*
    dependence of, 89
    differentiation in, 88
    nature of, *23*
    sexual abuse, 257
    stages of, 129
children's rights movement, 191
Chinese medicine, 205
choice fatigue, 226
Chosen People, 134
Christ. *See* Jesus Christ
Christian theology, 148
Christianity
    after Jesus, 146–152
    brotherhood and, 145
    Church. *See* Catholic Church
    Constantine and, 150, *334*
    crimes against humanity. *See* crimes against humanity
    Dark Ages of, 161–163
    development of, 142–143

dictatorial authority of, 155
dominance in world, 141–142
fear and order in, 162
focus of, 47
fourth chakra, 142–143, 145
Greece, 166
Heaven and Earth, gap between, 151
heretics, punishment of, 161
judgment and dogmatism of, 163
official religion of Roman Empire, *334*
original sin doctrine, 151–152, 154–155
Orthodox, 147, 150
power-over paradigm of, 179
Romanization of, 145, 147, 149
social message of, 144–145
stern Father God of, 227
teachings and life of Jesus, 142–147
time chart, *158–159*, *174–175*
unification of church and state, 150
unity and, 145, 282
chrysalises, 36, 41, 50, 51
Chrysostom, St. John, 162
circles, symbology of, 63, 74, 88, 99
Circus Maximus, 134
cities
Bronze Age, 99
consciousness in, focus of, 112
Iron Age, 110–111
social governance in, evolution of, 112, 113
citizen councils, 127
citizenship, origins of, 128
city-states, 121, 127–128, 130
civil disobedience, nonviolent, 204
Civil Rights movement, 191, 207, *339*
Civil War (U.S.), *337*
civilization. *See also* culture
adolescent rebellion of, 170
change, acceleration of, 226
common languages, spread of, 122
complexity of today's, 222
conflict resolution and, 93
converging paths of Nature and, 311
course of, steering the evolutionary,
293–294
cradle of, 109
cultural introversion in Dark Ages, 163
economies of ancient, 122

emergence from the old body politic,
320–321
future of. *See* future
galactic, 298
global, 221, 301
globally conscious, 226
humans as heartbeat of planetary, 319
infant phase, 60. *See also* culture
interrelatedness of, 302–305
leaders of early, 114
oil crisis impact on, 321, 323
relationships foundation of, 265
roots in Neolithic era, 78
sins of our, 315–316
synthesis in history of, 299–302
writing invention and, 93–94
civilization, planetary, 319
class society, development of, 94
Clement of Rome, Bishop, 161
Cleopatra, *333*
Clinton, William, *340*
closed systems, 241
Clottey, Kokoman, 294
co-creation, movement from procreation to,
300–301
co-hearts, 318–319, 327
Coffin, Zachary, 201
cogito ergo sum, 182
Cold War, end of, *340*
Coliseum, 135
collective attention, global focus of, 18
collective, death and resurrection of, 315
collective intelligence, 305
collective reality, ignorance of our, 26
collective unconscious, 57
collective vision, transformation and, 35
Columbus, Christopher, 168, 173, *335*
comfort, second chakra and, 223
coming of age, society's, 26, 32–34, 36, 313
common purpose, finding, 301
commonalities of dualities, seeking, 277
communal living, Middle Ages and, 187
communication
authentic, 266–267
chakras and, 28, 31, 189, 233–234
digital, 204
global, 189, 233–234, 295

high speed, 209–210

communities, 203, 322

community
Jesus' vision of, 145
loss of, 193
political left and right and the global, 323

compassion
awakening, 41–42
blindness to, 253
cerebral cortex and, 305
Christian belief in, 143
fourth chakra and, 28
practice of, 291

competition, 184, 185

condoning vs forgiveness, 292

Confessions (St. Augustine), 153, 154

conflict
birth of, 74
heroes and, 120
language of, 232

conformity
emergence of, 129–133
enforced, 65
fundamentalism and, 243

Confucius, *332*

coniunctio, 268

conscience, Darwin on, 185

Conscious Evolution, 263

consciousness
arrestment of, 120
brain levels and, 304–305
chakras as centers of, 268
chemical effects on, 273, 275
coalescence of, 305
of deep interior of self, 268
Descartes on, 182
divine, belief in, 143
eternal and omnipresent nature of, 252
evolution of, 81, 144
focus during golden age of Greece, 128
global network of, 304
heart as prime integrator of, 308
higher states of, 304
matter and, 275–276
as proof of existence, 183
relationship between outer world and, 270
self-reflective, 205, 267

senses as gateways to, 72–73
as source of questioning, 182
transcendent, 27–28
yoga postures, effect on, 273

consciousness-raising groups, 206

Conservative Right, 242–243

Constantine, Emperor, 150, *334*

Constitution, U.S., 245

consumer rights, 207

content vs process, 204

contribution, practice of, 289–290

control
fear and, 162
guilt and, 152
order and, evolvement of, 99
paradigm of the. *See* ruling paradigm

cooperation
fifth chakra and, 295
need for global, 301–302

Copernicus, 180–181, *335*

Corinthians, resurrection of Christ and, 148

corporatism
Dynamic Feminine and, 206
greed of, justification of, 185

cosmos, emergence of division of, 130

Council of Macon, 170

crafts, development of, 114, 122

creation
destruction and, 104, 226
perception of order in, 137

creativity, unconscious and, 190

Crick, Francis, *339*

crime, violent, 224–225

crimes against humanity, 165–167, 170, 173–174, 180

crisis, results of, 32, 220

Critique of Pure Reason (Kant), *336*

Cro-Magnons, 60

Cronos (Greek mythology), 128

cross, Christian symbol of, 147, 148, 270, 272

Crusades, 164–167, *335*

cult mentality, 65

cultural adolescents, 245

"Cultural Creatives", 209

cultural history, synopsis of, 299–300

cultural trance, society's, 308

culture

adolescence stage of, 20
ancestral beginnings of, 58–61
death of the parent, 221
dissociation of current, 193
environment and, 62
formation of values, 37
homogenization of, 118–119
pre-pubescence stage of, 180
rebellious differentiation stage, 89
rigidity of current, 122
separation from, 308
Static Feminine structure of, 65
synthesis of planet and, 206
time chart, *214–215*
curia council, 164
Cyrus the Great, 133, *333*

D

da Vinci, Leonardo, 168, *335*
Dalai Lama, 282, 291
Damkina (Babylonian), 101
dancing, Protestantism and, 173
Dark Ages, 156, 161–164, 184
Darwin, Charles, 184–185, 252, *337*
death
    avenging of, importance of, 122
    balance between birth and, 66
    fear of, 90
    glorification of, 91
    and resurrection, 147
    rites of passage and, 46
    transformation and, 46, 57, 66
debates of ideas, emergence of, 127
Declaration of Independence, U.S., *336*
"Declaration of Sentiments", 188
defenses, psychological, 191
Demeter (Greek mythology), 49, 98, 151
democracy
    Athenian, *333*
    origin of, 127–128
    participatory, 204, 263
depression, 39
Descartes, Rene, *175*, 182–183, 184, *336*
Descent of Man (Darwin), 184–185, *337*
Design for Evolution (Jantsch), 259
destiny, 39–43, 64

destruction
    creation and, 104, 226
    rebirth and, 220
detox, global, 34
Deus lo volt!, 164
devil, concept of the, 163, 173–174
The Dialogue of the Two Chief Systems of the World
    (Galileo), 181
Diana (Roman mythology), 135
differences, development of, 76
differentiation, cultural, 89
digital communications, 204
Dionysius (Greek mythology), 147
disabilities awareness, 207
disaster
    effects of, 34–35
    as form of initiation, 42, 43
    mitigation of, 35
    opening of the heart and, 34
disasters, natural, 34, 41
disease
    auto-immune, 53
    emotional causes of physical, 272–273
    sanitation to prevent, 186
    spreading of, 192
disequilibrium of systems, evolution and,
    241–242
dissent, danger of, 116
dissolution, society's, 50, 52, 53–54
distance, perspective and, 308
diversity, balance between unity, 282, 301
divine consciousness
    belief in, 143
    co-creation with the, 230
divine feminine realm, 143, 163, 188
Divine Mind, 253
divine realm, Dark Ages view of, 163
divine within, 144, 184
divorce, archetypal, 96
DNA structure revealed, *339*
dominator paradigm
    defending against, 325
    violence and, 228
Dominician order, establishment of, *335*
Donatists, 155
Dossey, Larry, 252, 275
doubt, 132, 182–183

downsizing, 24
drug culture, 224
dualism, ethical, 133
dualities
    attempts to resolve, 276
    commonalities of, seeking, 277
    differentiation, order and, 97
    Eros and, 74
    origins of, 97
    synthesis of, 301
dueling polarities, 232
Dumuzi (Sumerian), 98
Dutch Republic, *336*
Dynamic Feminine paradigm
    adolescence of human evolution and, 208
    Burning Man and, 202
    characteristics of, *279*
    comparison with other paradigms, 202
    contribution of, 280
    corporatism and, 206
    eroticism and, 204
    fight for all rights, 207
    freedom and, 208
    Internet and, 210
    men and, 202, 207
    Nature and, 205–206
    nature of, 202–203, 209, 210
    negative aspects, 208–209, *281*
    nonviolence and, 206
    origins of, 210
    progressive values and, 209, 264
    psychedelic revolution, 282
    redefinition of power, 209
    sacredness of life, 205
    self-determination and, 208
    sexuality and, 204
    spiral symbol of, 202, 272
    spirituality and, 205
    war and, 206
    women and, 202, 206–207
Dynamic Masculine paradigm
    awakening of the, 88
    characteristics of, *279*
    contribution of, 280
    evolution into Static Masculine, 280
    impact of, 122
    individuated identity and, 264

ruling paradigm of, 88–91, 122
terrible twos of human evolution and, 208

E

Ea (Babylonian), 101, 102
Earley, Jay, 234
Earth
    Dark Ages concept of, 162
    denigration and degradation of, 315
    divinity of, 274
    Gaia as, 261
    Heaven, integration with, 50, 267
    infusion with spirit, 274
    objectification of, 258
Earth Day, 205, *340*
Earth Mother, 96, 180
Earthlings, 318
East, material poverty and spiritual richness of, 282
Easterbrooke, Gregg, 222
Eastern traditions, upper chakras and, 282
eco-sustainability, 209, 250, 301
ecocide, ending, 269
ecology movement, 54, 65, 309–310
economics, evolutionary, 262
economies, community, 321–322
ecosystems, 239, 310
ecstasy, 161, 203, 205
Edict of Milan, *333*
Edison, Thomas, 190, *337*
educational institutions, Static Masculine and, 277
ego
    death and transformation of, 47, 51
    discovery of the, 190–192
    dissolution of exterior edges, 205
    evolution of, 81
    transcending the, 192
ego-centeredness, transforming, 29
ego development, 33
Egypt, unification of Upper and Lower, *331*
Egyptian Empire, *106–107*, 110, *124–125*
Egyptians, mythology of, 96–97, 98
Ehrlich, Paul, *340*
"eighth day of creation", 263
Einstein, Albert, 190, *338*
elections, emergence of, 127
electomagnetic forces, harnessing of, 190

electricity, discovery of, 189

electrons and photons, discovery of, 190

Eleusinian Mysteries/rites, 49, 151

Elgin, Duane, 21, 246, 275–276, 301

Eliade, Mircea, 81, 267

elite, ruling, 95

"emergent qualities", 234

emotional states, chemical correlates of, 275

emotions
    Dark Ages and repression of, 162
    effects of repression of, 72, 116–117, 119, 233
    mammalian (limbic) brain and, 304–305
    mythic system and, 260
    repression of male, origins of, 116
    as source of values, 116

empathy, practice of, 291

emperors, Roman, 119

empires
    chakras and, 28
    characteristics of, 121
    origins of, 106–107, 121
    war and, 302

empirical study, emergence of, 180

endangered species act, 339

endless void, 253

energy healing, 204

energy, matter and, 190

England, rebellion against, 245

Enkidu, 111

Enlightenment Age, 184–186, 189, 190

Enlil, Air God (Sumerian mythology), 96, 97

Enuma Elish (Babylonia), 99–104, 332

environment
    abuse of, 22, 29
    carcinogenic, creation of, 192
    culture and, 62
    destruction of, 224
    ethical dualism and destruction of, 133

environmental rights movement, 191, 207

environmentalism, 309

equality
    Christianity and, 145
    gender, 131
    Neolithic era male/female, 81

Ereshkigal (Sumerian), 48, 98

Eros, 73–74, 128, 203

eroticism, Dynamic Feminine paradigm and, 204

eschaton, 152

eternal Thou, 266, 287

ethical dualism, 133

ethical rationalism, 131

Euclidean geometry, 333

Euphrates-Tigris valley, 100, 109–110

European Dream, 303

The European Dream (Rifkin), 302

European economy, Papal Inquisition and, 167

European empires, 106–107, 124–125

European Union, 302

Eve and Adam, 154–155

evil, 132–133, 153

evolution. See also transformation
    adolescence of, Dynamic Feminine paradigm
      and, 208
    archetypal forces of, 62–63
    capacity to influence, 25
    chakras and, 27
    challenges of survival, 58
    Darwin on, 184–185
    disequilibrium of systems and, 241–242, 243
    end of hierarchy, 253
    fear and, 29
    fundamental ground of, 62
    God's way of making more gods, 144, 226, 306
    humans as agents of, 252
    infancy of, Static Feminine and, 208
    interrelatedness and, 302–305
    Jesus teachings and, 144
    limits and, 246
    love and, 29
    middle childhood of, Static Masculine and, 208
    mind's discovery of its own, 250
    principles required for, 243–253
    purpose/result of, 34
    relationships as crucible of, 264
    self-transcendence and, 252
    shift from power to love, 253
    stress and, 242, 243
    survival instinct and, 49, 57
    synthesis and, 299–302
    terrible twos of human, 208

evolutionary economics, 262

evolutionary system, 262–263, 263, 264–265

evolutionary wall, 246, 301–302

Exodus, Jewish, 332

experiments, influence of observer on, 275

extinction, species, 192, 224

F

Faraday, Michael, *337*

farming, Great Mother and, 78

fate, 39–43

Father, corrupt, 316–317

Father-Daughter motif, 143

Father God, Christian, 96, 227

Father, Son and Holy Ghost trinity, 150

Father Time (Zurvan), 132

Faust I (Goethe), *337*

fear

    causes of, 242

    evolution and, 29

    first chakra and, 162

    as means of control, 162

feedback mechanisms, 249, 254, 269

feelings. *See* emotions

females. *See* women

feminine and masculine paradigms. *See*
   paradigms, masculine and feminine

feminine symbols, Neolithic era and, 80, 82

feminine valences, 62–63, 88

feminine values, television and rebirth of, 206

feminism, rise in, 188

feminist movement, 210, *339*

Ferdinand, King, 173

fertility, worship of, 87

Feuerstein, Georg, 270

fifth chakra

    authentic communication and the, 266

    characteristics of, *31, 213*

    cooperation and, 295

    global communication and the, 189, 233–234

fire

    god of, 102

    power over Nature with, 92

first chakra

    autopoesis and, 244

    characteristics of, *30, 212*

    earth element of, 59

    fear and, 162

    Mother Nature and, 58–59

    movement to second chakra, 71–72

    need to reclaim, 234

    Static Feminine and, 63

    survival and, 59, 223

First World Nations, 225

fish, Christian symbol of, 147

Five Rhythms, 306

Florence, Italy, 168

Florentine Republic, *335*

force, as central organizing principle of society,
   228–229

forgiveness, practice of, 142, 292–293

four quadrant theory, 259, 275

fourth chakra

    air element of, 130–131

    characteristics of, *31, 212*

    Christianity and the, 142–143, 145

    compassion and, 28

    ethical rationalism, 131

    as integrator between upper/lower chakras, 234

    key archetypal symbol of, 283

    love and, 27, 28

    relationships and, 27, 28

    Sanskrit name of, 294–295, 297

Franklin, Benjamin, 318

free will

    Dark Ages and, 162

    development of, 93

    Martin Luther on, 170

    St. Augustine on, 154, 155

    suppresion of, 156

    third chakra and, 156

freedom

    Dynamic Feminine paradigm and, 208

    effects of repression of, 242

    external boundaries of, 245

    holon need for autonomy and, 244–246

    limitations to personal, 245–246

    maturation of power and, 246

    responsibility and, 248

    science and, 244

    stability and order in, 245

    third chakra, maturing of the, 246

    trend toward autonomy and, 244

    tyranny and, 42

French Revolution, *336*

Freud, Sigmund, 163, 190, *338*

Friedman, Thomas, 225
fundamentalism, 242–243, 245
future
    challenges of the, 193
    evolutionary system and the, 262
    fixed points, lack of, 222
    growth-based, 24
    guiding vision for the, 35, 221–222
    heroes, need for, 233
    myth of, 17, 313 ff
    navigating the complexity of, 226
    need to embrace, 243
    rites of passage for the, 221
    self-transcendence as organizing vision for, 250
    spiritual growth need for, 226
    uncertainty of, 243
    Z axis alignment of past and, 283

G

Gaea, 73
Gaia (Greek mythology), 96, 128, 261
Gaia Hypothesis, 340
Gaians, 318
Galileo, 33–34, 181, 336
Gandhi, Mahatma, 21, 34, 298
Ganges River, 261
garden, return to the, 326–327
gay liberation movement, 191, 207
Geb, Earth God (Egyptian mythology), 96, 97
Gen X and Y, 318
gender equality, 131
General Systems Theory, 339
A General Theory of Love (Lewis et al), 246, 264, 305
generosity, practice of, 288–289
genocide, 133, 269
Ghalib, 257
Gilgamesh, King, 111–112, 331
Gimbutas, Marija, 61, 340
give-aways, 289–290
global awakening, 221, 233
global brain, 234, 304, 305, 309, 319
global citizens, 318, 323
global communication, 189, 233–234
global feedback mechanism, 254
global heart
    absence of the, 234

awakening the, 265–266, 288–293
coordination and vitalization role of, 323
essential realms of the, 294
global warming, 220
Gnostics, 144, 147, 150
God
    anima mundi as, 269
    as divine architect, 182, 184
    of Love vs God of Hate, 172
    purity of Christian, 163
    transcendant unity of, 253
God and Goddess, integration of, 278
"God is Dead", 187
god-kings, worship of, 227
goddesses
    archaeological discoveries of, 206
    disappearance of, 150
    figurines, 80, 82, 331
    grieving, 97, 98
    Roman and Greek civilizations, 135
    worship of, 80. See also Great Mother
Goddesses and Gods of Old Europe (Gimbutas), 340
gods
    appeasing anger of, 99
    disappearance of, 150
    figurines of Neolithic era, 80
    fire, 102
    God's way of making more, 144, 226, 306
    Neolithic era, 82
    ordering of the, 128
    reduction of power and influence, 129
    sacrifices, ritual, 130
    sky, 91, 95, 96, 98
God's gifts to humanity, 151
gods-in-training, 320
God's way of making more gods, 144, 226, 306
Goethe, Johann, 189, 190, 299, 337
Good Mother/Bad Mother, 75
good vs evil, 132–133, 153
Goodman, Lion, 51
gospel of Jesus, 144–146
gratitude, practice of, 288–289
Graves, Robert, 339
Great Awakening, time of, 18
Great Father, daughter-wife and, 227
Great Mother
    Dark Ages obliteration of, 162

Dynamic Masculine overthrow of, 89–91,
113, 122, 280
era of the, 54, 60–62
farming and the, 78
loss of relevance, 113
as monster, 98
Mother Mary compared to, 143
Neolithic era and, 78–80
organic limits of, 227
primacy of, 89, 90
Roman and Greek civilizations, 135
shift of power to men, 118–119
slaying of, 96
son-lover motif, 102, 227
spirituality and, 90
Static Feminine and, 79, 80, 280
Great Reversal, 89, 162
"Great Turning", 221–222
Greek civilization
aqueducts, *333*
decline of, 134
goddesses of, 135
golden age of, 128–133
Great Mother and, 135
law and order, 129–133
mystery cults of death and rebirth, 148
mythology of, 96, 98
Olympic Games, *332*
poetry, *332*
polytheism, 135
rational system of, 259
reason and detachment, development of, 128
Roman conquest, *333*
time chart, *124–125*
women in, 135–136
Greek Empire
Alexander the Great, 114, 117–118, 133, *333*
slavery, 127
time chart, *106–107, 138–139*
Trojan War, *332*
Green level of Spiral Dynamics, 209
Gregory IX, Pope, 166
Gregory VIII, Pope, 164
"ground qualities", 234
group coordination, origins of, 113
group mind, global, 295
group rapture, 203

growth, measurement of, 24
guiding principles of systems, 239
guilds, formation of, 168
guilt
behavior and, 35
control with, 152
evolution and, 29
Guttenberg, Johan, 168–169, *335*

H

Hades (Greek), 49, 98
Harappa, 110, *332*
Harman, Willis, 308–309
Hawken, Paul, 237
Hayden, State Senator Tom, 234
healing
alternative practices of, 204
distant prayer and, 275
energy, 204
integration of mind and body and, 272
healing movement, alternative, 54
health insurance, lack of, 224
heart
blessing of the, 292
as center of chakra system, 308
coming of age in the, 27, 29
consciousness, prime integrator of, 308
defined, 18
disaster and opening the, 34
global, 221, 234, 278
integrator role of the, 323
joy and opening of the, 293
paradigm of the, 50, 323, 325, *329*
repression of the, 116–117
response to wounds of the, 297
Heart, Age of the, 301
heart chakra. *See* fourth chakra
Heaven and Earth
axis mundi core between, 267
gap between, Christianity and, 151
integration of, 50, 267
reuniting, 273–274
widening gap between, 151
Heaven on Earth
Jesus' promise of, 134, 145, 151, 152, 274
Hebrews, 99

Hegel, Georg, 299
heliocentric theory, *333*
Hellenic Greece, individualism in, 186–187
Hellenic world, 133
Henderson, Hazel, 229, 309
Henry IV, Emperor, 164
Hera (Greek mythology), 135
Heraclitus, 131
herbcraft, Middle Ages, 167
herbology, 204, 205
heretics, punishment of, 161, 164, 166–167
Heroic Age, 33, 119–121
Hero, Age of the, 119–121
hero-path, 313
The Hero with a Thousand Faces (Campbell), 120–121
Herod the Great, 141
heroes
    arrested consciousness of, 120
    conflict and, 120
    coopting of, 123
    dark and light side of, 120–121
    need for new, 232–233
    origins of male, 96, 117–121
    third chakra and, 119–120
    wealth of, 24
heroism
    definition, need for new, 232–233
    domination equation with, 265
    in earlier times, 232
    today's, 232
Hero's journey, 33–34, 37, 51
Hero's Quest, 119–121, 322–323
Hero's return, 33–34, 323
Hesiod, 128, *332*
Hexagrams, *273*, 273
"hi-tech-hi-touch", 234
hidden worlds, discovering, 41
hierarchical societies, anarchic vs, 114
hierarchies, development of, 93–94
hierarchy, death of, 253
hierosgamos, 278, 283, 323
Hill, Gareth, 62–63, 88, 148, 202, 203
Hippocrates, *333*
Hiroshima, 115, *339*
history, human. *See* human history, archetypes of
holarchy of self-organizing systems, 239, 253, 275
Holocaust, 133

Holocene Epoch, *85*
holons
    autonomy and freedom, need for, 244–246
    centering of, 305
    common identity in the, 301
    defined, 239
    mythic system and, 260
    relatedness, need for, 246–249
    self-organization of, conditions for, 243
    self-renewal of, capacity for, 244
    self-transcendence, need for, 249–253
Holy Duality, 143
Holy Trinity, 143, 150
homeless, 223
homeopathy, 205
homeorhesis vs homeostasis, 204
Homer, 128, *332*
Homo Erectus, *68*
Homo Habilis, 92
Homo Heidelbergensis, *68*
Homo Neanderthalensis, *68*
Homo Sapiens, 60, *68*, 69
horizontal (X) axis, 276–283
houses, Neolithic era and, 79
Houston, Jean, 25, 226
Hubbard, Barbara Marx, 263, 300
human history, archetypes of
    importance of understanding the, 26–28
    positive and shadow aspects of, 280
    social patterns among, *279*, 280
    synthesis and, 299–300
human potential movement, *339*
human rights protection, 191
humanism, civic, 168
humanities, *214–215*
humanity
    adolescence of, 21, 170
    awakening, 34
    crimes against, 165, 166–167, 170, 173–174
    global, 42
humans
    as agents of evolution, 252
    ancestors, 60
    awakening heart, need for, 25
    awakening of. *See* Dynamic Feminine
       paradigm
    awareness of self, 62

base instincts vs rational mind of, 131–132

binary conflict of, 75–76

brutality of, 257–258

childlike relationship to parental gods, 227

circular boundary of, 63–64

coming of age process, 26, 32–34, 36

as consumers, 35–36

cost of remaining as children, 316

dehumanization of, 258

developmental stages. *See* chakras; *indivdual chakras*

ego development of, 33

evil nature of, 155

evolution of. *See* evolution; transformation

feelings of disconnection, 225

fostering a new identity, 25

growth as a driving force of, 24

as heartbeat of planetary civilization, 319

hidden shadows of, 32, 54, 65

as holons, 253

identities of, changing, 317

ignorance of our collective reality, 26

individuation of, 33

initiation process. *See* rites of passage

innermost being, 39

interdependence of, 36

limits of, 112

magnificence of, 268

man against Nature, 95, 99

maturation of, 62

mature wisdom, need for, 25

moral development of, 291

needs, 39

next step for the species, 230

objectification of, 258

origins of the race of, 104

powerlessness of, origins of, 119

primal experiences, desire for, 53

reclaiming wholeness, 36

as redeemers, 317–318

renaming ourselves, 318

responsibility for macrosystem, 251

as servants to gods, 104

transformation of. *See* transformation

uniqueness of, 19

who we are, 19–26

Hume, David, 189

Hundred Years War (England and France), *335*

hurricanes, global warming and, 220

hypnotherapy, 204

I

I Ching, 273

I-it relationships, 258–260, 264–267, 269

I, sacred, 268

I-Thou relationships

    empathy and, 291

    mythic system and, 260

    nature of, 265–268

    profound love of, 288

    shift from I-it relationships to, 269, 301

    ultimate, 307

    Z axis and, 282

Ice Age, 58, 60, 76

id, 190

identity, 261, 264

    as co-hearts, 318-319

    new, need for, 317-319

identity crisis, collective adolescent, 25

idiotes, 186–187

The Iliad (Homer), 128

imaginal cells, 36, 323

immaculate conception, belief in, 188

immanence, transcendence and, 320

immortality, Jesus as figure of, 146

immune system, cultural, 53

imperialism, 265

Inanna (Sumerian), 47–48, 52, 97–98

incarcerated population, 225

incest, 102

individual rights, quest for, 191

individualism, 186–187, 248

individuality, third chakra and, 87–88

individuation, archetype of, 32

indulgences, selling of, 164, 169

industrial growth society, 24

Industrial Revolution, 186, 187, *197*

industry, *196–197*

infant mortality, global, 224

information, responsibility and, 248

information, transformation and, 54

initiation. *See also* rites of passage

    adolescent, 20–25

back door, 43
birth and, 57
character of, 45
death phase, 47
disaster as a form of, 42, 43
failure of, 43
feminine/watery, 71
fundamentalism as resistance to, 243
global, 220
Jesus teachings and, 145
levels of, *see individual chakras. See* chakras
masculine/fiery, 71
openness and, 46
psychological defenses against, 50
resurrection side of, 317
rites of, 267
separation and loss stages of, 268
shift from I-it to I-Thou relationships, 269
testing phase, 42
Underworld, 47–50
innate releasing mechanisms, 58
inner world and outer world, portal between, 268
innermost being, 39
Innocent VIII, Pope, 173
Inquisition, Papal, 166–167, *335*
Inquisition, Spanish, 166–167
instincts, overriding our, 308
instincts, survival, 49, 53, 57–58
integration
    Heaven and Earth, 50, 267
    masculine and feminine, 277–278
    mind and body, healing through, 272
    need for synthesis and, 301
    progress and sustainability, 301
    upper and lower chakras, 234
intellectual thinking, origins of, 103
intelligence
    collective, 305
    measurement of, 249, 304
intention, transformation and, 54
inter-dependency, 36, 319
Internet
    as autonomous self-organizing system, 295
    Dynamic Feminine paradigm and, 210
    evolution of, 269
    as feedback mechanism of global system, 249
    global brain of the, 319

information storage on, 304
as interactive information medium, 248
interconnectedness, global, 249
popularity based on networking, 303
social interactions on, 204
as social phenomenon, 249
super-consciousness of, 305
upper chakras and, 28
Interpretation of Dreams (Freud), *338*
Iraq
    invasion of, 229, 245, *340*
    killings and torture in, 53
    war, 42, 53, 229, 245, 296
Iron Age
    beginning of, *332*
    chakra of, *30*
    cities, 110–111
    mythology of, 99–104
    order, establishment of, 98, 128
    order in, establishment of, 98, 128
    temples, 110–111
    timeline, *124–125*
Isabella, Queen, 173
Isis (Egyptian), 98
Islam, 47, *159*, 166, 277, *333*
issues and problems, today's, 20, 208, 221, 223
Italian Renaissance, 167–169

J

Jantsch, Erich, 240, 243, 245, 250, 259
Japan, mythology of, 96
Jericho, 78, *331*
Jerusalem, 165, *334*
Jesuits, 171, *335*
Jesus Christ
    banning of mother-son images, 170
    birth of, *333*
    crucifixion of, *334*
    evolution and teachings of, 144
    as hero, 151
    initiation and, 145
    life and world of, 141–143
    message of love and glory on earth, 142,
        144–147, 149, 172
    original sin, without, 154
    as sacrificial scapegoat, 104

vision of synthesis, 319
Jesus movement, early, 146, 152
Jews
    belief about sin, 152
    Chosen People, 134
    covenant of the, 145
    crucifixion of, 145
    Crusades and, 165
    exile from Spain, 173
    Exodus from Egypt, *332*
    inclusion of gentiles, 152
    monotheism, 135
    Palestinian outreach, 317
    punishment for marrying, 161
    return to Palestine, *333*
    savior-king prophecy, 144
    Static Masculine principles of, 133–134
    tensions between Romans and, 145
    women rabbis, 277
Joan of Arc, *335*
John, Gospel of, *334*
Josephus, 145
journey to the Underworld, 47–50, 97–98
joy, signficance of, 293
Judaea, 141
judgment and damnation, Christian belief in, 152
Julian, Emperor, 150
"jump time", 226
Jung, Carl
    archetype of individuation, 32
    on chakras, 282
    on changes, 45
    on enlightenment, 161
    on feelings, 116
    Psychology of the Unconscious, *338*
    on that which can destroy itself, 46
    on unconscious, 163, 190
Juno (Roman mythology), 135

K

Kama, 73
Kant, Immanuel, 189, *336*
Keats, John, 189
Keen, Sam, 64
Keller, Catherine, 87
Kepler, Johannes, 181, *336*

Ki, Earth Goddess (Sumerian mythology), 96
kin-dom, 319
King, Martin Luther, 34
King of the Underworld (Hades), 49
"kingdom", 319
kingdom of God, accessibility of, 145
kingship, origins of, 118–119
Kingu (Babylonian), 102, 103–104
Koestler, Arthur, 239
Koran, 227
Kore (Greek), 49, 98
Kuhn, Thomas, *339*
kundalini yoga, 268
Kurgan invasion, 90, *331*

L

labor
    freedom from, 320
    slave, 94–95
    specialization of, 113
Land of the Dead, 49
language, spread of common, 122
Lannon, Richard, 246, 264, 305
law and order, 129–133, 135
leadership, 20, 114
Leadership and the New Science, 242
Leakey, Richard, 61
Leaves of Grass (Whitman), *337*
Leeuwenhoek, Antony van, *336*
Leo X, Pope, 171
Lewis, Thomas, 246, 264, 305
life expectancy, 224
life, sacredness of, 32, 205
lifestyles, 35, 187, 203
limbic brain, 264, 304–305
limitations by others, 74–75
literacy, Renaissance and, 169
literature, Renaissance, 168
lives, authentic, 32
lives, disembodied, 273
living systems theory, 204, 239
Locke, John, 189
logic and discourse, emergence of, 129–131
logic, objective masculine, 189
Logos (Greek mythology), 128, 131
longings

answering, 293
archaic, 73
    suppression of, 40, 233
    urge of human evolution through, 294
Lord of Death (Hades), 49
Lord's Prayer, 174
loss, transformation and, 51
love
    Darwin on, 185
    discounting of, 232
    elevation beyond personal relationships, 232
    evolution and, 29
    fourth chakra and, 27, 28
    inspirational capacity of, 247
    Jesus and message of, 142, 149
    meaning derived from serving what we, 250
    as potent source of power, 248
    power of, 18, 25, 323
    seeds of, 293
    struggle between power and, 230
    world, 265–266
love children, sixties, 206
Lovelock, James, *340*
lower chakras, 28, *30*, 191, 233–234, 282
Lower Paleolithic Era, *68*
Loye, David, 184–185
lugal (Sumeria), 118
Luther, Martin, 169, 170, 171, 181, *335*

M

machines, invention of, 186
macrosystem, responsibility for, 251
Macy, Joanna, 221–222
Maiden, rescue of the, 96
males. *See* men
Malleus Maleficarum (Pope Innocent VIII), 173
Malthus, Thomas, 22, *336*
mammalian brain, 304–305
man against man, 110
Mandela, Nelson, 34
Mani (Persia), 132
Manichaeism religion (Persia), 132, 153
manipulation, evolution and, 29
Maoris, mythology of, 96
Marduk (Babylonian mythology), 97, 101–104
Mark, Gospel of, *334*

markets vs networks, 303
marriage, 132, 325
The Marriage of Sense and Soul, 274
Mars, planet, 99
martyrdom, Christian, 149–151
Marx, Karl, 299
Mary Magdalene, 143
Mary, mother of Jesus. *See* Mother Mary
masculine and feminine archetypes, 27
masculine and feminine, balancing and
    integration of, 32, 277–278
Masculine and Feminine (Gareth), 62–63
"masculine birth", 182
masculine psyche
    erection of walls, 112
    ruling elite, development of, 95
masculine valences, 62–63, 88
masculine values, 232
mass distraction, story of, 26
mass production, 186, *336*
massage, 204
materialism, rise of, 188
mathematics, 114, 122, *332*
matrix, the basic creative, 270
matter
    consciousness and, 275–276
    energy and, 190
    as primal ground, 188
    relationship to spirit/mind, 131–132, 274, 275
    study of, 180
mature wisdom, crucial need for, 25
maturity, human, 62, 246
Mead, Margaret, 91
Meade, Michael, 66, 71
"mean green meme", 209
meaning, mythic system and, 261
mechanical medicine, 275
mechanical world view, 187
media, public, 28, 35, 51–52
medicine
    Chinese, 205
    Dynamic Feminine paradigm and, 204, 205
    Hippocrates, *333*
    mechanical, 275
    Middle Ages, 167
    non-local mind, 275
    psychosomatic, 275

three eras of, 275
meditation and yoga, 204, 205, 308–309
Medusa (Greek mythology), 135
megalithic sites, 82, *331*
memes, mainstream, 232
men
    blaming of, 278
    Dark Ages view of domination by, 163
    denial of feelings, 116–117
    differentiation, need for, 89
    Dynamic Feminine paradigm and, 202, 207
    equality with women, 208
    evil nature of, 155
    gender equality with women, 131
    groups for, importance of, 278
    gulf between women and, 152
    as heroes, origins of, 96, 117–121
    initiation of, 117
    as leaders, 114
    oppression of, 278
    sacred role of, 80–81
    shift of power to, 118–119
    Static Feminine and, 64
    symbols for, 80, 82, 99
mental health problems, 224
Mesopotamia, 93–94, 110, 111
Messiah, 134, 146
metal tools, 93
metamorphosis, caterpillars and, 53
metamorphosis, human, 35–36, 41, 50
Meyers, Hari, 114
Middle Ages, 164–168, *174*, 187
middle class, 127, 186
Middle East, 53
midwifery, Middle Ages, 167
"might makes right", 228
militarism, 94–95, 110, 114–117, 122, 134
Mill, John Stuart, 188
Millennials, 318
mind and body
    healing through integration of, 272
    severed connection between, 272–273
    synthesis of, 206
mind and matter, 131–132, 274, 275
mind medicine, non-local, 275
Minoan dynasties, *331*
Minos, King, 120–121

Modernity era, *214–215*
modernity, excesses of, 193
Mohenjo-Daro, 110
monotheism, masculine, 135, 150, 174, *332*
moon, cycle of the, 103
moral development, next stage of, 291
morality
    based on shared responsibility, 234
    cerebral cortex and, 305
    Dark Ages and, 161–162
    Darwin on, 185
    overhaul of, 233, 234
Morford, Mark, 199
Moses, commandments of, 134
Mother and Child archetype, 79
Mother, as archetype, 59–62, 98, 100, 103, 143
Mother Goddess, 60
Mother Mary
    Great Mother, compared to, 143
    immaculate conception of, belief in, 188
    Mother archetype of, 98
    status of, reduced, 143
    worship of, Protestant discouragement of, 170
Mother Nature
    bankruptcy of, 316
    Earth as, 61–62
    first chakra and, 58–59
    as nurturer and teacher, 227
    survival instinct and, 58
Mother-Son motif, 143
motion pictures, invention of, 189, 190, *338*
Muhammad, *333*
muladhara, 59
Mummu (Babylonian), 100–101
Murray, Judith Sargeant, 189
music, Renaissance, 168
Muslims
    Crusades and, 165, 166
    exile from Spain, 173
    peaceful, 317
mystery cults, Greek, 148
mystical practices, 267
myth and reason, separation of, 132
mythic system, 260–262, *263*, 264–265
myths
    Christian, 141–142
    divine order of Nature, destruction of, 163

emerging, 325
future, nature of, 17
power, 122
separation, 97
separation of reason and, 130, 132
myths of our civilization, 141, 315

N

Nagasaki, bombing of, 115, *339*
Nagler, Michael, 295, 298
Nammu, Goddess (Sumerian mythology), 96
natural disasters, 34, 41
natural order, end of, 114, 122
natural selection, 184, 185
Nature
    Aquinas on, 170–171
    association with witchcraft, 174
    Bacon on, 183
    converging paths of civilization and, 311
    cooperation with limits and laws of, 310
    cultivating relationship with, 310–311
    Descartes on, 183
    destruction of, 22, 24–25, 41
    destruction of myth of divine order in, 163
    dissociation and control of, 309
    Dynamic Feminine paradigm and, 205–206
    going backward, impossibility of, 310
    as guide, 269
    knowledge gained from observation of, 315
    Latin derivative for, 188
    man against, 95, 99
    as medium of our transformation, 309
    modeling of our living systems, 320
    objective study of, 180
    relationships foundation of, 265
    Static Feminine and, 264
    survival instinct of, 57
    symbiotic enmeshment with, 264
    synthesis with, 311
    walling against, 112
    womb of, 54
naval chakra. *See* third chakra
Nazism, 185
Neanderthals, *331*
neo-conservative politics, justification of, 185
Neolithic era, 76–82, *84–85*

Neopagan rituals, 80
Nesbitt, James, 234
Neti, 48
networks vs markets, 303
Neumann, Erich, 81, 97
New Age philosophies, 47
New Age platitudes, 208–209
new era, dawning of, 19
New Orleans, flooding of (2005), 34, 219–220, *340*
New World, discovery of, 168
new world, the, 323, 325
Newton, Sir Isaac, 183–184, *336*
Nicea, Council of, *333*
Nietzsche, Friedrich, 187, *337*, *338*
nomads, prehistoric, 24
non-linear dynamics, 204
nonviolence, 206, 298
nonviolent civil disobedience, 204
noosphere, 304, 305
North African civilization, 99
Northern Europe, 99, *158*, 169, *174*
now, focusing on, 222
nuclear arms race, 115–116
nuclear vs tribal family, 204
nudity, 204
Nut, Star Goddess (Egyptian mythology), 96, 97

O

obedience to authority, 228, 231, 233
objectification, human, 258
objectivity, 188, 259
The Odyssey (Homer), 128, *332*
Oedipus (Greek mythology), 96
Ohrmazd (Persian mythology), 132
oil crisis, 321, 323
Old Europe, 95
Omega Point, 305
open systems, 241
Orange level of Spiral Dynamics, 209
order, establishment of, 98, 99
organic food, 205
Origin of Species (Darwin), 184, *337*
original sin, 151–152, 154–155
The Origins and History of Consciousness
    (Neumann), 97
orphans, AIDS, 224

Orpheus, rites of, 151
Osiris (Egyptian mythology), 98, 147
Other, archetypal, 73
Ouranos (Greek mythology), 96
outer world and inner world, portal between, 268
outer world, consciousness and, 270

P

pacifists, origin of anger towards, 116
Pagans
 Dark Ages and, 162
 festivals, 204
 temples, destruction of, 150, *333*
 time chart, *158*
Pagels, Elaine, 154
Paleolithic era, *30*, 66, *68–69*, 76–77, 80–81
Palmieri, Matteo, 168
Pan, 173
Papal Inquisition, 166–167
The Parable of the Tribes (Shmookler), 115
paradigms, masculine and feminine
 characteristics of, *279*
 complimentary behavior of, 280
 dominator, 228
 Dynamic Feminine. *See* Dynamic Feminine paradigm
 Dynamic Masculine. *See* Dynamic Masculine paradigm
 positive and negative characteristics of, *281*
 power. *See* power paradigm
 ruling/control. *See* ruling paradigm
 Static Feminine. *See* Static Feminine paradigm
 Static Masculine. *See* Static Masculine paradigm
 submissive, 229
 synthesis among, 299–302
"parental" domination, freedom from, 227
"parental imperialism", 265
participation mystique, 62
participatory democracy, 204, 263
partnership, archetype of sacred, 32
passages. *See* rites of passage
passion and intimacy, sin of, 156
passive obedience, threat of violence and, 228
past, alignment with future, 283
Pater familias, 136
Paul, apostle, 148, 153–154, 170, *334*

Pax Romana, 136
peace, 42, 226, 294–298
peace march, 296
peace movement, 53, 54, 207, *339*
peak oil, 321
Pelagius, 155
"people of the parentheses", 25
persecutions, *334*
Persian Empire, 133
Persian mythology, 132
personal power, awakening of, 88
personal will, social responsibility and, 246, 248
personality, breakdown of, 48
perspective, distance and, 308
perspectives, archetypal, 27
Petrarch, Francesco, 168, *335*
phallic forms, Neolithic era and, 82
The Phenomenon of Man (Teilhard), *339*
Philip of Macedon, 133, *333*
philosophical poles of Enlightenment Age, 189
photons and electrons, discovery of, 190
physical heart, 18, 29
physical pleasure, sin of, 152
physical vs spiritual growth, 193
planet, synthesis of culture and, 206
planetary motion, laws of, 181
Plato, 131–132, 153, *333*
platonic ideals (Roman Empire), 135
Pleistocene Epoch, *84*
plurality, convergence of, 301
poetry, 168, *332*
Poland, invasion of, *338*
polarities
 continuum and unification of, 276
 dueling, 232
 origins of, 104
polarized thinking, 276
polis, development of the, 127–128
political ambition, third chakra and, 134
political left and right, global community and, 323
politics
 fundamentalism, 65
 of the left and right, essential values of, 323
 time chart, *214–215*
pollution, 192, 223
polytheism, 100, 135
Pope, power of, 164

Poppa, Mother (Maori mythology), 96
The Population Bomb (Ehrlich), *340*
population(s)
    cultural sophistication and large, 249
    fertility worship and growth of, 87
    global, size of, 22
    growth of, impact of, 93
    high casualties and dense, 41
    Industrial Revolution and growth of, 186
    limits to, 34
    Malthus on, *336*
    size, impact of, 34
    stabilization of, need for, 193
poverty, 42, 133
power
    age of, 113
    collaborative use of, 254
    freedom and maturation of, 246
    for global impact, 234
    god-like, 34
    Heroic Age and, 33
    hierarchical, evolution of, 118
    love and, struggle between, 230
    love as potent source of, 248
    love of, 18, 227–229
    maximization, in society, 122
    myth of, 122
    redefinement of, Dynamic Feminine
      paradigm and, 209
    relationship quality and, 247–248
    shadow side of our, 33
    shift of locus, 97–98, 118
    social development of, 121
    survival equated with, 122
    third chakra and, 27, 28, 87–88, 121, 223
    transformation of, 21
    wisdom/grace and, 34
The Power of Love to Transform Our Lives and Our
    World, 227
Power of Now, 253
power-over paradigm, 179
power paradigm
    current, 50
    dissolving/overthrowing the, 210, 232–233
    lack of heart in the, 231
power structures, imperial, 28
powerlessness, 208

Pre-Socratic philosophers, 130, *332*
predictions, dire, 322–323
prehistoric art, 60
priests, 118, 161–162
primal experiences, desire for, 53
primal thesis, 61–67
primary forces, making sense of, 104
Principia (Newton), 183
printing press, 169, *335*
privacy, Industrial Revolution and, 187
privatization, shame and, 187
problem-solving, peaceful, 295
problems and issues, today's, 20, 208, 221, 223
problems, systemic, 240
process vs content, 204
procreation, movement to co-creation from,
    300–301
progress
    Industrial Revolution and, 186
    integration with sustainability, 222, 301
    measurement of, 24
    results of, 222
The Progress Paradox (Easterbrooke), 222
Progressive Left, 242–243
progressive values, Dynamic Feminine paradigm
    and, 209, 264
proliferation, worship and, 87
proof of existence, consciousness as, 183
prosperity, poverty and, 42
protection of human rights, 191
Protestant Reformation, 169–174, *175, 335*
Protestantism, 170–173, 185, 315
psyche, study of the, 190–192
psychedelic revolution, 205, 281, *339*
psychoanalysis, development of, 191
psychology, development of, 190
The Psychology of Kundalini Yoga (Jung), 281
Psychology of the Unconscious (Jung), *338*
psychosomatic medicine, 275
psychotherapy, 207
public squares, emergence of, 127
purpose, awakening to our, 251–252
purpose, finding common, 301
purusha, 269
pyramids, Egyptian, 118

Q

quality of life, threat to, 224
quantum mechanics, 190, *338*
quantum physics, 204, 260–261, 275, *338*
questions, essential, 19

R

racism, 133, 207
radio, 189, 190, *338*
Rafael, 131–132
Rainbow Gatherings, 204
Ramakrishna, 280
Ramses II, 114
rape of women, 94–95
rational mind vs base instincts, 131–132
rational system, 259–260, *263*, 264–265
rationalism, 131, 183
raves, 204
Ray, Paul, 209
Raymond of Aguilers, 165
reason
    detachment and, development of, 128
    logic, 128–129, 130–131
    Luther on, 181
    myth and, separation of, 130, 132
    triune brain and, 305
rebellions and destruction, 90–91
rebellious differentiation, 88, 89
rebirth, destruction and, 220
Recovering the Soul: A Scientific and Spiritual Search
    (Dossey), 252
redemption, human
    Jesus' promise of, 142, 149
    suffering and, 152
refugees, displaced, 223
relatedness, holon need for, 246–249
relational holism, 238
relationships
    between anima and axis mundi, 270
    authentic, 231, 266–267
    autonomous, 231
    changing nature of, 225
    crucible of evolution, 264
    crucible of new paradigm, 234
    of divine feminine and divine masculine, 323
    dynamic web of, 204

egalitarian, requirements for, 143
    equality of, 230
    examination of, 190
    foundation of civilization, 265
    fourth chakra and, 27, 28
    I-It, 258–260, 264–267, 269
    I-Thou. *See* I-Thou relationships
    most basic of, 270
    narcissitic, 259
    participatory nature of, 247
    power and the quality of, 248
    as self-organizing webs, 247
    shift from I-it to I-Thou, 269
    shifting framework of our, 266
    spirit and matter, 274
    systems and, 238, 239, 259, 264
    We, 262–263
relativity, theories of, 190, 210, *338*
releasing mechanisms, innate, 58
religion
    ancient mystery of Jesus and, 147
    first, 61
    fundamental, 65
    meaning without empirical truth, 275
    revealed, 97
    science and, 184, 274–275
religious experience, Dark Ages and, 161–162
Remus (Roman mythology), 135
Renaissance, *31*, 167–169, *175*, 180
Renaissance, new, 325
repression, Dark Ages and, 163
repression, emotional. *See* feelings
reptilian brain, 304
resources, consumption of, 186
responsibility, 21, 248, 251
restlessness, 39, 40
resurrection, death and, 147
return home, Hero's, 33–34, 323
revolution(s)
    time chart, *214–215*
rhetoric, 130–131, 168
Rifkin, Jeremy, 187, 302–303
rights for all, 207–210
Rilke, Rainer Maria, 39
rites of passage
    adolescent, 45
    beginnings, 39, 43

death and, 46
destiny and, 39
future and, 221
global, 19, 20, 25–26
nature of, 33–34
preparing for, 45–54
purpose of, 45–46
rituals, 45
threshold, 57
today's, 221
tribal, 26, 42
unpredictability of, 46
ritual sacrifices, 99, 130
rivalries, archetypal generational, 101
Rolfing, 205
Roman baths, 134–135
Roman Empire
    age of, 133–136
    art, 135
    Christianity and the, 145, 146, 149–150, *333*
    class distinctions in, 151
    collapse of, 156
    conquest of Greece, *333*
    control of Galilee, 141
    emperor, deposition of last, *333*
    end of western, *333*
    reign of terror, 145
    slavery, 135, 136
    time chart, *138–139, 158–159*
    violence and, 135
    wars, 136
    women, repression of, 151
Roman Republic, *333*
Romantics, 189
Romulus (Roman mythology), 135
Rongi, Father (Maori mythology), 96
root chakra. *See* first chakra
Roth, Gabrielle, 306
Rousseau, Henri, 189
ruling elite, 95
ruling paradigm
    Dynamic Masculine, 88–91, 122
    overthrowing the current, 234
    overwhelm of the, 242
    Static Masculine, 129–130

S

sacral chakra. *See* second chakra
sacred, finding entrance into the, 46
sacred I, the, 268
Sacred Marriage archetype, 278, 283
Sacred Other, 29, 76
sacred partnership, archetype of, 32
sacredness of life, 32, 205
sacrifices, ritual, 99, 130
Sahtouris, Elizabet, 35, 310, 318
salvation, promise of, 163
sanitation to prevent disease, 186
satyagraha, 21
saving vs serving, 251
savior-messengers, 132, 144
Schiller, Friedrich, 190
The School of Athens, 132
science
    aim of, 183
    attack on, 52, 181
    doubt and development of, 182–183
    focus on understanding the parts, 238
    freedom and, 244
    history of, 238
    mythic reality of, underlying, 264
    as the new religion, 182
    religion and, 274–275
    roots in mystical traditions, 274
    Spanish Inquisition and, 174
    technology and, *196–197, 214–215*
    truth without personal meaning, 275
scientific method, 182
Scientific Revolution, 180–186, 192, 259, 315
sea levels, Neolithic era and, 78
The Search for a Nonviolent Future (Nagler), 295
second chakra
    autopoesis and, 244
    characteristics of, *30, 72, 212*
    comfort and, 223
    differences, development of, 76
    Good Mother/Bad Mother, 75
    movement from first chakra to, 71–72
    need to reclaim, 234
    sexuality and, 74, 75
    urge to expand, 74
    urge to merge, 73–74, 76

water element of, 72
second enlightenment, 269
seeds, discovery of, 77
self
    authentic connection to, 267
    as causative agent, 88
    losing the, 267
    uniting Heaven and Earth within the, 267
    vertical core (axis mundi) of the, 272
self-awareness, 62, 307
self-determination, 208
self-examination, crisis and, 32
self-help groups, 207–210
self-improvement, imperative of, 306
self-interest, transforming, 29, 254
self-organizing systems, 239–253, 275
The Self-Organizing Universe (Jantsch), 240
self-reflection, 207, 251, 267
self-renewal, capacity for, 243
self-transcendence, 249–253
Seneca Falls Conference, 188, *337*
senses, as gateways to consciousness, 72–73
sensitivity to initial conditions, 326
separation
    from culture, need for, 308
    myths of, 97
    of spirit and matter, 183
    Static Masculine paradigm and, 148
service, practice of being in, 288
serving vs saving, 251
Set (Egyptian), 98
seventh chakra, *30–31*, *213*, 234
sex before marriage, 173
sexism, overcoming, 207
sexual abuse, childhood, 257
sexuality
    binary conflict of, 75
    Christian attitudes toward, 153–156
    cultural taboos, 75–76
    Dynamic Feminine paradigm and, 204
    laws restricting, *331*
    laws restricting women's, 95, 331
    Protestantism and, 172
    reptilian brain and, 304
    second chakra and, 74, 75
    spirituality and, 208
shadows, our hidden, 32, 54, 65, 232–233

Shakespeare, *336*
shame, privatization and, 187
Shelley, Percy, 189
Shiva, 51
Shlain, Leonard, 94, 206
Shmookler, Andrew Bard, 109, 113, 115–116, 122
"A Shot in the Light", 51
Shu (Egyptian mythology), 97
simony, buying of, 164
sin
    buying off, 164
    Dark Ages concept of, 162
    Martin Luther on, 170
    original, 151–152, 154–155
    passion and intimacy, 156
    physical pleasure, 152
Singer, June, 227
singing, Protestantism and, 173
sins, humanity's, 315–316
sisterhood, emergence of, 206
sixth chakra, *31*, *213*, 234
Sixtus IV, Pope, 169
skin as a spiritual liability, 172
Sky Father, 96, 180
sky gods, 91, 95, 96, 98
slavery
    abolishment of, 193, *336*, *337*
    in ancient civilizations, 119
    anti-slavery convention, World, *337*
    Greek Empire, 127
    institutionalization of, 94, 114, 118
    Roman Empire, 135, 136
social equality, Christian belief in, 143
social groups, basis of, 61–62
social hierarchy, origins of, 114, 122
social justice, 250
social responsibility, balance of personal will and, 246
social systems, self-organization of, 237
society. *See also* civilization
    adolescent, 43
    anarchic vs hierarchical, 114
    archetypal dynamics of birth of, 57
    attack of new structures, 52
    avoidance and denial of, 52
    balancing of masculine and feminine in, 277–278

chakras and wholeness of, 27–28
class, development of, 94
co-creative, 199
collective rite of passage, 40
collective unconscious, 57
coming of age, 29, 32–34, 36
conformity, enforced, 65
cultural immune system, 53
cultural trance of, 308
cultural values, formation of, 37
development of class, 94
disembodied lives of our, 273
dissolution of, 50, 52, 53–54
evolution of. *See* evolution
force and violence as organizing principle
of, 228
force as central organizing principle of,
228–229
fragmentation of, 28
freedom and responsibility in, 230
hierarchical, evolution of, 114, 118
ills of, 316
law and order emergence in, 129–133
men as leaders of, 114
militarization, origins of, 94–95, 110,
114–117
organizing principle for, 28
polis, development of the, 127–128
power maximization in, 122
primal thesis of, 61–67
self-organizing systems as model for, 240
shaping of, Darwin's theories and, 185
shift from feminine to masculine values, 122
sovereign individuals vs master/servants in, 246
submission as the dominant paradigm, 229
transformation of, limits to, 51
violence, proclivity toward, 52, 53–54
women as leaders of natural order, 114
Socrates, 131, 299, *333*
solar plexus chakra. *See* third chakra
soldiers, origins of, 114
son archetype, maturation of, 143
son-lover motif, 102, 227
Spanish Inquisition, 173–174, 179, *335*
species extinction, 192, 224
species, mature vs immature, 310
Spencer, Herbert, 184

Spiral Dynamics, 209
spiral symbol, Dynamic Feminine, 202, 272
spirit
relationship to matter, 131–132, 274, 275
as teacher, 269
spiritual growth vs physical, 193
spiritual heart, 18
spiritual maturity, achieving, 104
spiritual paths, Dark Ages view of, 163
spiritual salvation, 144
spirituality
ascendant, 47
beauty and, 73
chakras and, 28
current trends in, 21, 28
Dark Ages and repression of, 156
descendent, 47–48
diversity of, attacks on, 52
Dynamic Feminine paradigm and, 205
ecstatic, in Dark Ages, 163
emerging era of, 308
equal opportunity, 144
evolution of worship, 90
Great Mother and, 90
Industrial Revolution and, 187
as industry, 307
pre-dawn, 307
revolutionary Christian, 144–147
sexuality and, 208
today's, 307
transcendant aspect of, 308
standard of living, 186, 222–223
Stanton, Elizabeth Cady, 189
Static Feminine paradigm
characteristics of, *279*
contribution of, 280
culture, structure of, 65
enclosing circle symbol of the, 62–66, 74
ending of the, 102
first chakra and, 63
Great Mother and, 79, 80, 280
inertia of, 76
infancy of human evolution and, 208
men and, 64
Mother and Child archetype of, 79
Mother-Son motif of, 143
Nature, symbiotic enmeshment with, 264

opposition to, 99
Static Masculine compared to, 130
women and, 64, 65
Static Masculine era
Inquisition and, 133
Static Masculine paradigm
battle between good and evil, 133
central myth of, 141
characteristics of, *279*
contribution of, 280
cross as initiation symbol of, 148, 270, 272
educational institutions and, 277
Enlightenment Age and impact on, 190
Father -Daughter motif of, 143
fundamentalism and, 242–243
middle childhood of human evolution and, 208
origins of, 122
rational system replacement of mythic
system, 264
ruling paradigm of, 129–130
separation and, 148
separation of spirit and matter, 183
Static Feminine era compared to, 130
static systems, outgrowth of, 222
steam engines, 186, *336*
Stewart, R. J., 48, 49–50
Stonehenge, 82
stories we tell ourselves, 313–317
story
ancestor's, 314–315
creating a new, 264
human, 19, 21
mass distraction, 26
mythic system and, 261
our new, 314
stress, evolution and, 242, 243
Structure of Scientific Revolutions (Kuhn), *339*
structures, dissipative, 245
struggle, third chakra and, 184
subatomic particles, 190, 239
subjectivity, mythic system and, 260
submissive paradigm of society, 229
success, measurement of, 24
suffering, Christian belief in, 148, 152
suffrage, women's, *337*
Sumeria, mythology of, 96–97
Sumer, unification of, *331*

Sumerian civilization, 109, 118
Summer, William Graham, 185
superego, 190
superstition and persecution of Dark Ages,
161–163, 184
superstition, replacement by rationalism, 183
survival
anarchy and, 113
balance between birth and death, 66
evolution and challenges to, 58
first chakra and, 59, 223
imperative of global peace for, 297–298
instincts for, 49, 53, 57–58
keys to, 24, 25, 54
man against man, origins of, 110
man against Nature, origins of, 95, 99
militarization for, 94–95, 110, 114–117
power equated with, 122
reptilian brain and, 304
rules of, 58
"survival of the fittest", 184–185
Susanowo (Japanese mythology), 96
sushumna, 268
symbolic thinking, evolution of, 60
synthesis
cultural history and, 299–300
of dualities, 301
human history archetypes of and, 299–300
thesis, antithesis and, 299–302
systemic problems, 240
system(s)
closed, 241
corruption of current, 231
defined, 239
destruction of, causes of, 241–242
evolution and disequilibrium of, 241–242, 243
evolutionary, 262–263, *263*
guiding principles of, 239
internal organization of, 239
Internet and global, 249
levels of, 259, 264–265
mythic, 260–262, *263*
nested holarchy of, 253
non-equilibrium of open, 241
open vs closed, 241
rational, 259–260, *263*, 264–265
self-organizing nature of, 240

shift from rational to mythic, 269
strengthening of, information and the, 248
systems theory, 239, 245

T

taboos, cultural, 75–76
Taliban (Afghanistan), 277
Tannen, Deborah, 232
Tao, 253, 269
The Tao of Physics (Capra), 274, 340
technology. See also science
    capability of today's, 20
    Enlightenment Age, 189
    focus of, 320
Tefnut (Egyptian mythology), 97
Teilhard de Chardin, Pierre
    best guarantee, 327
    on elements of the organized whole, 299
    on mind's discovery of its own evolution, 250
    on noosphere layer of conscious connection,
        304, 305
    on patterns of the whole, 237
    on personalized vs abstract love, 270
    The Phenomenon of Man, 339
    on reflective exercise, meaning of the, 323
    on remaining true to oneself, 302
telegraph, invention of, 189, 190, 337
telephone, invention of, 189, 190, 337
television, 206, 210, 338
temple bureaucracies, 95
temples
    Bronze Age, 99
    Iron Age, 110–111
    Neolithic era and, 79
Terrible Mother, awakening of the, 102
terrorism, ending, 296
Tertullian, 170
text messaging, 204
Thales, 131
theocratic rule, origins of, 118
Theodosius, Emperor, 150, 333
Theogony (Hesiod), 128, 332
therapies, body-based, 205
thermodynamics, second law of, 239
thesis, antithesis and synthesis, dance of, 299–302
thinking. See reason

third chakra
    awakening of personal power and will, 87–88
    Babylonian mythology and, 101–104
    Bronze Age and, 30, 93
    characteristics of, 30, 212
    Darwin's theories and, 184
    emergence of individuality, 87–88
    finding autonomy, 192
    fire element of the, 92
    free will and, 156
    freedom and, 246
    harnessing of electomagnetic forces and, 190
    heroes and, 119–120
    impact on world of, 120
    obedience to authority, 233
    origins of, 109
    political ambition and, 134
    power and the, 27, 28, 87–88, 121, 223
    struggle and competition of, 184
    supremacy battle with second chakra, 102
    will and the, 92
Third World Nations, 225
Thou, eternal, 269
throat chakra. See fifth chakra
Tiamat (Babylonian mythology), 97, 99–104, 332
Tigris-Euphrates valley, 100, 109–110
time, counting of, 103
Tolle, Eckhart, 219, 222
tool-making, 92
tools, metal, 93
Torah, 152
torus, 270
trade, Neolithic era and, 79
tragedies, 41, 220
traitors, origins of punishment of, 116
transcendence, 308–309, 320
Transcendental Meditation society, 309
transformation
    body politic, 36
    collective vision and, 35
    death and, 46, 57, 66
    intention, information and, 54
    limits to cultural, 51
    loss and, 51
    meaning of, 46
    metaphor for, 35–36, 40
    Nature as medium of our, 309

Treatise on Electricity and Magnetism (Maxwell), *337*
tribal societies, 26, 42
tribal vs nuclear family, 204
triune brain, 305
truth without personal meaning, 275
Tsunami, South Asian (2004), 34, 220, *340*
Turner, Nick, 298
"Turning", 267
tyranny, freedom and, 42
tyrant-monsters, 121

U

uncertainty, embracing, 243
unconscious
    collective, 57
    creativity and, 190
    discovery of the, 190, 191
Underworld
    initiation, 50
    journey to the, 47–50, 97–98
The Underworld Initiation, (Stewart), 48
unions, development of, 191
United Nations, founding of, *339*
unity, 145, 282, 301
Universal Spirit, 253
universe as mechanical system, 184
University of California, Berkeley, 298
upper chakras, 28, *31*, 233–234, 254, 282
Upper Paleolithic era, 60, *69*, *84*
Ur-Nammu (Mesopotamia), 114, *332*
Urban II, Pope, 164, *335*
Uroboros, 63
Urshanabi, 111–112
Uruk, 111–112
Urukagina, 95, *331*
U.S. government, hidden agenda of, 245
Utopia, 297

V

valences, masculine and feminine, 62–63, 88
values
    alignment of larger purpose with, 250
    Dynamic Feminine paradigm and
        progressive, 264
    feelings as source of, 116

formation of cultural, 37
    importance of, 243
    overhaul of, 233
    restriction from, 243
    shift from feminine to masculine, 122
    shift from material to mental, 132
Venus (Roman mythology), 135
vertical Y axis of self, 272
Vietnam War, 53, 206, *339*
violence
    dominator paradigm, and, 228
    as organizing principle of society, 228
    overcoming, 295–296
    overcoming language of, 295–296
    Roman Empire, 135
    roots of, 117
    society's proclivity toward, 52, 53–54
    threat of, passive obedience and, 228
Virgin Mary. *See* Mother Mary
Visigoths, *333*
vision, chakras and, 28
visions, guiding, 35, 54, 250
Vivikenanda, Swami, 280
void, endless, 253
vote, women's right to, *338*

W

wake up calls, tragedies as, 41
Walden Pond (Thoreau), *337*
walls, 112, 121–122, 187, 323
war games, adolescent, 24
warrior class, development of a, 93
wars
    ending, 269
    ending belief in inevitability of, 297
    evolution of, 114–115
    impact of, 296–297
    overcoming language of, 295–296
    peace and, 42
    time chart, *214–215*
    trend away from, 296
    wealth and, 94
waste pollution, 223
water, 72, 102
water chakra. *See* second chakra
water pollution, 223

Watson, James, *339*
Watt, James, *336*
wave equation, *338*
wax cylinder recording, first, *337*
We relationship, 262–263, 266, 269, 301
wealth
    distribution of, 94
    isolation of people with, 187
    rationalizations for, 151–152
    war and, 94
webs, unity and diversity of, 247
WELL (Willits Economic LocaLization),
    321–322
Weller, Brian, 322
West, material richness and spiritual poverty
    of, 282
Western civilization
    Christian myth and, 141–142
    Hellenic influence of, 133
    intellectual foundations of, 128
Western culture, 27
Western lifestyles, lower chakras and, 282
Wheatley, Margaret, 242, 247–248
Wheatley, Phyllis, 189
The White Goddess (Graves), *339*
Whitehead, Alfred North, 89
WHO (World Health Organization), 224
wholeness
    integration of axes for, 283
    loss of, 81
    path toward, 32
    reclaiming, 36
Wilber, Ken
    on convergence of science and religion,
        274–275
    "dignity of modernity", 193
    "flatland", 116–117
    four quadrant theory, 259
    on interior world, society's ignoring of, 232
    "mean green meme", 209
    on separation from matter, need for, 308
will, development and mastery of, 75, 87–88,
    91, 92, 93
Willits Economic LocaLization (WELL),
    321–322
wisdom/grace, power and, 34
wisdom, source of, 270

witch hunts/burnings, 173, 180, 183
witchcraft, 173, 174
witchcraft laws, repeal of (England), *339*
Wittenberg, 171
Wollstonecraft, Mary, 189
women
    blaming of, 278
    body as temple, 79–80
    control of sexuality of, 95
    covering of the body, 172
    denial of citizenship to, 128
    as devil's gateway, 170
    Dynamic Feminine paradigm and, 202,
        206–207
    enslavement of, 94–95
    equality with men, 208
    feminism, rise of, 188
    gender equality for, 131
    groups for, importance of, 278
    gulf between men and, 152
    influence, waning of, 103
    Inquisitions and, 174, 180
    lack of soul in, 170
    laws restricting sexuality, 95
    as leaders of natural order, 114
    Martin Luther on, 171
    between men and, 152
    oppression of, 278
    Papal Inquisition and, 166
    Protestantism and, 170, 173, 180
    rape and enslavement of, 94–95
    rebellion against oppressors, 207
    repression in the Roman Empire, 151
    right to vote, 188–189, 191, *338*
    Roman and Greek civilizations, 135–136
    Roman Catholic Church and, 277
    sacred role of, 80, 81. *See also* Great Mother
    sexual desire blame on, 170
    Static Feminine and, 64, 65
    suffrage, *337*
    as weaker vessel, 170
women-only environments, 207
Women's Liberation movement, 206, *339*
women's rights movement, 191
Woodward, Charlotte, 189
workouts, aerobic, 205
world

magnificence of the, 268

mechanical view of, 187

soul (anima mundi) of the, 267–270, 293

World anti-slavery convention, *337*

World Health Organization (WHO), 224

The World is Flat (Friedman), 225

World Navel, 121

World Parents, separation of, 96, 148

World Parliament of Religions, 280

World Trade Center, destruction of, 34, 41, *340*

World Tree, 47

World Wars, 133, *338*

World Wide Web, 225, 304

worship

evolution of, 90

god, 82

goddess, 80

Great Mother. *See* Great Mother

proliferation and, 57, 87

sky god, 91, 95

wounds

collective initiatory, 41

importance of healing, 292

result of healing, 297

Wright, Orville, *338*

writers, rise of feminist, 189

writing

cuneiform, 93–94

development of, 122

first, *331*

invention of, 93–94, 114

Renaissance, 168

Wurm Glaciation, 60, *68*, *69*, *84*, *331*

X

X axis, 276–283

X, Y, Z axes, unification of, *284*

Y

Y axis, 272, 299

Yahweh (Hebrew), 134

Yellow River, 110

yoga

chakras and, 27

effect on consciousness, 273

focus of, 47

kundalini, 268

meditation and, 204, 205, 308–309

United States introduction to, 280–281

Yoga Sutras, *334*

youth

concerns of, 18

responsibility of, 21, 248

Z

Z axis, 282–283, 299

Zen, 47

Zeus (Greek), 98

ziggurats, Mesopotamian, 118

zodiac, signs of the, 103

Zoroastrianism (Persia), 132, *332*

Zurvan (Persian mythology), 132

Books by Anodea Judith, Ph.D.

Wheels of Life

Eastern Body, Western Mind

Chakra Balancing

The Chakra System (audio series)

The Illuminated Chakras (video)

The Sevenfold Journey (with Selene Vega)

Contact: The Yoga of Relationship (with Tara Guber)

For more information:

www.SacredCenters.com

Notes

Notes

Notes

Notes

Notes

Notes

Notes

Notes

Notes